Influence of Natural and/or Vaccine Immunity on the Dynamics of SARS-CoV-2

Influence of Natural and/or Vaccine Immunity on the Dynamics of SARS-CoV-2

Guest Editor

Chloé Dimeglio

MDPI

Basel • Beijing • Wuhan • Barcelona • Belgrade • Novi Sad • Cluj • Manchester

Guest Editor
Chloé Dimeglio
Virology Laboratory
Toulouse University Hospital
Toulouse
France

Editorial Office
MDPI AG
Grosspeteranlage 5
4052 Basel, Switzerland

This is a reprint of the Special Issue, published open access by the journal *Vaccines* (ISSN 2076-393X), freely accessible at: https://www.mdpi.com/journal/vaccines/special_issues/Influence_Natural_Vaccine_Immunity.

For citation purposes, cite each article independently as indicated on the article page online and as indicated below:

Lastname, A.A.; Lastname, B.B. Article Title. *Journal Name* **Year**, *Volume Number*, Page Range.

ISBN 978-3-7258-6830-8 (Hbk)
ISBN 978-3-7258-6831-5 (PDF)
https://doi.org/10.3390/books978-3-7258-6831-5

Contents

About the Editor . . . vii

Preface . . . ix

Chloe Dimeglio
Natural and Vaccine-Induced Immunity in the Post-Pandemic Era: Convergence, Divergence, and Unfinished Challenges
Reprinted from: *Vaccines* **2025**, *13*, 1251, https://doi.org/10.3390/vaccines13121251 . . . 1

Gian Luca Salvagno and Giuseppe Lippi
Correlation between Anti-SARS-CoV-2 Total Antibodies and Spike Trimeric IgG after BNT162b2 Booster Immunization
Reprinted from: *Vaccines* **2022**, *10*, 890, https://doi.org/10.3390/vaccines10060890 . . . 5

Buchhorn Reiner
Dysautonomia in Children with Post-Acute Sequelae of Coronavirus 2019 Disease and/or Vaccination
Reprinted from: *Vaccines* **2022**, *10*, 1686, https://doi.org/10.3390/vaccines10101686 . . . 8

Vivek P. Chavda, Gargi Jogi, Srusti Dave, Bhoomika M. Patel, Lakshmi Vineela Nalla and Krishna Koradia
mRNA-Based Vaccine for COVID-19: They Are New but Not Unknown!
Reprinted from: *Vaccines* **2023**, *11*, 507, https://doi.org/10.3390/vaccines11030507 . . . 16

Emma Chang-Rabley, Menno C. van Zelm, Emily E. Ricotta and Emily S. J. Edwards
An Overview of the Strategies to Boost SARS-CoV-2-Specific Immunity in People with Inborn Errors of Immunity
Reprinted from: *Vaccines* **2024**, *12*, 675, https://doi.org/10.3390/vaccines12060675 . . . 44

Ali Alsuheel Asseri and Abdullah Alsabaani
Seroprevalence of SARS-CoV-2 among Children Visiting a Tertiary Hospital during the Prevaccination Period, Southwest Region, Saudi Arabia
Reprinted from: *Vaccines* **2022**, *10*, 1344, https://doi.org/10.3390/vaccines10081344 . . . 76

Chloé Dimeglio, Marion Migueres, Naémie Bouzid, Sabine Chapuy-Regaud, Caroline Gernigon, Isabelle Da-Silva, et al.
Antibody Titers and Protection against Omicron (BA.1 and BA.2) SARS-CoV-2 Infection
Reprinted from: *Vaccines* **2022**, *10*, 1548, https://doi.org/10.3390/vaccines10091548 . . . 85

Eline Meyers, Evelien De Smet, Hanne Vercruysse, Steven Callens, Elizaveta Padalko, Stefan Heytens, et al.
No Significant Association between 25-OH Vitamin D Status and SARS-CoV-2 Antibody Response after COVID-19 Vaccination in Nursing Home Residents and Staff
Reprinted from: *Vaccines* **2023**, *11*, 1343, https://doi.org/10.3390/vaccines11081343 . . . 95

Hyerin Gim, Seul Lee, Haesook Seo, Yumi Park and Byung Chul Chun
Effects of Severe Acute Respiratory Syndrome Coronavirus Vaccination on Reinfection: A Community-Based Retrospective Cohort Study
Reprinted from: *Vaccines* **2023**, *11*, 1408, https://doi.org/10.3390/vaccines11091408 . . . 106

Monikaben Padariya and Umesh Kalathiya
Single Ferritin Nanocages Expressing SARS-CoV-2 Spike Variants to Receptor and Antibodies
Reprinted from: *Vaccines* **2024**, *12*, 446, https://doi.org/10.3390/vaccines12050446 . . . 119

Carmen-Daniela Chivu, Maria-Dorina Crăciun, Daniela Pițigoi, Victoria Aramă, Monica Luminița Luminos, Gheorghiță Jugulete, et al.
Hybrid Immunity and the Incidence of SARS-CoV-2 Reinfections during the Omicron Era in Frontline Healthcare Workers
Reprinted from: *Vaccines* **2024**, *12*, 682, https://doi.org/10.3390/vaccines12060682 . . . . **131**

Jae-Hoon Ko, Choon-Mee Kim, Mi-Seon Bang, Da-Yeon Lee, Da-Young Kim, Jun-Won Seo, et al.
Risk Factors for Impaired Cellular or Humoral Immunity after Three Doses of SARS-CoV-2 Vaccine in Healthy and Immunocompromised Individuals
Reprinted from: *Vaccines* **2024**, *12*, 752, https://doi.org/10.3390/vaccines12070752 . . . . **146**

Gerald Kevin Oluka, Jackson Sembera, Joseph Ssebwana Katende, Violet Ankunda, Laban Kato, Ashwini Kurshan, et al.
Long-Term Immune Consequences of Initial SARS-CoV-2 A.23.1 Exposure: A Longitudinal Study of Antibody Responses and Cross-Neutralization in a Ugandan Cohort
Reprinted from: *Vaccines* **2025**, *13*, 143, https://doi.org/10.3390/vaccines13020143 . . . . **158**

About the Editor

Chloé Dimeglio

Chloé Dimeglio is a biostatistician and researcher affiliated with the Virology Laboratory at the Centre Hospitalier Universitaire (CHU) de Toulouse and with the Toulouse Institute for Infectious and Inflammatory Diseases (INFINITy), a joint INSERM–CNRS research unit in Toulouse, France. She holds a PhD in applied mathematics and has developed a research profile at the intersection of quantitative modeling, infectious disease dynamics, and immunology.

Her scientific work focuses on the statistical modeling of viral transmission, the analysis of serological and immunological data, and the evaluation of natural and vaccine-induced immune responses to SARS-CoV-2. Drawing on her expertise in biostatistics, she has contributed to key studies quantifying the durability of antibody responses following infection and vaccination, helping to clarify how immune protection evolves over time and differs by exposure history.

Dimeglio has also modeled SARS-CoV-2 transmission dynamics in the Toulouse metropolitan area to assess the impact of non-pharmaceutical interventions, such as social distancing and lockdowns, providing insights relevant to regional public health strategies. She has co-authored multiple peer-reviewed publications in high-impact journals, including *Clinical Infectious Diseases*, notably on neutralizing antibody responses in previously infected healthcare workers after mRNA vaccination, thereby contributing to the understanding of hybrid immunity.

Throughout her career, she has combined rigorous mathematical methods with real-world epidemiological data, strengthening the interpretation of complex immune responses and the forecasting of epidemic trends. Her work continues to inform researchers, clinicians, and policymakers involved in managing SARS-CoV-2 and guiding vaccination strategies.

Preface

The global spread of SARS-CoV-2 has profoundly reshaped scientific understanding of infectious diseases, immunity, and vaccination strategies. As the pandemic evolved, it became increasingly evident that immunity to SARS-CoV-2 is complex, heterogeneous, and dynamic, influenced by prior infection, vaccination, viral evolution, and host-specific factors. This Special Issue, "Influence of Natural and/or Vaccine Immunity on the Dynamics of SARS-CoV-2", is devoted to examining these interactions and their implications for individual protection and population-level disease dynamics.

The scope of this Special Issue encompasses a broad range of disciplines, including immunology, virology, epidemiology, public health, and vaccinology. It brings together experimental, clinical, and population-based studies that explore immune responses elicited by natural infection, vaccination, or their combination, often referred to as hybrid immunity. Particular attention is given to the durability and quality of immune protection, immune waning, reinfection, breakthrough infections, and the impact of emerging variants of concern. By integrating mechanistic insights with real-world data, this collection provides a comprehensive perspective on how immunity shapes the trajectory of SARS-CoV-2 circulation.

The primary aim of this Special Issue is to advance scientific understanding of how different forms of immunity influence viral transmission, disease severity, and long-term pandemic control. While vaccines have proven highly effective in reducing severe disease and mortality, the continuous emergence of immune-evasive variants highlights the need to reassess assumptions about protective immunity. Through rigorous peer-reviewed contributions, this Special Issue seeks to inform future vaccine development, booster strategies, and public health policies that are grounded in evidence rather than extrapolation.

The motivation for assembling this scientific work arises from both urgency and opportunity. The pandemic has generated an unprecedented volume of data on immune responses across diverse populations, yet translating this information into coherent knowledge remains a challenge. Differences in immune outcomes based on exposure history, vaccine platforms, host characteristics, and viral evolution underscore the necessity of a dedicated forum to critically examine these variables. This Special Issue was conceived to foster dialogue across disciplines and to synthesize findings that may otherwise remain fragmented.

This Special Issue targets a wide audience, including researchers in immunology and infectious diseases, clinicians, epidemiologists, vaccine developers, and public health professionals. It is also intended for policymakers and health authorities seeking a deeper scientific basis for vaccination strategies and long-term COVID-19 management. By bringing together diverse perspectives, this collection aspires to contribute meaningfully to ongoing efforts to understand and control SARS-CoV-2 and to better prepare for future emerging pathogens.

Chloé Dimeglio
Guest Editor

vaccines

MDPI

Editorial

Natural and Vaccine-Induced Immunity in the Post-Pandemic Era: Convergence, Divergence, and Unfinished Challenges

Chloe Dimeglio

Toulouse Institute for Infectious and Inflammatory Diseases (INFINITY), Institut National de la Santé et de la Recherche Médicale (INSERM), Unité Mite de Recherche 1291, Centre National de la Recherche Scientifique (CNRS), Unité Mite de Recherche 5051, 31300 Toulouse, France; dimeglio.c@chu-toulouse.fr

The global response to SARS-CoV-2 has advanced at unprecedented speed: vaccines developed in record time, mass immunization campaigns, and real-world data confirming reductions in severe disease and death [1,2]. Yet, as we mark a shift into a more endemic phase of the pandemic, the central question is no longer whether we can provide immunity, but rather how well, how durably, and how equitably we can deliver it. The Special Issue of *Vaccines* titled "Influence of Natural and/or Vaccine Immunity on the Dynamics of SARS-CoV-2" was launched precisely to interrogate this complexity—how natural infection and vaccination, alone or in combination, shape immunity in the face of evolving viral dynamics.

This collection offers crucial insights into three interlinked domains: the heterogeneity of immune acquisition and waning, the operational significance of hybrid immunity, and the threat posed by viral evolution in undermining protection. While the fundamental tenets—vaccination is key [3], immunity wanes [4], variants matter [5]—are well established, the contributions to this Special Issue refine our understanding and signal new strategic imperatives.

Several contributions emphasize that the quality of immune memory varies markedly with the variant first encountered. Oluka et al. [6] followed individuals in Uganda initially exposed to A.23.1 and revealed durable yet uneven cross-neutralization against other strains over 427 days. This provides rare evidence that immune imprinting—beneficial or limiting—depends on the immunological "first impression". Hybrid immunity remains a critical asset among those at highest occupational risk. In healthcare workers, Chivu et al. [7] reported lower reinfection rates during Omicron dominance among individuals with mixed infection and vaccination history, emphasizing the sustaining role of repeated antigenic stimulation. These findings not only align with established global observations but also extend them by variant-specific granularity—a cornerstone for future vaccine guidance. Community-scale evidence from Gim et al. [8] clarifies that vaccination reduces both symptomatic reinfections and the speed of recurrence, confirming its population benefit despite immune evasion by Omicron sublineages. Yet heterogeneity remains a decisive factor. Through immune profiling after three vaccine doses, Ko et al. [9] identified age, compromised immunity, and specific comorbidities as critical predictors of impaired humoral and cellular responses—reinforcing the need for stratified booster policies rather than universal schedules. The study by Meyers et al. [10] further challenges assumptions: Vitamin D levels—long suspected to impact vaccine response—showed no significant correlation with antibody generation in nursing home residents and staff, suggesting that routine supplementation is not a proxy for immune optimization in vaccination. Dimeglio et al. [11] provide one of the most actionable contributions: quantitative antibody thresholds required to protect against Omicron BA.1/BA.2. Although higher than for previous variants, such correlates remain essential tools for public health decision-making, booster deployment, and clinical risk stratification. Sero-surveillance among children in Saudi Arabia by Asseri and Alsabaani [12] underlines that immunity levels were substantial in the pre-vaccination era, revealing widespread silent transmission and the need for child-focused monitoring strategies. Chang-Rabley et al. [13] synthesize evidence on individuals with inborn errors of immunity and call for bespoke vaccination strategies, including monoclonal antibodies and adjuvant-enhanced formulations—a still-underfunded horizon in global immunization equity. Padariya & Kalathiya [14] advance the future of vaccine engineering through ferritin nanocage platforms displaying variant RBDs—a versatile tool for pan-variant vaccine development. Meanwhile, Buchhorn [15] sheds light on dysautonomia in children following infection and, more rarely, vaccination—a reminder that post-acute sequelae remain a critical frontier requiring multidisciplinary research rather than dismissal. Finally, Salvagno & Lippi [16] present a pragmatic contribution: spike IgG measurements strongly correlate with total antibody responses, streamlining sero-monitoring protocols for large cohorts. Chavda et al. [17] offer a timely perspective on mRNA vaccine technology, reminding the reader that despite recent deployment, the platform is founded on decades of immunobiology research—a narrative crucial to counter vaccine skepticism.

Crucially, this Special Issue adds value over the extant evidence base in three ways. It expands the focus on under-served populations (immunocompromised and hybrid immunity cohorts), it underscores improvements in methodology (linking immunologic and epidemiologic data; variant-specific neutralization), and it advances an operational lens: how immune trajectories can inform policy (boosting schedules, variant-adapted vaccines, and equity of access). While the previous literature laid the groundwork for waning immunity and variant impact [18] on durability of natural and vaccine-mediated immunity), this collection elevates it into a more actionable domain.

On the basis of these insights, this Special Issue offers the following strategic recommendations:

1. Refined Immunological Surveillance

Surveillance systems should measure both humoral (neutralizing antibodies; binding IgG) and cellular immunity (T-cell responses; memory B cells), particularly in populations with increased vulnerability. Evidence demonstrating variability in neutralization breadth and durability across exposure histories supports the need for immune history stratification [6,7,9]. Moreover, variant-specific immune escape requires the integration of updated neutralization assays into public health practice [6,11].

2. Tailored Vaccination and Booster Strategy

Booster policies must incorporate prior infection profiles: hybrid immunity confers enhanced resistance against reinfection in frontline workers [7], while vaccination alone remains protective against recurrent disease at the community level [8]. Individuals with underlying immune impairment exhibit suboptimal vaccine-induced responses [9,13], justifying enhanced regimens and frequent monitoring. Vaccine antigen updates must reflect the dynamic variant landscape to avoid mismatches in immune recognition [14,17].

3. Dynamic Modeling and Planning

Epidemiological models should integrate waning immune markers, variant evolution, and repeated antigen exposure, as supported by longitudinal evidence showing altering neutralization profiles over time [6] and changes in reinfection risk during Omicron waves [7,8]. Incorporating such parameters will better guide booster deployment and resource prioritization.

4. Focused Research on Immune Correlates and Special Populations

The establishment of quantitative correlates of protection remains essential [11]. Long-term follow-up is needed across age and exposure groups, including children—who demonstrated substantial pre-vaccination seropositivity [12]—and individuals with inborn errors of immunity, who may benefit from tailored immunization strategies and alternative biologics [8]. Emerging observations regarding post-acute sequelae, including dysautonomia in pediatric cases after infection and/or vaccination, highlight an ongoing need for protective strategies that minimize both short- and long-term harm [15].

5. Equity in Access and Implementation

Global control of SARS-CoV-2 requires the prevention of immunity gaps between well-resourced and underserved populations. Hybrid immunity must not become a privilege tied to inequitable infection and vaccine access [7,8]. Efforts to expand variant-adapted vaccine availability, reinforce genomic and immunologic surveillance, and sustain public communication are imperative to ensure that vaccination remains a universal benefit rather than a selective advantage [10,14,17].

In conclusion, the body of work compiled in this Special Issue confirms that immunity to SARS-CoV-2 is not merely a milestone but a journey—one characterized by complexity, variation, and evolution. The scientific community has moved from demonstrating what is possible to grappling with what is optimal. The ambition now must be to translate this rich evidence into resilient, adaptive, and equitable immunization systems: systems that do not just cover populations but protect them durably across viral variants, immunological histories, and global settings.

The path ahead remains challenging—but the tools, the data, and the strategic clarity are now in hand. Our collective responsibility is to deploy them effectively so that immunity against SARS-CoV-2 becomes not a variable state but a sustained reality.

Conflicts of Interest: The author declares no conflict of interest.

References

1. Polack, F.P.; Thomas, S.J.; Kitchin, N.; Absalon, J.; Gurtman, A.; Lockhart, S.; Perez, J.L.; Pérez Marc, G.; Moreira, E.D.; Zerbini, C.; et al. Safety and Efficacy of the BNT162b2 mRNA Covid-19 Vaccine. *N. Engl. J. Med.* **2020**, *383*, 2603–2615. [CrossRef] [PubMed]
2. Thompson, M.G.; Stenehjem, E.; Grannis, S.; Ball, S.W.; Naleway, A.L.; Ong, T.C.; DeSilva, M.B.; Natarajan, K.; McEvoy, C.; Bozio, C.H.; et al. Effectiveness of COVID-19 Vaccines in Preventing SARS-CoV-2 Infection among Frontline Workers Before and During Delta Variant Predominance—Eight U.S. Locations, December 2020–August 2021. *MMWR Morb. Mortal. Wkly. Rep.* **2021**, *70*, 1167–1171.
3. Levin, E.G.; Lustig, Y.; Cohen, C.; Fluss, R.; Indenbaum, V.; Amit, S.; Doolman, R.; Asraf, K.; Mendelson, E.; Ziv, A.; et al. Waning Immune Humoral Response to BNT162b2 COVID-19 Vaccine over 6 Months. *N. Engl. J. Med.* **2021**, *385*, e84. [CrossRef] [PubMed]
4. Crotty, S. Hybrid Immunity. *Science* **2021**, *372*, 1392–1393. [CrossRef]
5. Cao, Y.; Wang, J.; Jian, F.; Xiao, T.; Song, W.; Yisimayi, A.; Huang, W.; Li, Q.; Wang, P.; An, R.; et al. Omicron Escapes the Majority of Existing SARS-CoV-2 Neutralizing Antibodies. *Nature* **2022**, *602*, 657–663. [CrossRef] [PubMed]
6. Oluka, G.K.; Sembera, J.; Katende, J.S.; Ankunda, V.; Kato, L.; Kurshan, A.; Graham, C.; Seow, J.; Doores, K.J.; Malim, M.H.; et al. Long-Term Immune Consequences of Initial SARS-CoV-2 A.23.1 Exposure: A Longitudinal Study of Antibody Responses and Cross-Neutralization in a Ugandan Cohort. *Vaccines* **2025**, *13*, 143. [CrossRef] [PubMed]
7. Chivu, C.-D.; Crăciun, M.-D.; Pițigoi, D.; Aramă, V.; Luminos, M.L.; Jugulete, G.; Nițescu, V.G.; Lescaie, A.; Apostolescu, C.G.; Streinu Cercel, A. Hybrid Immunity and the Incidence of SARS-CoV-2 Reinfections during the Omicron Era in Frontline Healthcare Workers. *Vaccines* **2024**, *12*, 682. [CrossRef] [PubMed]
8. Gim, H.; Lee, S.; Seo, H.; Park, Y.; Chun, B.C. Effects of Severe Acute Respiratory Syndrome Coronavirus Vaccination on Reinfection: A Community-Based Retrospective Cohort Study. *Vaccines* **2023**, *11*, 1408. [CrossRef] [PubMed]

9. Ko, J.-H.; Kim, C.-M.; Bang, M.-S.; Lee, D.-Y.; Kim, D.-Y.; Seo, J.-W.; Yun, N.-R.; Yang, J.-Y.; Peck, K.-R.; Lee, K.-W.; et al. Risk Factors for Impaired Cellular or Humoral Immunity after Three Doses of SARS-CoV-2 Vaccine in Healthy and Immunocompromised Individuals. *Vaccines* **2024**, *12*, 752. [CrossRef] [PubMed]
10. Meyers, E.; De Smet, E.; Vercruysse, H.; Callens, S.; Padalko, E.; Heytens, S.; Vandekerckhove, L.; Cools, P.; Witkowski, W. No Significant Association between 25-OH Vitamin D Status and SARS-CoV-2 Antibody Response after COVID-19 Vaccination in Nursing Home Residents and Staff. *Vaccines* **2023**, *11*, 1343. [CrossRef] [PubMed]
11. Dimeglio, C.; Migueres, M.; Bouzid, N.; Chapuy-Regaud, S.; Gernigon, C.; Da-Silva, I.; Porcheron, M.; Martin-Blondel, G.; Herin, F.; Izopet, J. Antibody Titers and Protection against Omicron (BA.1 and BA.2) SARS-CoV-2 Infection. *Vaccines* **2022**, *10*, 1548. [CrossRef] [PubMed]
12. Asseri, A.A.; Alsabaani, A. Seroprevalence of SARS-CoV-2 among Children Visiting a Tertiary Hospital during the Prevaccination Period, Southwest Region, Saudi Arabia. *Vaccines* **2022**, *10*, 1344. [CrossRef] [PubMed]
13. Chang-Rabley, E.; van Zelm, M.C.; Ricotta, E.E.; Edwards, E.S.J. An Overview of the Strategies to Boost SARS-CoV-2-Specific Immunity in People with Inborn Errors of Immunity. *Vaccines* **2024**, *12*, 675. [CrossRef] [PubMed]
14. Padariya, M.; Kalathiya, U. Single Ferritin Nanocages Expressing SARS-CoV-2 Spike Variants to Receptor and Antibodies. *Vaccines* **2024**, *12*, 446. [CrossRef] [PubMed]
15. Buchhorn, R. Dysautonomia in Children with Post-Acute Sequelae of Coronavirus 2019 Disease and/or Vaccination. *Vaccines* **2022**, *10*, 1686. [CrossRef] [PubMed]
16. Salvagno, G.L.; Lippi, G. Correlation between Anti-SARS-CoV-2 Total Antibodies and Spike Trimeric IgG after BNT162b2 Booster Immunization. *Vaccines* **2022**, *10*, 890. [CrossRef] [PubMed]
17. Chavda, V.P.; Jogi, G.; Dave, S.; Patel, B.M.; Vineela Nalla, L.; Koradia, K. mRNA-Based Vaccine for COVID-19: They Are New but Not Unknown! *Vaccines* **2023**, *11*, 507. [CrossRef] [PubMed]
18. Townsend, J.P.; Hassler, H.B.; Sah, P.; Galvani, A.P.; Dornburg, A. The durability of natural infection and vaccine-induced immunity against future infection by SARS-CoV-2. *Proc. Natl. Acad. Sci. USA* **2022**, *119*, e2204336119. [CrossRef] [PubMed]

vaccines

MDPI

Letter

Correlation between Anti-SARS-CoV-2 Total Antibodies and Spike Trimeric IgG after BNT162b2 Booster Immunization

Gian Luca Salvagno and Giuseppe Lippi *

Section of Clinical Biochemistry, University of Verona, 37126 Verona, Italy; gianluca.salvagno@univr.it
* Correspondence: giuseppe.lippi@univr.it

Abstract: Objective: In this work we monitored both total and IgG anti-SARS-CoV-2 antibodies responses after BNT162b2 vaccine booster immunization in a cohort of ostensibly healthy healthcare workers. Methods: The study population consisted of 266 subjects (median age, 46 years and interquartile range (IQR), 35–52 years; 168 females) undergoing homologous 30-μg BNT162b2 booster administration. Serum samples were collected immediately before the booster dose and 1 month after. Results: The concentration of anti-SARS-CoV-2 RBD total antibodies and anti-SARS-CoV-2 spike trimeric IgG increased by 31 (IQR, 16–53) and 22 (IQR, 11–43) folds, respectively, after receiving the BNT162b2 vaccine booster. A highly significant Spearman's correlation was found between the relative increase (i.e., ratio of post-booster and pre-booster serum values) of anti-SARS-CoV-2 RBD total antibodies and anti-SARS-CoV-2 spike trimeric IgG ($r = 0.86$; $p < 0.001$). Conclusion: These results suggest that monitoring of post-BNT162b2 booster immunization for purposes of identifying "low responders" could be conducted almost interchangeably with either total or IgG anti-SARS-CoV-2 antibodies.

Keywords: COVID-19; SARS-CoV-2; vaccination; antibodies; booster

1. Introduction

In a recent article published in this journal, Skrzat-Klapaczyńska and colleagues [1] showed that a booster dose of the mRNA-based BNT162b2 vaccine was effective at increasing the serum values of SARS-CoV-2 IgG antibodies measured with the MAGLUMI SARS-CoV-2 S-RBD IgG assay over the maximum measurable level according to the method used by the authors (i.e., >433 BAU/mL). To provide further insights on this important aspect in terms of limiting SARS-CoV-2 infection and lowering the risk of developing serious complications from coronavirus disease 2019 (COVID-19), we monitored both total and IgG anti-SARS-CoV-2 antibodies response after BNT162b2 vaccine booster immunization in a cohort of ostensibly healthy healthcare workers, with a specific focus on emphasizing the potential correlation between the post-booster variation of these two antibodies classes.

2. Materials and Methods

This serosurveillance observational study is based on a cohort of ostensibly healthy workers of Pederzoli Hospital (Peschiera del Garda, Verona, Italy), who volunteered to undergo COVID-19 vaccination with the mRNA-based Pfizer/BioNTech BNT162b2 vaccine (Pfizer Inc., New York, NY, USA; double 30-μg dose with 3 weeks interval), followed by homologous 30-μg booster dose >8 months thereafter. Nucleic acid amplification tests were carried out at 2–4 weeks interval throughout the study period with Altona Diagnostics RealStar SARS-CoV-2 RT-PCR Kit (Altona Diagnostics GmbH, Hamburg, Germany) or Seegene Allplex SARS-CoV-2 Assay (Seegene Inc., Seoul, South Korea) to rule out incident SARS-CoV-2 infections, that would lead to eliminating these subjects from the study, since booster vaccination is not normally given to people with a history of recent infection. Blood was drawn throughout the study period, including the same day as receiving the BNT162b2 vaccine booster and 1 month afterwards. Serum was used for assaying anti-SARS-CoV-2 RBD total antibodies with Roche Elecsys Anti-SARS-CoV-2 S on Roche Cobas 6000 (Roche Diagnostics, Basel, Switzerland), a method which measures total anti-SARS-CoV-2 anti-RBD (receptor binding domain) antibodies [2], as well as with anti-SARS-CoV-2 spike trimeric IgG with DiaSorin Trimeric spike IgG immunoassay on Liaison XL (DiaSorin, Saluggia, Italy) [3]. Results exceeding the upper linearity limit of both immunoassays (i.e., >25,000 kBAU/L for anti-RBD total antibodies and >108,160 kBAU/L for anti-trimeric spike IgG, respectively) were excluded, in order to allow for more accurate estimation of the relative post-booster increase in anti-SARS-CoV-2 antibodies. The measurement of anti-SARS-CoV-2 spike trimeric IgG antibodies was chosen since they sufficiently differ from anti-RBD antibodies, where a good correlation is obviously anticipated. Statistical analysis was carried out with Analyse-it (Analyse-it Software Ltd., Leeds, UK). All participants signed an informed consent for participating to the study, which was conducted in accordance with the Declaration of Helsinki and approved by the Ethics Committee of Verona and Rovigo Provinces (59COVIDCESC; 3 November 2021).

3. Results

The final study population consisted in 266 healthcare workers (median age, 46 years and interquartile range (IQR), 35–52 years; 168 females). The main results of this study are shown in Figure 1.

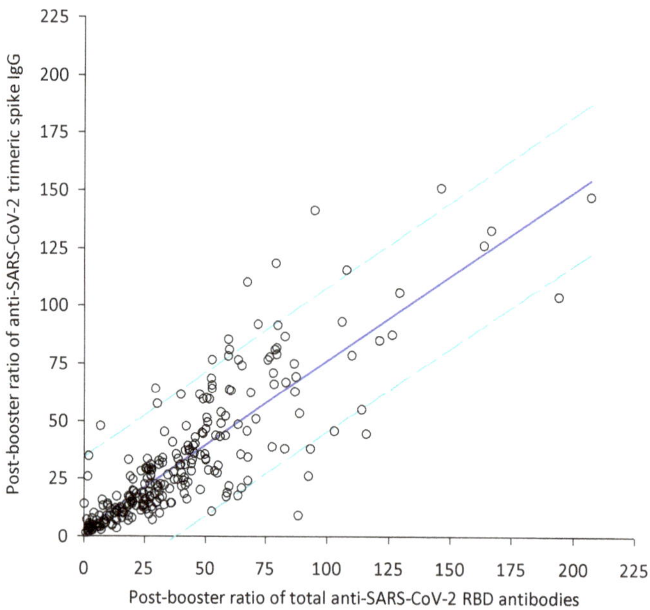

Figure 1. Correlation between relative increase (i.e., ratio of BNT162b2 post-booster and pre-booster serum values) of anti-SARS-CoV-2 total antibodies and anti-SARS-CoV-2 spike trimeric IgG.

After receiving the BNT162b2 vaccine booster, the serum concentration increased by a median of 31 folds (IQR, 16–53), from 463 (IQR, 271–882) kBAU/L to 15,280 (IQR, 11,773–19,447) kBAU/L for anti-SARS-CoV-2 RBD total antibodies, and by a median of 22 (IQR, 11–43) folds, from 662 (IQR, 339–1255) kBAU/L to 13,624 (IQR, 9939–19,019) kBAU/L for anti-SARS-CoV-2 spike trimeric IgG, respectively. The absolute values of anti-SARS-CoV-2 antibodies assayed with the Roche immunoassay were predictably much higher than those obtained with the DiaSorin method, since the former technique measures total anti-SARS-CoV-2 antibodies, whilst the latter only detected IgG. A highly significant Spearman's correlation was found between the relative increase (i.e., ratio of post-booster and pre-booster serum values) of anti-SARS-CoV-2 RBD total antibodies and anti-SARS-CoV-2 spike trimeric IgG (r = 0.86; 95%CI, 0.83–0.89; $p < 0.001$), as shown in Figure 1. This correlation was described by the following equation:

$$[\text{Anti-SARS-CoV-2 spike trimeric IgG}] = [\text{Anti-SARS-CoV-2 total antibodies}] \times 0.73 + 2.70$$

Such correlation remained highly significant both in males (r = 0.88; 95%CI, 0.82–0.92; $p < 0.001$) and females (r = 0.85; 95%CI, 0.80–0.89; $p < 0.001$), as well as in subjects aged <50 (r = 0.86; 95%CI, 0.81–0.89; $p < 0.001$) or ≥50 (r = 0.85; 95%CI, 0.78–0.90; $p < 0.001$) years.

4. Discussion

The results of our analysis were aimed to complement those published earlier by Skrzat-Klapaczyńska and colleagues [1] on elucidating the effect of BNT162b2 booster immunization on anti-SARS-CoV-2 antibodies. For this purpose, we measured both total and IgG anti-SARS-CoV-2 antibodies, showing that both classes of antibodies considerably increased (by 31 and 22-fold, respectively) 1 month after receiving the BNT162b2 vaccine booster. Besides providing an accurate measure of such increment in subjects with precisely measurable anti-SARS-CoV-2 antibodies values, we also demonstrated a very high correlation (i.e., $p < 0.001$) between the increase in anti-SARS-CoV-2 RBD total antibodies and anti-SARS-CoV-2 spike trimeric IgG, thus potentially reflecting a similar trend of humoral immune response despite the antigen target of these classes of immunoglobulins is different (i.e., trimeric spike protein vs. RBS). This is inherently important for demonstrating that even distinct class of antibodies, targeting different antigenic moieties on the spike protein, could be reliably used for purposes of monitoring COVID-19 vaccination.

5. Conclusions

The results of this study suggest that monitoring of post-BNT162b2 booster immunization for purposes of identifying "low responders" to vaccine boosters could be performed almost interchangeably with either total or IgG anti-SARS-CoV-2 antibodies.

Author Contributions: Conceptualization, G.L.S. and G.L.; methodology, G.L.S.; formal analysis, G.L.; resources, G.L.S.; data curation, G.L.; writing—original draft preparation, G.L.; writing—review and editing, G.L.S. All authors have read and agreed to the published version of the manuscript.

Funding: This research received no external funding.

Institutional Review Board Statement: The study was conducted in accordance with the Declaration of Helsinki, and approved by the Ethics Committee of Verona and Rovigo Provinces (59COVIDCESC; 3 November 2021).

Informed Consent Statement: Informed consent was obtained from all subjects involved in the study.

Data Availability Statement: Data are available upon reasonable request to the corresponding author.

Acknowledgments: The authors are thankful to the entire staff of the Pederzoli Hospital of Peschiera del Garda (Verona, Italy) for accepting to participate to this study.

Conflicts of Interest: The authors declare no conflict of interest.

References

1. Skrzat-Klapaczyńska, A.; Bieńkowski, C.; Kowalska, J.; Paciorek, M.; Puła, J.; Krogulec, D.; Stengiel, J.; Pawełczyk, A.; Perlejewski, K.; Osuch, S.; et al. The Beneficial Effect of the COVID-19 Vaccine Booster Dose among Healthcare Workers in an Infectious Diseases Center. *Vaccines* **2022**, *10*, 552. [CrossRef] [PubMed]
2. Riester, E.; Findeisen, P.; Hegel, J.K.; Kabesch, M.; Ambrosch, A.; Rank, C.M.; Pessl, F.; Laengin, T.; Niederhauser, C. Performance evaluation of the Roche Elecsys Anti-SARS-CoV-2 S immunoassay. *J. Virol. Methods* **2021**, *297*, 114271. [CrossRef] [PubMed]
3. Bonelli, F.; Blocki, F.A.; Bunnell, T.; Chu, E.; De La, O.A.; Grenache, D.G.; Marzucchi, G.; Montomoli, E.; Okoye, L.; Pallavicini, L.; et al. Evaluation of the automated LIAISON®SARS-CoV-2 TrimericS IgG assay for the detection of circulating antibodies. *Clin. Chem. Lab. Med.* **2021**, *59*, 1463–1467. [CrossRef] [PubMed]

vaccines

MDPI

Brief Report

Dysautonomia in Children with Post-Acute Sequelae of Coronavirus 2019 Disease and/or Vaccination

Reiner Buchhorn

Praxis für Kinder- und Jugendmedizin, Kinderkardiologie und Erwachsene mit Angeborenen Herzfehlern, Am Bahnhof 1, 74670 Forchtenberg, Germany; buchrein@gmail.com

Abstract: Long-term health problems such as fatigue, palpitations, syncope, and dizziness are well-known in patients after COVID-19 (post-acute sequelae of coronavirus (PASC)). More recently, comparable problems have been noticed after the SARS-CoV-2 vaccination (post-VAC). The pathophysiology of these problems is not well-understood. Methods: In 38 children and young adults, we tested if these health problems were related to dysautonomia in an active standing test (Group 1: 19 patients after COVID-19; Group 2: 12 patients with a breakthrough infection despite a vaccination; and Group 3: 7 patients after a vaccination without COVID-19). The data were compared with a control group of 47 healthy age-matched patients, as recently published. Results: All patients had a normal left ventricular function as measured by echocardiography. Significantly elevated diastolic blood pressure in all patient groups indicated a regulatory cardiovascular problem. Compared with the healthy control group, the patient groups showed significantly elevated heart rates whilst lying and standing, with significantly higher heart rate increases. The stress index was significantly enhanced in all patient groups whilst lying and standing. Significantly decreased pNN20 values, mostly whilst standing, indicated a lower vagus activity in all patient groups. The respiratory rates were significantly elevated in Groups 1 and 2. Conclusion: The uniform increase in the heart rates and stress indices, together with low pNN20 values, indicated dysautonomia in children with health problems after COVID-19 disease and/or vaccination. A total of 8 patients fulfilled the criteria of postural orthostatic tachycardia syndrome and 9 patients of an inappropriate sinus tachycardia, who were successfully treated with omega-3 fatty acid supplementation and pharmacotherapy.

Keywords: SARS-CoV-2 virus; COVID-19; dysautonomia; heart rate variability; vaccination; long COVID

1. Introduction

Coronavirus disease 2019 (COVID-19) is caused by a SARS-CoV-2 virus infection. After the acute disease, ongoing health problems of COVID-19 are now being identified with the most common being fatigue, shortness of breath, chest pain, and palpitations that may indicate cardiovascular disease. Furthermore, patients can suffer from difficulty concentrating, arthralgia, low-grade fever, and headaches that may indicate ongoing inflammation. These ongoing health problems have been termed Post-Acute Sequelae of Coronavirus 2019 Disease (PASC) [1]. However, as most symptoms of PASC are not clearly defined, the number of affected patients cannot be clearly stated. However, PASC is an increasing health problem in adults and children. Recently, among SARS-CoV-2-positive children, the most common long-term symptom was fatigue or weakness (1.1%) [2].

Additionally, the impact of the SARS-CoV-2 vaccination on PASC is controversial. Most physicians speculate that the vaccination may protect against long-term health problems [3] and can even be used for therapy [4]. Recent findings suggest that a vaccination before an infection confers only a partial protection against PASC. In addition, new data have been published that show that the SARS-CoV-2 vaccination may cause PASC [5].

Dysautonomia has been found in patients who suffer from PASC [6]. Moreover, dysautonomia may be linked to long-term health problems after COVID-19 as well as the

SARS-CoV-2 vaccination [7]. Currently, there are no established therapies for PASC and the concept of "dysautonomia" could open up therapeutic approaches to which there is already a guideline recommendation [8].

We now introduce our data of 38 children who suffered from PASC after COVID-19 (N = 19), a breakthrough infection after a vaccination (N = 12), or PASC-like long-term health problems after the SARS-CoV-2 vaccination (N = 7).

2. Methods

The study was a retrospective analysis of 38 consecutive children and adolescents who had an active standing test of the cause of ongoing health problems for more than 11 weeks on average after COVID-19 disease or vaccination. In Group 1, there were 19 patients after COVID-19, Group 2 contained 12 patients with a breakthrough SARS-CoV-2 infection despite a vaccination, and Group 3 had 7 patients after a vaccination without COVID-19. After excluding other clearly defined diseases, we did not assess the subjective clinical problems and included all patients who displayed ongoing health problems after COVID-19 and/or SARS-CoV-2 vaccination. The most common symptoms were fatigue or weakness as well as palpitations, chest pain, dizziness, shortness of breath, inattention, and gastrointestinal problems. COVID-19 disease was proven by a PCR in all patients. All patients had a complete cardiovascular check-up with ECG, a fully automatic photoplethysmography blood pressure test, and echocardiography.

The healthy control group included 47 healthy adolescents (mean age = 14.2 ± 3.8 years) with a normal body mass index and without any somatic or psychosomatic diseases. These data were collected prior to the pandemic. The groups were stratified according to their age, height, weight, and gender (Table 1).

Table 1. Basic data and HRV analysis of the active standing test.

	Healthy Control	Post-COVID-19	Post-COVID-19 + VAC	Post-VAC
Patients	47	19	12	7
Gender (female/male)	30/17	13/6	8/4	4/3
Age (years)	14.2 ± 3.8	13.3 ± 2.9	17.1 ± 3.7	14.9 ± 1.5
Height (cm)	160.1 ± 14.2	154.8 ± 10.9	166.4 ± 10.3	161.9 ± 5.5
Weight (kg)	52.6 ± 14.3	47.9 ± 13.1	60.1 ± 11.3	49.7 ± 7.2
Systolic BP (mmHg)	114.5 ± 9.2	115.4 ± 13.7	119.1 ± 9.7	120.7 ± 9.7
Diastolic BP (mmHg)	61.7 ± 11.2	67.2 ± 9.1 *	75.4 ± 8.6 ***	71.0 ± 6.3 *
Fractional shortening (%)	>30	37.4 ± 4.1	40.6 ± 3.7	35.40 ± 1.80
Myocardial Performance Index	<0.4	0.14 ± 0.06	0.13 ± 0.10	0.18 ± 0.13
Heart Rate Increase (bpm)	16.2 ± 7.1	25.3 ± 11.7 **	26.2 ± 14.2 **	29.6 ± 12.8 **
		Lying		
Mean Heart Rate (bpm)	71.9 ± 8.1	80.7 ± 15.9 *	76.7 ± 16.5	85.4 ± 15.4 **
Stress Index (pt)	97.8 ± 85.1	150.7 ± 202.7 *	183.6 ± 140.4 ***	201.7 ± 213.6 **
SDNN (ms)	89.1 ± 38.4	68.7 ± 26.4 *	71.8 ± 64.7	75.3 ± 50.4
pNN20 (%)	78.6 ± 10.8	68.8 ± 26.6	56.0 ± 28.5 ***	53.3 ± 32.9 ***
RMSSD (ms)	85.1 ± 56.2	68.7 ± 38.5	77.2 ± 94.6	64.7 ± 66.8
Power HF Band (ms^2)	2920 ± 2229	2097 ± 2442	2376 ± 5298	3301 ± 6482
Power LF Band (ms^2)	1518 ± 2795	794 ± 774	1132 ± 1800	788 ± 674
Power VLF Band (ms^2)	1553 ± 2182	1099 ± 764	2612 ± 4472	1907 ± 2385
Power Total (ms^2)	5819 ± 6203	3990 ± 3260	6119 ± 11,289	5997 ± 7248
LF/HF Ratio	0.97 ± 1.1	0.98 ± 1.23	1.48 ± 1.52	1.61 ± 1.69

Table 1. *Cont.*

	Healthy Control	Post-COVID-19	Post-COVID-19 + VAC	Post-VAC
		Standing		
Mean Heart Rate (bpm)	89.8 ± 13.2	106.0 ± 13.1 ***	102.9 ± 10.8 ***	115.1 ± 12.8 ***
SDNN (ms)	58.0 ± 22.7	43.9 ± 19.4 **	62.9 ± 48.8	38.8 ± 16.1
pNN20 (%)	45.8 ± 18.6	27.5 ± 17.4 ***	20.6 ± 13.5 ***	15.6 ± 13.6 ***
RMSSD (ms)	40.4 ± 22.7	26.7 ± 22.2 *	30.9 ± 48.9	22.4 ± 22.3
Stress Index (pt)	168 ± 116	343 ± 292 ***	319 ± 219 **	494 ± 340 ***
Power HF Band (ms^2)	949 ± 1222	939 ± 2334	642 ± 1905	1184 ± 2640
Power LF Band (ms^2)	1331 ± 1115	1623 ± 5006	785 ± 762	1276 ± 1725
Power VLF Band (ms^2)	1299 ± 1506	1058 ± 2197	1309 ± 1926	948 ± 848
Power Total (ms^2)	3579 ± 3012	3611 ± 9437	2737 ± 4144	3409 ± 4895
LF/HF Ratio	2.54 ± 1.95	3.13 ± 2.96	9.41 ± 9.63	4.20 ± 3.50 *
Respiratory Rate (1/min)	16.3 ± 3.3	18.8 ± 2.1 **	19.1 ± 4.0 *	17.7 ± 1.8
Number of Beats	792 ± 111	902 ± 139 **	883 ± 168 *	895 ± 192 *
Quality (%)	82.7 ± 18.5	82.5 ± 15.0	[illegible] ± 24.7	79.1 ± 17.0

The *t*-test between healthy control group and patient groups: * *p*-value < 0.05; ** *p*-value < 0.01; *** *p*-value < 0.001.

2.1. Active Standing Test

All patients had at least one active standing test with a continuous measurement of their heart rate during 5 min in a supine position and 5 min during active standing using an HRV Scanner™ (BioSign GmbH, Ottenhofen, Germany). We performed the blood pressure tests in the supine position.

2.2. HRV

The measurement and interpretation of the HRV parameters in the current sample were standardised according to the task force guidelines.

- A short-time HRV analysis was performed using the HRV Scanner™ (BioSign GmbH, Ottenhofen, Germany) at two time periods: (1) in a supine position; and (2) 5 min of active standing. The HRV measurements were based on the RR intervals of normal QRS complexes (NN intervals) of the two 5 min intervals.

2.2.1. Time Domain HRV

- Average heart rates in beats per minute = mean heart rates of each 5 min interval.
- SDNN in milliseconds = standard deviation of NN; this reflected the general variability of the heart rate influenced by the autonomic nervous system and also the endocrine and thermoregulatory mechanisms.
- pNN50 and pNN20 in percent = percent of NN intervals that differed more than 50/20 ms from the prior interval; this mainly reflected the parasympathetic influence.
- RMSSD in milliseconds = root mean square of the differences between successive NN intervals; this mainly reflected the parasympathetic influence.

2.2.2. Stress Index

$$Stressin\ dex = \frac{Amo}{2 \times Mo \times MxDMn}$$

Where *Mo* is the modal value, the most common value of the RR intervals; *Amo* is the number of RR intervals corresponding with the mode as a percentage of the total number of all readings; and *MxDMn* is the variability width, the difference between the maximum and minimum RR intervals.

The stress index is becoming increasingly popular because it reacts sensitively to shifts in the vegetative balance between the sympathetic and parasympathetic nerves.

2.2.3. Frequency Domain HRV

The Fourier transformation shows that HRV signals are concentrated into three different frequency bands:

- Very low frequency power (VLF = 0.00–0.04 Hz) in ms^2: an uncertain physiological meaning.
- Low frequency power (LF = 0.04–0.15 Hz) in ms^2: this is mediated by a sympathetic tone; however, the interpretation is controversial and may represent both sympathetic and parasympathetic activity.
- High frequency power (HF = 0.15–0.4 Hz) in ms^2: "sinus arrhythmia" mediated by alternating levels of a parasympathetic tone.
- LF/HF ratio: often referred to as the balance between the sympathetic and parasympathetic tones.
- Total power (TP) in ms^2: this measures the total variance in HRV.

2.3. Statistics

All analyses were performed using IBM SPSS Statistics software, (IBM Corp. IBM SPSS Statistics for Windows, Version 26.0, Armonk, NY, USA). For the descriptive statistics, the data were expressed as the mean ± standard deviation. The study population was divided into three diagnosis groups and one healthy control group. An unpaired *t*-test was used to compare the differences between the healthy control group and each patient group (Table 1). Significant group differences were anticipated if the *p*-value was <0.05.

3. Results

The time line, as illustrated in the Figure 1, showed that the initial COVID-19 infection of our study group had a peak in November 2021 when the Delta variant of the SARS-CoV-2 virus was dominant in Baden Württemberg (BW), a state of origin of our patients in southern Germany. Despite the high increases in new infections due to the Omicron variant of the SARS-CoV-2 virus up to February 2022, the number of initial infections in our analysis decreased. The first visit for ongoing health problems of our patients after COVID-19 or vaccination had a peak in February 2022, two months after the initial infection peak. There were only a few infections and first visits prior to November 2021. This mostly depended on the low infection rates of children in Germany due to a hard school lockdown.

The following results of our analysis are displayed in Table 1.

The age was not significantly different between the patient groups and the healthy control group (healthy control: 14.2 ± 3.8 years; Group 1: 13.3 ± 2.9 years; Group 2: 17.1 ± 3.7 years; Group 3: 14.9 ± 1.5 years). There were a few young adults up to 21 years of age in all groups. The body weight and height were not significantly different between the groups. The systolic blood pressure was normal and not significantly different. However, the diastolic blood pressure was significantly enhanced in the three patient groups (Group 1: 67.2 ± 9.1 mm Hg *; Group 2: 75.4 ± 8.6 mm HG ***; Group 3: 71.0 ± 6.3 mm Hg *) compared with the age-matched healthy control group (61.7 ± 11.2 mm Hg). The myocardial function, measured by fractional shortening and the left ventricular performance index, were normal in all patients and not significantly different between the patient groups.

The heart rate increase during the 5 min standing was significantly higher in all patient groups (Group 1: 25.3 ± 11.7 bpm **; Group 2: 26.2 ± 14.2 bpm **; Group 3: 29.6 ± 12.8 bpm **) compared with the healthy controls (16.2 ± 7.1 bpm). The average heart rates were enhanced whilst lying and standing in all patient groups. However, the heart rate increase depended on significantly higher heart rates whilst standing (Group 1: 106.0 ± 13.1 bpm ***; Group 2: 102.9 ± 10.8 bpm ***; Group 3: 115.1 ± 12.8 bpm ***) compared with 89.8 ± 13.2 bpm in the healthy controls. The stress index was enhanced whilst lying in all patient groups, but was more pronounced whilst standing (Group 1: 343.0 ± 292.0 ***; Group 2: 319.2 ± 219.3 **; Group 3: 494.1 ± 340.8 ***) compared with the healthy controls (168.5 ± 116.5). Our HRV data indicated that the heart rate increase whilst standing in children with dysautonomia after COVID-19 depended on a collapse of the vagus, with significantly lower pNN20 values (Group 1: 27.5 ± 17.4% ***; Group 2: 20.6 ± 13.5% ***; Group 3: 15.6 ± 13.6% ***) compared with the healthy control group (78.6 ± 10.8%). However, the RMSSD as well as the high frequency power data, which also depend on the vagus activity, were not clearly different in the patient groups compared with the healthy controls. This uncertainty depended on the high standard deviations of the frequency domain data. The respiratory rates were significantly increased in patient Groups 1 and 2 (healthy control: 16.3 ± 3.3/min; Group 1: 18.8 + 2.1/min **; Group 2: 19.1 ± 4.0/min *; Group 3: 17.7 ± 1.8/min). The quality of measurement, shown as analysable heart beats per measurement, was not significantly different between the groups (healthy control: 82.7 ± 18.5%; Group 1: 82.5 ± 15.3%; Group 2: 80.8 ± 24.7%; Group 3: 79.1 ± 17.0%).

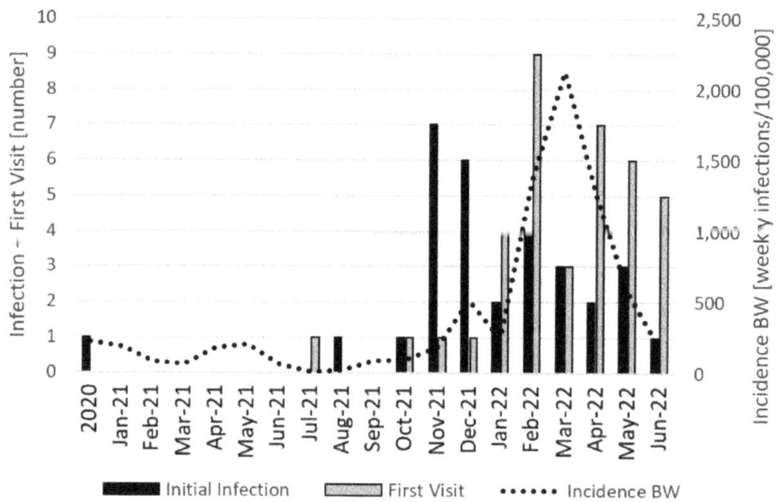

Figure 1. Timeline between initial SARS-CoV-2 infection/vaccination and first visit of cause of post-acute sequelae (PASC). **X-axis:** time; **left Y-axis:** number of initial infections and first visits in this month. **Right Y-axis:** Monthly new SARS-CoV-2 infections in Baden-Württemberg (State in southern Germany, BW).

4. Discussion

Persistent health problems after COVID-19 and longer than 11 weeks on average in our patient group of children and young adults up to 21 years of age overlapped with many symptoms that were difficult to specify. What they all had in common was a deterioration in physical and/or mental performance, with a significant impact on school performance. These problems were well-known prior to the COVID-19 pandemic, but have now increased further; perhaps due to the disease, but probably also as a consequence of health policy measures to prevent the spread of the pandemic such as lockdowns or vaccinations. As the perception of the burden of illness of our patients was influenced by a controversial public discussion about these political interventions, we looked for methods that could make an objective assessment possible.

The analysis of heart rate variability is an established method to calculate work performance [9]. Based upon our experience with the HRV analysis in children, we have used HRV monitoring since the beginning of the pandemic; thus, we were able to describe in detail the effects of the SARS-CoV-2 infection on the autonomic nervous system. We now present the first analysis of HRV data in children with long-term health problems after COVID-19 and its vaccination.

The results showed comparable highly significant effects on the heart rate whilst lying and standing in all patient groups who shared the fact that their immune system had been confronted with the spike protein of the SARS-CoV-2 virus, either through the infection and/or the vaccination. In summary, exactly half of our patient group had two mRNA vaccinations on average, which agreed well with the current vaccination rate of 67% for this age group in Baden-Württemberg, Germany.

Interestingly, the elevated heart rate in our children proceeded with elevated diastolic blood pressure, as recently shown in adults with PASC [10]. A subclinical diastolic impairment without a systolic involvement may be observed in patients with COVID-19, measured with the myocardial performance index [11]. However, our data clearly indicated a complete myocardial recovery in all our patients.

Together with many publications about dysautonomia in adults with PASC [12], there seems to be no question that the clinical symptoms of PASC are an expression of dysautonomia with elevated heart rates; however, the underlying pathophysiology seems to be unclear. The interpretation of the HRV data with elevated heart rates together with low pNN20/50 values may indicate a vagus weakness [13]. However, our RMSSD data and the frequency domain analysis were difficult to interpret due, in part, to the high standard deviations.

It has been shown that autoantibodies against G-coupled receptors have an impact on HRV and may cause dysautonomia. These autoantibodies are elevated in adults with PASC [14]. It seems plausible that autoimmunity has an impact on the heart rate and blood pressure independent of the sympatico vagal balance.

Therapeutically, it seems necessary to decrease elevated heart rates primarily to improve the clinical symptoms. However, eight patients fulfilled the criteria of postural orthostatic tachycardia syndrome and nine patients of an inappropriate sinus tachycardia, who were treated according the current guidelines [8]. Many other patients had heart rates just below our limits of a heart rate increase with average heart rates whilst lying and standing of more than 35 bpm or a lying heart rate of more than 90 bpm. Three athletes had low heart rates whilst lying but suffered from a heart rate increase whilst standing, as recently published in a case report [15].

In addition to a clinical improvement, there is increased evidence to treat elevated resting heart rates that are related to cardiovascular disease, cancer, and all-cause mortality [16]. This prognostic impact was even shown in adolescents by Swedish register data [17]. In the first step, we advise to increase sports [18] and supplement with omega-3 fatty acids, which significantly reduce the heart rate [19] and cardiovascular mortality [20]. Many of our patients required pharmacotherapy with low-dose propranolol, ivabradine, or midodrine; several of the children had to take this pharmacotherapy for up to one year after several unsuccessful attempts to exit.

It is not possible to make any recommendations for the SARS-CoV-2 vaccination based upon our data. However, vaccinations do not safely protect against PASC. Current publications suffer from significant methodological limitations such as a vaccination rate of only 1.6% in one publication of big data [3]. The apparently lower incidence of PASC after a natural infection with the Omicron variant could be an indication that a mucosal immunity is better protection against PASC than the systemic immunity of the current vaccinations. A number of such intranasal vaccines against SARS-CoV-2 are being tested in clinical trials [21].

5. Limitations

This retrospective analysis had a few limitations. First of all, the data of the healthy control grouped were measured prior to the pandemic. We are aware that the lockdown had an effect on heart rate variability, as recently published [22]. We used our published healthy control group and proved the matching according to age, height, weight, and gender. Patients with somatic and psychosomatic problems were carefully excluded.

Funding: This research received no external funding.

Institutional Review Board Statement: Ethical review and approval were waived for this study due to the fact that the data are collected from clinical routine in our pediatric practice.

Informed Consent Statement: Informed consent was obtained from all children and/or their parents for diagnostics and therapy.

Data Availability Statement: Anonymized data are available from the author.

Acknowledgments: I would like to thank Luise Hessing for editorial support.

Conflicts of Interest: The authors declare no conflict of interest.

Abbreviations

BW: Baden-Württemberg; HF: high frequency power; HF/LF: ratio of HF to LF; HRV: heart rate variability; LF: low frequency power; PASC: post-acute sequalae of SARS-CoV-2 infection; pNN20: percent of NN intervals that differed more than 20 ms from the prior interval; SDNN: standard deviation of all NN intervals; RMSSD: the square root of the mean of the sum of the squares of the differences between the adjacent NN intervals; VLF: very low frequency power.

References

1. Hope, A.A.; Evering, T.H. Postacute Sequelae of Severe Acute Respiratory Syndrome Coronavirus 2 Infection. *Infect. Dis. Clin. North Am.* **2022**, *36*, 379–395. [CrossRef] [PubMed]
2. Funk, A.L.; Kuppermann, N.; Florin, T.A.; Tancredi, D.J.; Xie, J.; Kim, K.; Finkelstein, Y.; Neuman, M.I.; Salvadori, M.I.; Yock-Corrales, A.; et al. Post-COVID-19 Conditions among Children 90 Days after SARS-CoV-2 Infection. *JAMA Netw. Open* **2022**, *5*, e2223253. [CrossRef]
3. Zisis, S.N.; Durieux, J.C.; Mouchati, C.; Perez, J.A.; McComsey, G.A. The Protective Effect of Coronavirus Disease 2019 (COVID-19) Vaccination on Postacute Sequelae of COVID-19: A Multicenter Study from a Large National Health Research Network. *Open Forum Infect. Dis.* **2022**, *9*, ofac228. [CrossRef] [PubMed]
4. Mumtaz, A.; Sheikh, A.A.E.; Khan, A.M.; Khalid, S.N.; Khan, J.; Nasrullah, A.; Sagheer, S.; Sheikh, A.B. COVID-19 Vaccine and Long COVID: A Scoping Review. *Life* **2022**, *12*, 1066. [CrossRef]
5. Said, K.B.; Al-Otaibi, A.; Aljaloud, L.; Al-Anazi, B.; Alsolami, A.; Alreshidi, F.S.; Ha'il COM Research Unit Group. The Frequency and Patterns of Post-COVID-19 Vaccination Syndrome Reveal Initially Mild and Potentially Immunocytopenic Signs in Primarily Young Saudi Women. *Vaccines* **2022**, *10*, 1015. [CrossRef]
6. Eldokla, A.M.; Mohamed-Hussein, A.A.; Fouad, A.M.; Abdelnaser, M.G.; Ali, S.T.; Makhlouf, N.A.; Sayed, I.G.; Makhlouf, H.A.; Shah, J.; Aiash, H. Prevalence and patterns of symptoms of dysautonomia in patients with long-COVID syndrome: A cross-sectional study. *Ann. Clin. Transl. Neurol.* **2022**, *9*, 778–785. [CrossRef] [PubMed]
7. Finsterer, J. Small fiber neuropathy underlying dysautonomia in COVID-19 and in post-SARS-CoV-2 vaccination and long-COVID syndromes. *Muscle Nerve* **2022**, *65*, E31–E32. [CrossRef] [PubMed]
8. Sheldon, R.S.; Grubb, B.P., 2nd; Olshansky, B.; Shen, W.K.; Calkins, H.; Brignole, M.; Raj, S.R.; Krahn, A.D.; Morillo, C.A.; Stewart, J.M.; et al. 2015 heart rhythm society expert consensus statement on the diagnosis and treatment of postural tachycardia syndrome, inappropriate sinus tachycardia, and vasovagal syncope. *Heart Rhythm* **2015**, *12*, e41–e63. [CrossRef]
9. Tomes, C.; Schram, B.; Orr, R. Relationships Between Heart Rate Variability, Occupational Performance, and Fitness for Tactical Personnel: A Systematic Review. *Front. Public Health* **2020**, *8*, 583336. [CrossRef] [PubMed]
10. Mahmoud, Z.; East, L.; Gleva, M.; Woodard, P.K.; Lavine, K.; Verma, A.K. Cardiovascular symptom phenotypes of post-acute sequelae of SARS-CoV-2. *Int. J. Cardiol.* **2022**, *366*, 35–41. [CrossRef] [PubMed]
11. Kaya, H.; Asoglu, R.; Afsin, A.; Tibilli, H.; Kurt, E.; Kafadar, S.; Gulacti, U.; Kafadar, H. Evaluation of myocardial performance index in patients with COVID-19: An echocardiographic follow-up study. *Rev. Port. Cardiol.* **2022**, *41*, 455–461. [CrossRef] [PubMed]
12. Shah, B.; Kunal, S.; Bansal, A.; Jain, J.; Poundrik, S.; Shetty, M.K.; Batra, V.; Chaturvedi, V.; Yusuf, J.; Mukhopadhyay, S.; et al. Heart rate variability as a marker of cardiovascular dysautonomia in post-COVID-19 syndrome using artificial intelligence. *Indian Pacing Electrophysiol. J.* **2022**, *22*, 70–76. [CrossRef] [PubMed]
13. Acanfora, D.; Nolano, M.; Acanfora, C.; Colella, C.; Provitera, V.; Caporaso, G.; Rodolico, G.R.; Bortone, A.S.; Galasso, G.; Casucci, G. Impaired Vagal Activity in Long-COVID-19 Patients. *Viruses* **2022**, *14*, 1035. [CrossRef] [PubMed]
14. Wallukat, G.; Hohberger, B.; Wenzel, K.; Fürst, J.; Schulze-Rothe, S.; Wallukat, A.; Hönicke, A.S.; Müller, J. Functional autoantibodies against G-protein coupled receptors in patients with persistent Long-COVID-19 symptoms. *J. Transl. Autoimmun.* **2021**, *4*, 100100. [CrossRef] [PubMed]
15. Hottenrott, L.; Gronwald, T.; Hottenrott, K.; Wiewelhove, T.; Ferrauti, A. Utilizing Heart Rate Variability for Coaching Athletes During and After Viral Infection: A Case Report in an Elite Endurance Athlete. *Front. Sports Act. Living* **2021**, *3*, 612782. [CrossRef]
16. Aune, D.; Sen, A.; ó'Hartaigh, B.; Janszky, I.; Romundstad, P.R.; Tonstad, S.; Vatten, L.J. Resting heart rate and the risk of cardiovascular disease, total cancer, and all-cause mortality—A systematic review and dose-response meta-analysis of prospective studies. *Nutr. Metab. Cardiovasc. Dis. NMCD* **2017**, *27*, 504–517. [CrossRef]

17. Lindgren, M.; Robertson, J.; Adiels, M.; Schaufelberger, M.; Åberg, M.; Torén, K.; Waern, M.; Åberg, N.D.; Rosengren, A. Resting heart rate in late adolescence and long term risk of cardiovascular disease in Swedish men. *Int. J. Cardiol.* **2018**, *259*, 109–115. [CrossRef]
18. Reimers, A.K.; Knapp, G.; Reimers, C.D. Effects of Exercise on the Resting Heart Rate: A Systematic Review and Meta-Analysis of Interventional Studies. *J. Clin. Med.* **2018**, *7*, 503. [CrossRef]
19. Zhang, W. Chronotropic effects and mechanisms of long-chain omega-3 polyunsaturated fatty acids on heartbeat: The latest insights. *Nutr. Rev.* **2021**, *80*, 128–135. [CrossRef]
20. Khan, S.U.; Lone, A.N.; Khan, M.S.; Virani, S.S.; Blumenthal, R.S.; Nasir, K.; Miller, M.; Michos, E.D.; Ballantyne, C.M.; Boden, W.E.; et al. Effect of omega-3 fatty acids on cardiovascular outcomes: A systematic review and meta-analysis. *EClinicalMedicine* **2021**, *38*, 100997. [CrossRef]
21. Karczmarzyk, K.; Kęsik-Brodacka, M. Attacking the Intruder at the Gate: Prospects of Mucosal Anti SARS-CoV-2 Vaccines. *Pathogens* **2022**, *11*, 117. [CrossRef] [PubMed]
22. Bourdillon, N.; Yazdani, S.; Schmitt, L.; Millet, G.P. Effects of COVID-19 lockdown on heart rate variability. *PLoS ONE* **2020**, *15*, e0242303. [CrossRef] [PubMed]

vaccines

MDPI

Review

mRNA-Based Vaccine for COVID-19: They Are New but Not Unknown!

Vivek P. Chavda [1,*], Gargi Jogi [1], Srusti Dave [2], Bhoomika M. Patel [3], Lakshmi Vineela Nalla [4] and Krishna Koradia [5]

[1] Department of Pharmaceutics and Pharmaceutical Technology, L M College of Pharmacy, Ahmedabad 380009, India
[2] Department of Pharmacology, Institute of Pharmacy, Nirma University, Ahmedabad 382481, India
[3] School of Medico-legal Studies, National Forensic Sciences University, Gandhinagar 382007, India
[4] Department of Pharmacy, Koneru Lakshmaiah Education Foundation, Vaddeswaram 522302, India
[5] Department of Pharmaceutics, Saurashtra University, Rajkot 360005, India
* Correspondence: vivek.chavda@lmcp.ac.in

Abstract: mRNA vaccines take advantage of the mechanism that our cells use to produce proteins. Our cells produce proteins based on the knowledge contained in our DNA; each gene encodes a unique protein. The genetic information is essential, but cells cannot use it until mRNA molecules convert it into instructions for producing specific proteins. mRNA vaccinations provide ready-to-use mRNA instructions for constructing a specific protein. BNT162b2 (Pfizer-BioNTech) and mRNA-1273 (Moderna) both are newly approved mRNA-based COVID-19 vaccines that have shown excellent protection and efficacy. In total, there are five more mRNA-based vaccine candidates for COVID-19 under different phases of clinical development. This review is specifically focused on mRNA-based vaccines for COVID-19 covering its development, mechanism, and clinical aspects.

Keywords: COVID-19 vaccine; mRNA vaccines; vaccine development; vector-based vaccines

1. Introduction

Coronavirus disease-19 (COVID-19) pandemic caused by severe acute respiratory syndrome coronavirus-2 (SARS-CoV-2) has spread worldwide. As of now, globally, there have been 662 million confirmed cases of COVID-19, including 6.6 million deaths reported to the World Health Organization (WHO) [1]. The virus affects more than 200 countries worldwide, with the bulk of cases reported in Brazil, Russia, and the United States [2]. The first report of an outbreak of COVID-19 was from Wuhan city, Hubei Province of China on 30 December 2019. Clusters of cases of pneumonia were recorded in Wuhan. Later on 7 January 2020, a novel coronavirus (2019-nCoV) was found to be the causative agent. The WHO eventually named the disease COVID-19 [3,4]. The estimated case fatality rate ranges from 0.5–1.5%. SARS-CoV-2 belongs to the family *Coronaviridae* and the order *Nidovirales*. SARS-CoV-2 belongs to Betacoronavirus having a close genomic relation with two viruses, SARS-CoV and Middle Eastern respiratory syndrome coronavirus (MERS-CoV). As compared to SARS and MERS, SARS-CoV-2 is highly contagious. COVID-19 is a serious illness of global significance. The illness cannot be treated with a specific antiviral medication, the key to preventing the spread of the disease is to break the chain of transmission [5]. To decrease the prevalence and mortality rates, mass immunization against the pandemic is used [6,7]. Since the SARS-CoV-2 genome sequence was released on 11 January 2020, more than 150 authority immunization projects were studied. The main goal of vaccination is to induce an immune response that provides long-term protection against severity of the disease [8]. As evaluated by Paddy Ssentongo and colleagues [9], vaccine efficacy (VE) against all SARS-CoV-2 infections fell from 83% in the first month after completion of the first immunisation series to 22% after 5 months or more. Similarly, VE against symptomatic COVID-19 decreased from 94% in the first month to 64% during the fourth month following immunisation. Overall, VE against severe COVID-19 was strong at all ages, with a level of 90% (95% CI, 87–92%) five months or more after being completely vaccinated.

Coronavirus has spiked (S) protein on its surface; this S protein will interact with the receptor-binding domain of the angiotensin-converting enzyme (ACE) receptor [10,11]. Most of the vaccine candidates are targeting this S protein of the virus [12]. The Pfizer-BioNTech COVID-19 Vaccine-BNT162b2 is the first immunization approved by the Food and Drug Administration (FDA). It is based on messenger RNA (mRNA) made by Pfizer which received emergency use authorization for 12–15 years of age or older for the prevention of the COVID-19 disease. US food and drug administration (USFDA) approved the Pfizer vaccine on 23 August 2021 [13]. Various studies have reported that immunization is having an efficiency of 89.1% to prevent the SARS-CoV-2 infection; additionally, vaccines have also decreased COVID-19-related hospitalization, deaths, and prevention of ICU admission. Controllable spread of SARS-CoV-2 can be accomplished earlier when a large proportion of the population is immunized (e.g., 70–80%). Immunization significantly reduces the incidence of COVID-19. The vaccine provides a robust and effective immune response to eradicate the SARS-CoV-2 infection from the human body. People who were infected had a potent T-cell response to the virus, which may aid in their ability to recover from the infection [14,15]. Neutralisation remained strongly correlated with protection from symptomatic infection with SARS-CoV-2 variants of concern [16]. Thus, vaccination is the strategy to control the pandemic.

COVID-19 vaccines are being developed on a variety of platforms. A live attenuated virus, inactivated vaccines, non-replicating viral vectors, RNA, and DNA are examples of these. Different types of vaccines with examples are listed in the Figure 1. A strategy for vaccine development is of using the killed SARS-CoV-2 virus, it is not able to replicate but it can remain intact in the body. The immune system will trigger its response against the virus by making antibodies against it. COVAXIN® (BBV152) manufactured by Bharat Biotech, Hyderabad, India, and CoronaVac also known as sinovac® developed by Sinovac Biotech, Beijing, China has used inactivated virus approach to develop the vaccine [17]. The nonreplicating viral vector is also a technique adopted by companies for vaccine production. The adenovirus (Ads) is a widely used viral vector that has a double-stranded genome acting as a causative agent for a common cold. CanSino Biologics Tianjin, China has developed Ad5-nCoV (Convidecia®) which encodes the full length of S-protein of the SARS-CoV-2 virus. The viral vector does not possess replicating properties and hence does not cause actual disease. Once entered into the body the viral DNA is presented on antigen-presenting cells and an immune response is generated against it. Oxford/Astrazeneca has used adenovirus from the chimpanzee (ChAdOx1) which possesses the potential to minimize interaction with prevalent antibodies against adenovirus. The vaccine is named AZD122 (Vaxzevria™). The Gamaleya Research Institute, Moscow, Russia developed the Sputnik V™ vaccine is also a viral vector having recombinant human Ad26 serotype. The Janssen vaccine was manufactured by Johnson and Johnson, New Jersey, USA using the same approach [18].

mRNA is also considered a new approach to formulating a vaccine. mRNA vaccines are new to the public, but scientists have been researching them for a long time. These mRNA vaccines are synthesized from the DNA template which encodes the spike protein and is packed into the lipoprotein-based carrier to speed up the entry of the mRNA inside the body and prevent degradation [19]. When the vaccine is given through the intramuscular route, it is injected into deeper tissues and the mRNA molecules will enter inside the cell, facilitating the translation process [20]. Upon entering the body, mRNA will be recognized as an antigen and a humoral immune response will be activated which will stimulate B cells to develop into memory B cells. Thereby on secondary exposure to the antigen; memory B cells will neutralize and block the antigens [21]. FDA has approved mRNA-based vaccines, one of which is Pfizer-BioNTech's, New York, NY, USA BNT162b2 (Comirnaty®) and another one is Moderna™, Cambridge, MA, USA mRNA-1273 also known as Spikevax. The

FDA approved mRNA-1273 for emergency use authorization (EUA) for use in people aged 18 years and over. The current review will provide detailed information about vaccinology and facts about COVID-19, mRNA-based vaccine development, how mRNA vaccines work, the formulation and ingredients used, safety and efficacy, and the regulatory challenges for vaccines.

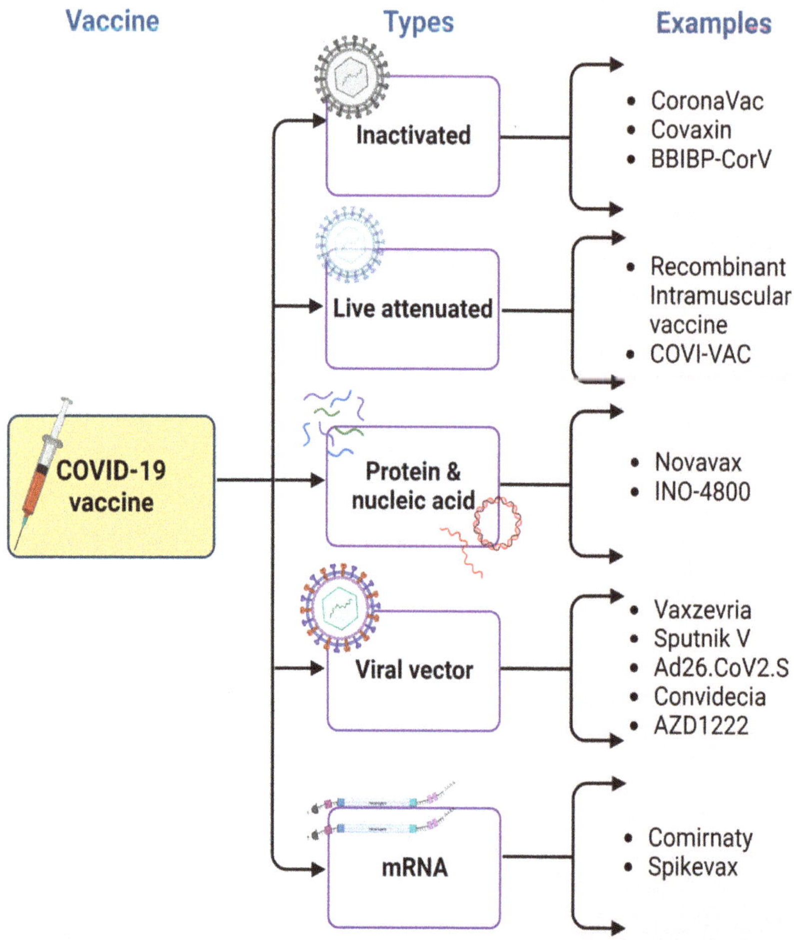

Figure 1. Different types of vaccine for COVID-19 infection. (Created with BioRender.com accessed on 31 December 2022).

2. Vaccinology and Facts about COVID-19

In December 2019, a group of individuals suffering from lung disorders for an unidentified reason was reported in China. The Chinese Centre for Disease Control and Prevention (CDC) then investigated the uncertainty in pneumonia-related cases and their origin by collecting specimens from the patient's body which were detected using real-time polymerase chain reaction [22]. Later, the cause of the lung disorder was known and it was found to be caused by a coronavirus, which was further named SARS-CoV-2 (severe acute respiratory syndrome) or COVID-19. Since then, it has turned into a global pandemic. It belongs to a group of β-coronaviruses. Structurally, it is an enveloped, non-segmented, belonging to the subgenus of *Sarbecovirus*, and *Orthocoronavirinae* subfamily. The genomic material present in its structure is the single-stranded positive-sense RNA sequence [23]. They are found primarily in avian and mammal hosts. The genomic structure of coronavirus has been depicted in Figure 2, which represents that the viral structure possesses spike proteins, having subunits, S1 and S2, on the outer membrane. The RNA viral genome is encapsulated inside the membrane along with the nucleocapsid. Thus, we can say that there are four structural proteins, i.e., the spike protein (S), nucleocapsid protein (N), membrane protein (M), and envelope protein (E) [24]. In addition to this, non-structural proteins (Nsp) are also present which are sixteen in total. The spike proteins are the prominent receptor binding sites, where the proteins can interact with receptors present in the body [25]. The S1 subunit includes the receptor binding domain (RBD), wherein the angiotensin-converting enzyme II binds to the spike protein. It also consists of the N-terminal domain (NDT). The S2 subunit possesses the fusion proteins (FP) and transmembrane proteins (TM) [26]. Upon entry of the virus into the host cells, it leads to fusion and uncoating of the viral membrane, followed by transcription and translation of mRNA, which is essential for the formation of viral assembly, which then exoduses out of the host via exocytosis to infect other cells. The entry of viral particles into the other cells of the body leads to stimulation of the immune response and generation of antibodies [27].

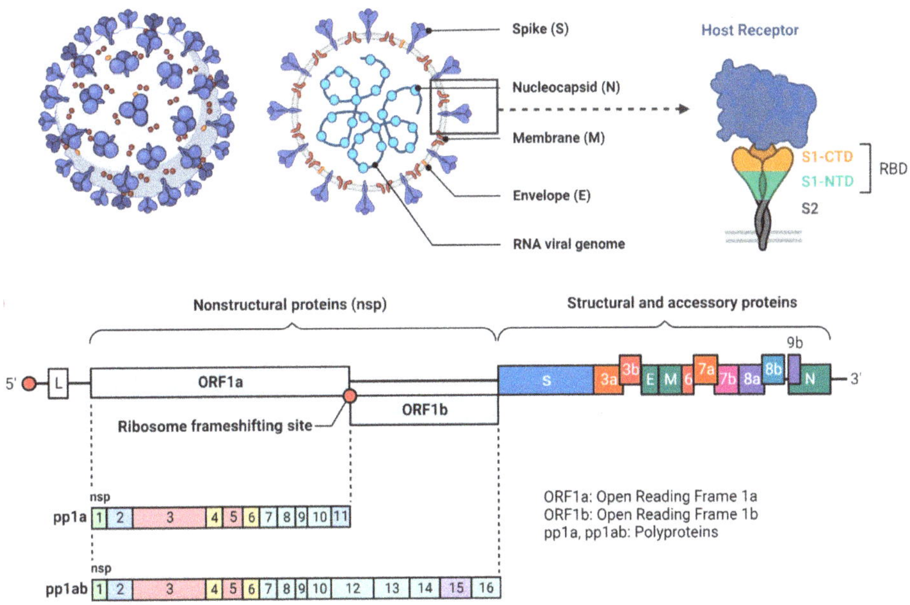

Figure 2. Genomic structure of coronavirus. (Created with BioRender.com accessed on 31 December 2022).

Globally, immunizations have been widely used and are efficient to decrease mortality rates. Based on sound science and knowledge, the assessment of the safety and efficacy of vaccines and their uptake evaluation can be enhanced [28]. Vaccines have evolved from traditional vaccines such as live attenuated or killed vaccines to subunit vaccines and lastly, homologous or heterologous prime-boost immunization strategies [29]. Different vaccine strategies have been depicted in Figure 3. In antiquity, live attenuated vaccines have been proved to be a saviour against various pathogenic viruses and are considered to be safe against millions of populations, but they are often neglected. Many vaccines including MMR (measles, mumps, rubella) and chicken pox vaccines are live-attenuated vaccines [25,30]. The weakened forms of the virus can be attained by its exposure to adverse conditions or by genetic modifications. This type of vaccine, specifically the oral polio vaccine (OPV) can be administered via non-invasive routes. In contrast, killed vaccines, which are the inactivated versions of the viruses, have limited application in terms of immunological response but the currently used Indian vaccine, COVAXIN®, manufactured by Bharat Biotech International Limited, Hyderabad, Telangana, India uses the inactivated version of the virus in its vaccine formulation [31]. The inactivated virus is capable enough to retain its epitome conformity that aids in modulating the humoral immune response [32].

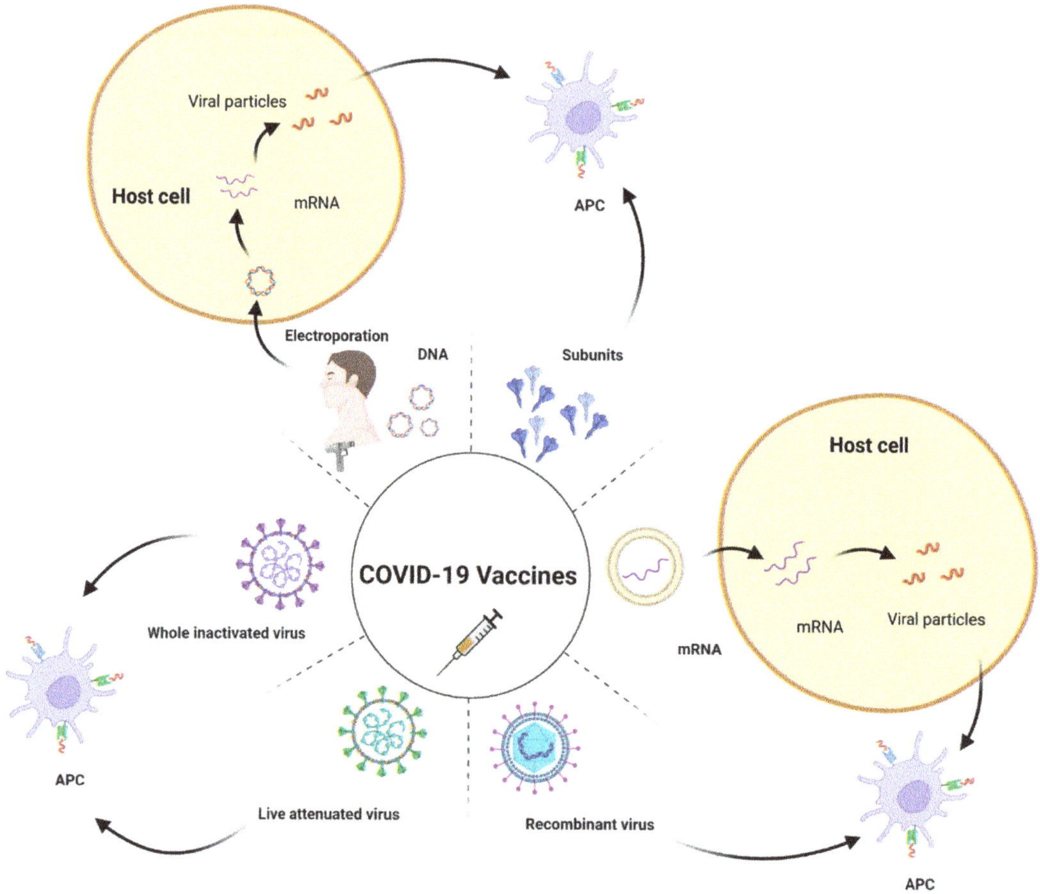

Figure 3. Interaction of vaccines with the host cells and viral particle. (Created with BioRender.com accessed on 31 December 2022).

Recent technologies such as mRNA-based vaccines or vector-based vaccines make the most of it for the safety and efficacy of COVID-19 vaccines [33]. The vector-based vaccines are also known as heterologous prime-boost vaccination, which helps in inducing both cellular and humoral immune responses, whereas the live sub-unit vaccines provoke a humoral response only [34–39]. According to a study, a 5–10 times increase in T cell-mediated immune response in case of a heterologous vector-based vaccine in comparison to the same formulation, prepared using a homologous approach [40]. Hence, the vector-based vaccines, namely DNA and RNA based are more preferred over sub-unit based, often considered more robust as compared to RNA vaccines, and effective as they encode the spike protein of the virus structure. In the case of the Chikungunya virus, the co-immunization strategy using DNA and virus-like particles generated a better immune response in animal studies [41]. Sometimes, DNA vaccines require specialized delivery systems such as electrophoresis, microneedle arrays, and carrier-based systems such as liposomes to enhance the permeability. Polylactic-co-glycolic acid-based microspheres were formulated for HIV-1 DNA vaccine delivery via the intramuscular route [42]. However, DNA-based vaccines generate a meager immune response and often require another dosing. This can be overcome by the use of mRNA-based vaccines [25,43].

3. mRNA-Based Vaccine Development

Formerly, different forms of RNA were used for the vaccine formulation, including in vitro transcribed mRNA, siRNA (small interference RNA), RNA based aptamers, riboswitches, antisense molecules and later-on, mRNA. The awareness of messenger ribonucleic acid, i.e., mRNA originates from its basic, furthermore, economical creation, its transient movement and slow breakdown in the target cells, and its security benefits contrasted with DNA therapeutics as it does not coordinate the human genome, inhibiting insertional mutagenesis, and is promptly accessible for interpretation into protein in the cell cytoplasm [44].

In the early 1990s, researchers worked abundantly to succeed in the development of mRNA-based vaccines. Various experiments were performed in vitro and the results showed a subsequent production of desired proteins; therefore, it was concluded that since mRNA is capable enough to produce proteins, then it can be a probable therapeutic regimen to treat the ailment [45]. According to Martinon et al., the nucleoprotein-based mRNA vaccine for the treatment of influenza was synthesized by in vitro transcription and was incorporated into liposomal vesicles. The results demonstrated the induction of cytotoxic T-cells and antibodies, in vivo [46]. Since then, there has been a progressive development in the use of mRNA as a therapeutic tool due to its significant effectiveness, easy scale-up, and cost-effectiveness, which is a primary requirement for the treatment of highly contagious diseases and cancer therapy. Recent research studies revealed that mRNA-based therapies significantly protected mice from Chikungunya symptoms and maintained desirable levels of antibodies after two doses [47]. RNA-based vaccines target the immune cells of the body by alteration of their functions, targeting the ribosomes for translation, thereby generating an immune response [19].

mRNA-based immunizations comprise single-stranded mRNA, which encodes the antigen desired. They can be conveyed as naked mRNA or encapsulated into suitable carrier systems to facilitate delivery into the cells. Once the mRNA enters the cell, it is translated into protein-based structures by the cell's natural mechanisms. It is further subjected to post-translational modifications to obtain a protein of interest and generates an immune response as determined by the signal peptides [44,48]. mRNA-based vaccines face a minimum of two hurdles: nuclear degradation when injected into animals and innate immunogenicity similar to that of antigen [49]. To outrange this problem, pseudo-uridine (Ψ) is a well-known RNA modification. Ψ replace uridine with in vitro transcribed (IVT) mRNA, which is highly prevalent, and naturally occurring nucleotide in all the cells with RNAs. Vaccination against COVID-19, produced by both, Moderna and Pfizer-BioNTech consist of novel modified Ψ having efficacy up to 90% against symptoms [50]. Wherein, a vaccine developed by CureVac NV lacked Ψ-modified mRNA and clinical trials confirmed the efficacy of 48% only [51].

During the translation process, primarily, two different categories of mRNA vaccines exist, namely, non-amplifying mRNA (NMR) and self-amplifying mRNA (SMR). The working mechanism of non-amplifying mRNA and self-amplifying mRNA is explained in Figure 4. Structurally, as shown in Figure 5, both the structures possess a CAP, 5′ and 3′ untranslated regions (UTR), an opening frame (ORF), and a ponytail in common [52,53].

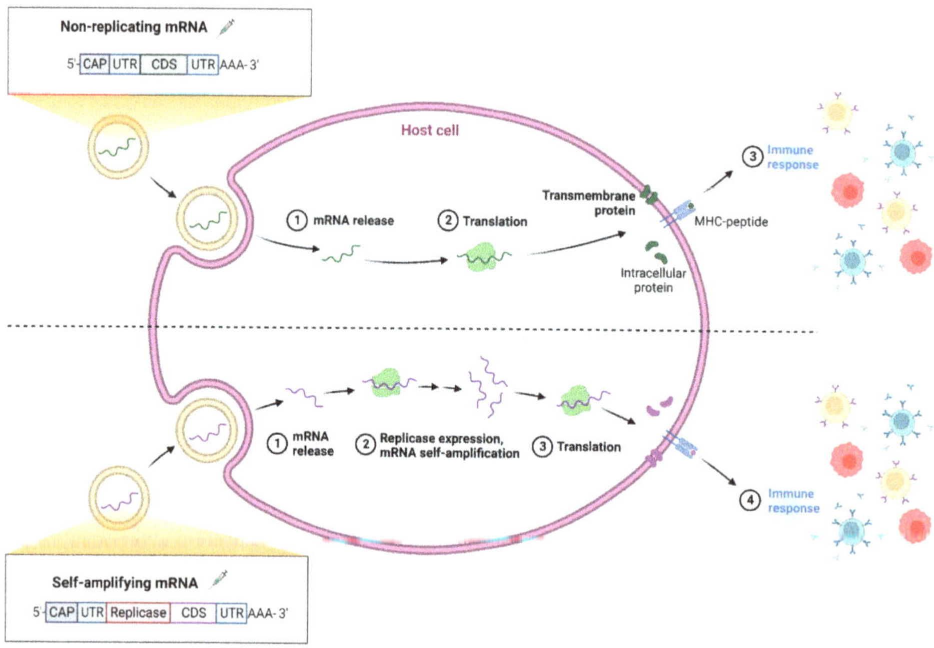

Figure 4. Categories of mRNA. (Created with BioRender.com accessed on 31 December 2022).

In addition to this, the SMR possess replicase as a segment which helps in amplification of mRNA intracellularly. Further, the segments are translated by ribosomes in order to produce proteins of interest. The proteins secreted lead to generation of immune response [54]. SMRs are comparatively larger than NMRs and anionic molecules. Recent studies of self-replicating RNA showed better in vitro sub-genome expression of non-structural proteins of Venezuelan equine encephalitis (VEE) replicon when different mutations were observed. A similar clinical trial study was conducted to target the Rabies glycoprotein using VEE-Sindbis virus self-amplifying RNA formulated into nano-emulsions is currently ongoing [55]. The major critical quality attributes (CQAs) which define efficacy of mRNA therapies are summarized in the Table 1 [54].

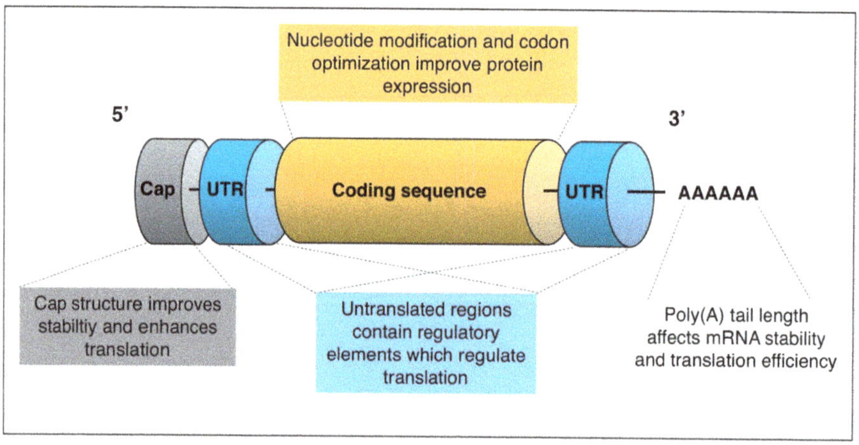

Figure 5. Optimization of mRNA sequence. (Adapted from [56] with rights and permissions).

Table 1. CQAs for mRNA vaccines.

CQA	Key Features	Optimization	References
5′ and 3′ Untranslated regions (UTR)	Both 5′ and 3′ UTRs are evident for recognition by the ribosomes and for initiation of translation process and mRNA stability.	• Canonical and non-canonical start codons such as AUG and CUG, respectively, must be avoided, which has its influence on the translation process. • In an arbitrarily conducted study by Sample et al., 0.3 million random 5′ UTR based predictive model was identified and used to fabricate a new model for optimal protein expression and efficiency.	[57–59]
5′ CAP	For effective vaccination mechanisms, 5′ CAP of the mRNA holds as a backbone along with N7-methylated guanosine sidechain. Capped or uncapped mRNAs are identified by Pattern recognition receptors (PRR), which may lead to destruction of mRNA.	• Natural capping of the mRNA evades destruction by the PRRs. Dithiodiphosphates are presented in the phosphate bridge, which declines the CAP sensitivity and enhances translation potential. • According to a study conducted by Ryzdik, substitution of oxygen in PO4−3 moieties by CCl2 or CF2 resist decapping without diminishing the translation process.	[58,60–62]
Poly (A) tail	Usually consists of 15–250 units of adenosine ribonucleotide. It enacts a critical role in regulation of translation and protein expression. The 3′ stretch of the poly tail when attached to a poly(A)-binding protein (PABP) interacts with eukaryotic translation initiation factors (EIFs) and forms a closed-loop assembly.	• Addition of a poly-U sequence synergizes the translation process. • Pfizer COVID-19 vaccine utilizes a 110-Poly (A) tail consisting of 30 adenosine residues, 10-nucleotide linkers, and 70 adenosine residues. While, Curevac utilizes 64-Poly(A) tail.	[56,63,64]

The manufacturing of mRNA is a two-step process, which includes production and purification. No impurities are present in mRNA manufacturing systems as it does not contain any animal or cell-derived raw materials, the production is relatively safer [65]. The production of mRNA sequence may be a single-step enzymatic process or a two-step enzymatic process. A capping analog is used in the case of one-step production process, which is generally used at a laboratory scale. The process is then accomplished by purification, which involves separation using chromatographic techniques as shown in Figure 6. The two-step enzymatic reaction for the production of mRNA encompasses in vitro transcription of the DNA template to form an RNA polymerase sequence [66]. The mRNA template so formed can be capped using vaccinia capping enzyme and methyl donor. The production of mRNA is relatively high and at an industrial scale, it is difficult to achieve reproducibility [67].

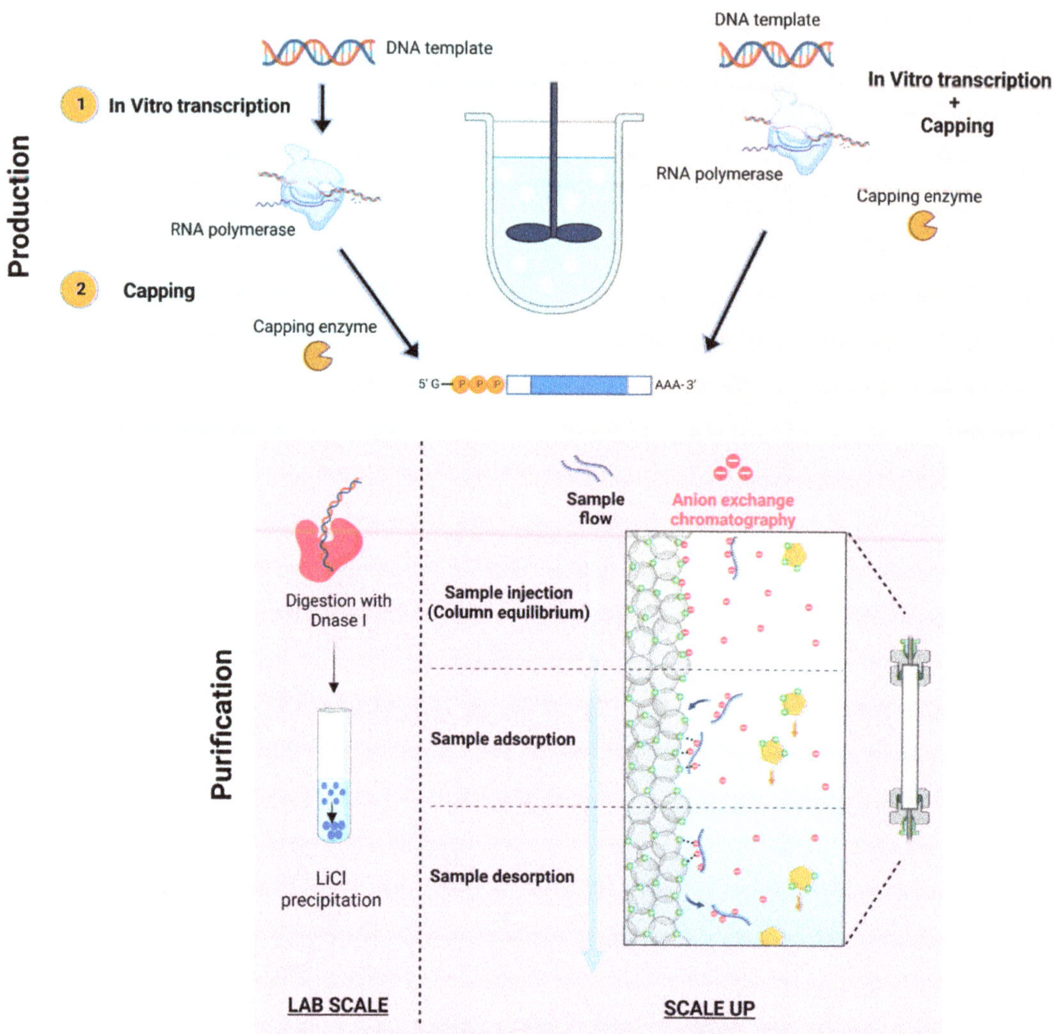

Figure 6. Manufacturing process of mRNA sequence. (Created with BioRender.com accessed on 1 January 2023).

4. How do mRNA Vaccines Work?

mRNA is unstable negatively charged molecule which is encapsulated in lipidic nanoparticles. Through endocytosis, these lipidic nanoparticles enter cells. Once enter the cytoplasm these endosomes are immediately directed to lysosomes for degradation. Studies reveal that ionizable lipids play an important role in endosomes' escape and release of mRNA. The head group of lipids is protonated within the acidic environment of endosomes, and this cationic state is subsequently attached to the anionic head of the phospholipid in the endosomal membrane. The hydrophobic tail of cationic lipid and phospholipid then extends, disrupting the bilayer phospholipid structure and allowing mRNA to escape into the cytoplasmic compartment. Ribosomes transform mRNA into proteins when it is released. This protein can activate an immune response in two ways: (1) The proteasome degrades these proteins into peptides, which are then presented as an antigen on the cell surface by MHC (major histocompatibility complex) class I molecules, which bind to TCR (T cell receptor) to activate CD8+ T cells, which kill infected cells; the protein itself can activate an immune response in two ways. (2) Extracellularly secreted proteins are engulfed by APCs (antigen-presenting cells) and degraded into peptides that are presented on the cell surface by MHC class II and recognised by CD4+ T cells, which secrete cytokines to produce a cellular response and co-activate B cells to produce a humoral immune response, as shown in Figure 7. Furthermore, mRNA vaccines delivered double-stranded and single-stranded RNA that binds to TLR (Toll-like receptor) in the endosome, resulting in the stimulation of numerous IFN-1 (type I interferon) stimulated genes, hence activating antiviral innate immune responses.

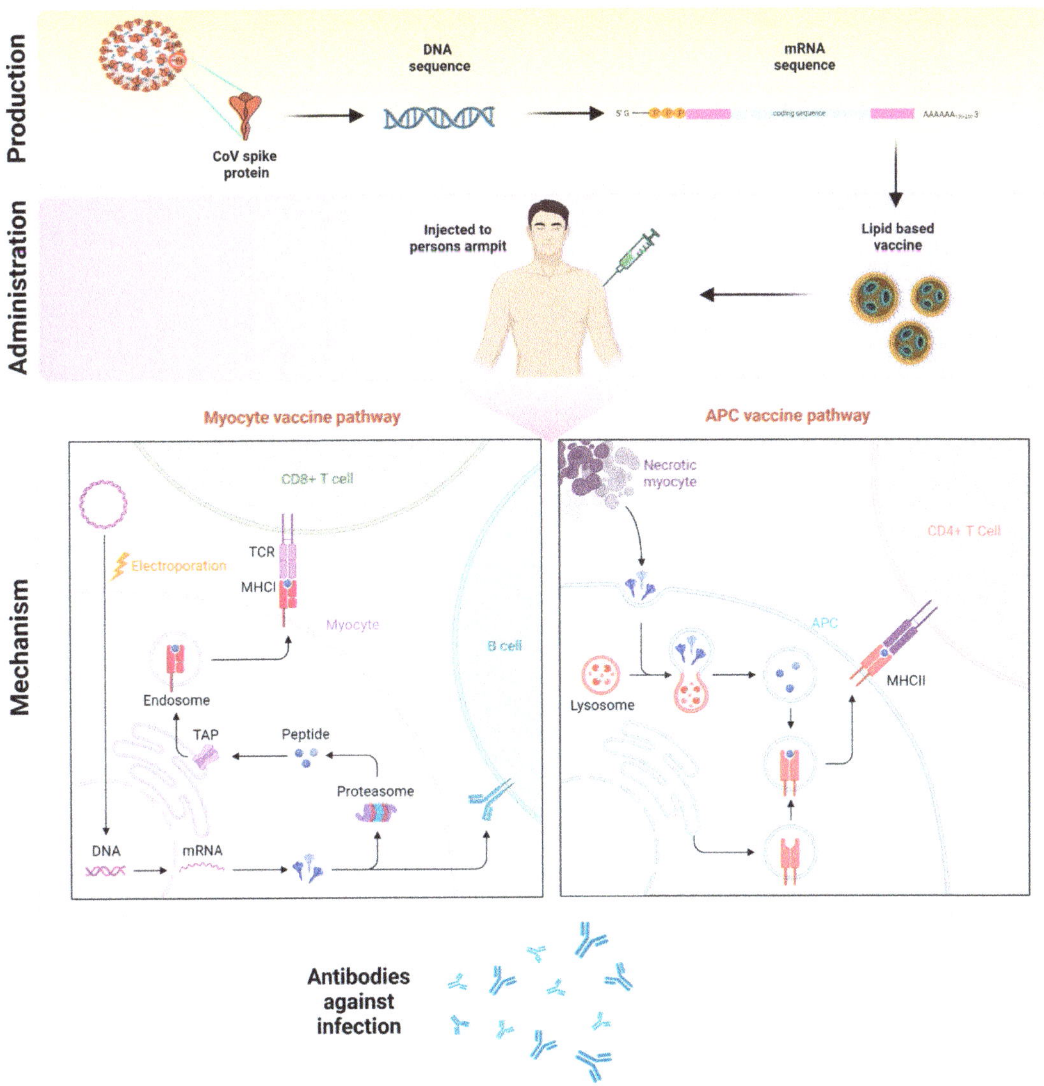

Figure 7. Mechanism through which mRNA Vaccine elicit immunity to the host. (Created with BioRender.com accessed on 1 January 2023).

5. Formulation Aspects of mRNA-Based Vaccines

Once the transcribed mRNA is injected, it will express proteins inside the body. An immunological response is observed due to the expressed protein from the mRNA. This process is predominantly the basis of mRNA vaccine development [68].

5.1. DNA Template

Identification of the antigen from the target pathogen is the foremost step. The development of mRNA immunisation needs the addition of the encoded antigen in a DNA template, which will help in the translation of mRNA in vitro. The specific antigen will be produced in vivo by the transcription of the transcribed mRNA, which will only reach the cytoplasm; this will help in eliciting an immune response. The plasmid DNA (pDNA) contains a promoter sequence with strong affinity to a DNA dependent RNA polymerase, such as T7, SP6, or T3, as well as the appropriate sequence for the mRNA construct. The enzyme will pass along the template, extending the RNA transcript until it reaches the template's end [69].

5.2. Capping Enzyme

For efficient translation of mRNA from the DNA template capping at the 5′ end of the mRNA is very much important. Furthermore, 5′ capping in mature mRNA is required for mRNA protection from degradation, gene expression, and ribosome recruitment. A 5′-5′-triphosphate bridge connects the 5′ cap of eukaryotic mRNA to 7-methylguanosine (m7G) (m7GpppN). A novel co-transcriptional technique that employed a clean cap kit to precisely add a natural 5′ cap1 structure to the start site during IVT reactions has made the generation of 5′ capped mRNA by T7 polymerase a commonly used capping method with good translation and minimal reactogenicity. In the COVID-19 BNT162b1 mRNA vaccines, 5′ caps were added using the clean cap method [70]. The cap analog-transcribed mRNA has a poly 1 tail and a 3′(poly A) tail is present at the 3′ end of eukaryotic mRNA. This poly A tail is performing functions of transport, translation, and stability of mRNA. The 3′ poly A tail and 5′ cap will create a stable closed loop structure with the eIF4F complex for the start of the translation process. Because of its 120 nucleotides (nt) in the 3′ poly(A) tail, the BioNTech mRNA vaccine has superior stability and translation efficiency [71].

5.3. Nucleotide Triphosphate Substrates (NTPs)

When DNA plasmids are integrated with T7 polymerase and nucleotide triphosphates, mRNA is translated more efficiently and more yields are produced. After administration of the vaccine a concern raised is immunogenicity. On activation of the downstream signaling, the body will recognize and responds to viral RNAs. This recognition of single and double-stranded RNA is by endosomal receptors such as Toll-like receptors (TLR3), TLR7, and TLR8. Double-stranded and 5′-triphosphate modified RNA is recognized by the cytosolic receptor's retinoic acid-inducible gene-I (RIG-1) and melanoma differentiation-associated protein 5 (MDA-5). Allergic reactions and anaphylactic shock were reported when the body's immune system is activated in an uncontrolled manner. This overstimulation of the immune system on a molecular level will limit the protein translation, expression of antigens, and vaccine efficacy. This limitation can be overcome by nucleobase modifications. N1-methylpseudouridin, a modified nucleobase, will increase the protein output and decrease the activation of TLR3. Modified nucleotides through RIG-1 not only affect protein-RNA interaction but also decrease the ability of mRNAs to disseminate immunological signals. Translation efficiency of mRNA into protein is improved because of N1-methylpseudouridin. Translation initiation occurring rapidly will coordinately increase the half-life of mRNA [50].

5.4. Lipid Nanoparticle Components for mRNA Delivery

As compared to all other vaccines, mRNA vaccines are developed relatively fast and are more efficacious. However, the greatest challenge in the manufacturing of mRNA vaccines is their poor stability. The vaccine's stability and capacity to treat the COVID-19 infection are reduced because the vaccine is rapidly broken down by ribonucleases after delivery, producing broken-down components that are eliminated through the kidney. To address this challenge, mRNA can be formulated with lipid nanoparticles (LNPs). The mRNA-LNP vaccine will protect the mRNA from premature degradation and will facilitate cytoplasmic delivery to antigen-presenting cells [72]. Lipids are perfect agents to deliver mRNA at the cytosolic site, as their fusion is compatible with lipid cell membranes; leading to the targeted and effective release of the mRNA. LNPs are nanosized particles with a diameter of less than one micron that contain two or more lipids in varying proportions. LNPs differ from liposomes because of the presence of lipids components in the core as a discontinuous mix. The LNPs that underwent formulation have a multilamellar vesicular structure, a homogeneous core-shell, and a nanostructured core [73]. There is the presence of water inside the core of the LNPs, which exposes mRNA for interaction with an aqueous medium. As shown in Figure 8, mRNA is located inside the LNPs, which protects it from the external environment. The most common composition, which makes up the mRNA-LNP systems are a cationic/ionizable lipid, a phospholipid ("helper lipid"), cholesterol, and a poly-ethylene-glycol (PEG). Physicochemical characteristics inside the LNP delivery system, such as encapsulation effectiveness, outer surface charge, particle size, and shape can be easily modified by adjusting the lipid composition. The components ratios are adjusted depending on the desired target tissue [74].

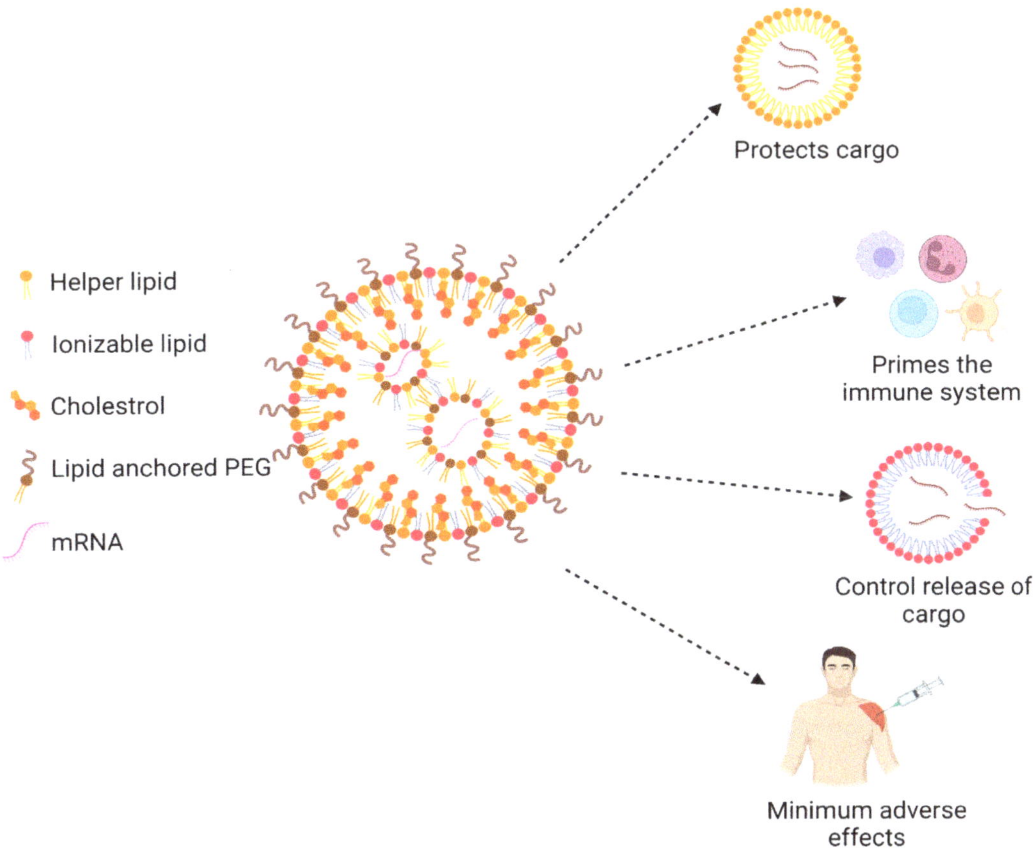

Figure 8. Structure of Lipid Nanoparticles used for efficient mRNA delivery. (Created with BioRender.com accessed on 1 January 2023).

5.4.1. The Cationic Lipids

With an amine group that imparts a net positive charge, a hydrophobic chain, and a linkage group that enables the attachment of the hydrophilic moiety to the hydrophobic chain, cationic lipids exhibit the amphiphilic property. They have a permanent positive charge at its polar head, which aids in interaction with negatively charged nucleic acids, enhancing the efficiency to entrap. Endosomal escape of the LNP system and cellular uptake is also increased because of the net positive charge. For mRNA administration, cationic lipids, ionizable lipids, and other lipid types have been investigated. As compared to non-ionizable cationic lipids, ionizable lipids, which are positively charged at low pH and at physiological pH remains neutral, are comparatively less toxic due to variations of pH. Inside the cell membrane they are charged positively and in the blood stream they possess uncharged property. BNT162b2 vaccine comprises cationic lipid ALC-0315 whereas mRNA-1273 comprises SM-102; at low pH both of the lipids are protonated which will easily form complex with mRNA. A stream of mRNA in water is combined with a lipid mixture in ethanol using a microfluidic device. In order to trap the negatively charged mRNA the components of these two streams combine quickly to generate nanoparticles [75]. For the BNT162b2 vaccine the molar ratios of the cationic lipid: PEG-lipid: cholesterol: DSPC are (46.3:1.6:42.7:9.4) and for the mRNA-1273 it is (50:1.5:38.5:10). The nanoparticles are having a diameter of 80–100 nm and approximately 100 mRNA molecules are there for one lipid nanoparticle [73].

5.4.2. The Polyethylene Glycol (PEG) Lipids

For stability of colloids and prevention of protein binding to the nanoparticle polyethylene glycol lipids are used. They impart longer systemic circulation by minimizing the clearance of the nanoparticles. LNPs may cause physical aggregation in the solution, this can increase the particle size of the LNPs and PEG lipids can overcome possibly even a premature release of the encapsulated mRNA, this problem. Moreover, the storage stability of the LNPs will also be enhanced [76].

5.4.3. Cholesterol

For transfection of cells and to stabilize LNPs cholesterol is having a vital role. A lower transition temperature is achieved when the contents of cholesterol is increased in LNPs, this will help in releasing mRNA from the LNP and its translocation across the endosomal membrane [77]. In a study conducted by Zhang et al., modified liposomes were formulated using cholesterol-modified cationic peptide DP7 along with Dioleoyl-3-trimethylammonium propane (DOTAP) as a carrier for mRNA delivery. The liposomes were prepared by film hydration technique and then, evaluated for its transfection efficiency. In vitro transfection studies revealed an increase in transfection efficiency with increase in the concentration of DP7 peptide. In addition to this, in vivo anti-tumour studies showed that the complex had better efficacy against the tumour [78].

5.4.4. Other Excipients

The mRNA vaccines are composed of stabilizers eg. Tromethamine, buffers to maintain pH of 7–8, Salts: Helping to balance the acidity in your body, Sugar: Helps the molecules maintain their shape during freezing acting as a cryoprotectant and maintains the long term stability of lipid nanoparticle-mRNA formulation [73]. A summary of key ingredients used in mRNA-based vaccines is provided in Tables 2 and 3.

Table 2. Key ingredients used in mRNA-based vaccines.

Ingredients	Functions	References
DNA template	For encoding antigens which will help in transcription of mRNA in the cell.	[66]
Vaccinia-capping enzyme	5′ capping-To cap the mRNA	[67]
Polymerase	T7, SP6 or T3 will mediate synthesis of targeted mRNA form the DNA template	[66]
Nucleotide triphosphates substrates (NTPs)	To improve translation efficiency of mRNA into protein	[69,70]
Lipid Nanoparticle Components	The lipid nanoparticles will enclose the mRNA, which eases uptake of mRNA and endo-cellular penetration to protect against degradation	[79]
Antigen	Full-length S protein with two proline substitutions (K986P and V987P) Wuhan-Hu-1 (GenBank: MN908947)	[75]
Polymerase co factor	$MgCl_2$	[75]
Stabilizers	Tromethamine	[75]
Buffer E.g. Potassium dihydrogen phosphate, Disodium hydrogen phosphate dehydrate, Tris (Tromethamine)	To maintain the pH 7–8	[75]
Other excipients A. Salts - Potassium chloride - Sodium chloride - Sodium acetate B. Sugar - Sucrose	Salts: Helping to balance the acidity in the body. Sugar: To maintain the shape of the molecules during freezing.	[75]

Table 3. Formulation ingredients of Pfizer and Moderna mRNA vaccines.

Ingredients		Pfizer mRNA Vaccine	Moderna mRNA Vaccine
Active moiety		• SARS-CoV-2 viral spike glycoprotein encoded by nucleoside-modified mRNA	• SARS-CoV-2 viral spike glycoprotein encoded by nucleoside-modified mRNA
Inactive	Lipids	• (4-hydroxybutyl)azanediyl)bis(hexane-6,1-diyl)bis(2-hexyldecanoate) • 2[(PEG)-2000]-N, N-ditetradecylacetamide • 1,2-Distearoyl-sn-glycero-3-phosphocholine • Cholesterol	• SM-102 (proprietary to Moderna)PEG 2000 dimyristoyl glycerol • 1,2-Distearoyl-sn-glycero-3-phosphocholine • Cholesterol
	Other ingredients (Buffers, sugar, diluent, salts)	• Potassium chloride, monobasic potassium phosphate, sodium chloride, dibasic sodium phosphate dihydrate, sucrose, sodium chloride	• Tromethamin, Tromethamin hydrocholoride, acetic acid, sodium acetate, sucrose

5.5. Other Delivery System for mRNA

5.5.1. Polymeric Nanoparticles

Polymeric nanoparticles can be synthesized from synthetic or natural polymers such as PLGA [poly (lactic-co-glycolic acid)], chitosan, PLA (polylactic acid), polycaprolactone, gelatin, and poly-alkyl-cyanoacrylates. These polymeric nanoparticles can encapsulate hydrophobic and hydrophilic compounds and proteins, long shelf life; and can modify the delivery of therapeutic compounds. RNA can be encapsulated in self-assembled cationic polymers with hydrophobic modification [80,81].

5.5.2. Cationic Nano-Emulsions

Cationic nano-emulsions have been proven as an effective delivery vehicle for the delivery of nucleic acids. Ccationic lipids present in the nano-emulsions are important for complexes with nucleic acid through electrostatic interactions and improve the transfection efficiency of nucleic acid and its stability. Studies reveal that the mRNA cationic nano-emulsions delivery system enhances immune response by recruiting immune cells and prompting cellular responses to antibodies and T-primates at comparatively low doses [80,82].

5.5.3. Silica Nanoparticles

Mesoporous silica nanoparticles consist of an amorphous silica matrix with well-arranged porosity in the mesoporous range. These nanoparticles have large surface areas with large pore volumes and its surface can be easily modified by certain positively charged moieties to effectively transport negatively charged RNA. Moreover targeted delivery of RNA can be possible by attaching specific ligands on the surface [81]. As per a study conducted by Adam et al., a modified porous silicon microparticle (mPSM)-based nasal vaccine was formulated for COVID-19. The formulation led to increase in helper T cells (Th1) and immune responses and mPSM caused uptake of antigen by nasal pathway. The viral load was found to be reduced significantly [83].

5.5.4. Carbon and Gold Nanomaterials

Carbon nanotubes, Gold nanoparticles, nanographene oxide, and quantum dots, are synthesized nanostructures that also have the potential to deliver RNA to the targeted site and also protecting it from degradation [81].

6. Challenges for Storage of Vaccine

The stability of and storage requirements are the major concern for mRNA vaccines. Stability depends on factors such as excipients, pH, and temperature. The COVID-19 vaccine from BioNTech/Pfizer needs to be stored at −80 °C and has a shelf life of up to 6 months, while the COVID-19 vaccine from Moderna needs to be stored at −20 °C and has the same shelf life. BioNTech/Pfizer vaccine requires packaging with dry ice while transporting. Distribution of both vaccines in poor countries of the world is challenging, as mRNA vaccines need to be stored at ultra-cold temperature. These requirements are expensive and in regions of the world with limited resources, arrangements are difficult. The development of a thermostable mRNA vaccine that is clinically efficacious and can be kept for a longer time without incurring large storage costs is one of the problems. According to EMA storage recommendations, mRNA vaccines made by Moderna and BioNTech are stable when frozen for up to 6 months at −25 °C, up to 30 days at refrigerator temperature (4 °C), and up to 6 h at room temperature [84].

7. Safety and Efficacy of mRNA Vaccines

7.1. Safety of mRNA-Based Vaccines

Assessment of safety related outcomes were carried out for mRNA vaccines. A phase 1 dose-escalation, open-label trial trials of mRNA-1273 was carried out on participants of age between 18 and70 years or older [85]. Study was carried out in two groups in which participants of 18–55 years of age received the vaccine dose of 250 µg and older subjects were given 25 µg or 100 µg of the dose. Solicited local and systemic adverse events, unsolicited adverse events, serious adverse events, and development of new chronic medical conditions were observed after vaccination. The results showed no development of serious adverse events. The most typical adverse reactions reported were headaches, weariness, myalgia, chills, and soreness at the injection site. Neutralizing antibody levels have been demonstrated to correlate with defence against a variety of viruses in humans and with defence against SARS-CoV-2 in animal challenges. The mRNA-1273 vaccine in older adults produced high levels of binding and neutralizing antibodies, and the time- and dose-dependent trends were similar to responses in younger adults. The responses following the second vaccination were comparable to those seen in patients who had recovered from COVID-19 and had donated convalescent serum, including some who were critically ill. Older patients receiving 100 μg dose showed higher antibody and T-cell responses in comparison to those who received 25 μg and the response was identical to the reaction in participants aged 18 to 55 who received the 100 μg dosage. Patients older than 56 years need to receive a second dose of the vaccine to attain neutralizing antibodies. On receiving a booster dose, antibody titers increase rapidly. The safety key results of Moderna and Pfizer vaccines observed during various clinical trials have been listed in Table 4.

Table 4. Safety and efficacy studies of mRNA vaccines in clinical trials.

Brand Name	Company	Clinical Trials Gov. Identifier	Phase of Clinical Trials	Study Design	Race of the Participants	Safety Key Results	Efficacy and Key Results	References
Spikevax (mRNA-1273)	Moderna	NCT04470427	3	Observer-blinded, placebo-controlled (30,000 participants)	High risk COVID-19 patients in the United States	No safety concerns were identified	94.1% efficacy in preventing COVID-19	[86]
		NCT04649151	2	Randomized, Parallel Assignment (4431 participants)	Healthy Adolescents (12 to <18 Years)	Injection-site pain, headache, and fatigue	Not Available	[87]
		NCT04860297	3	Open-label, single intervention study; no randomization (234 participants)	Adult Solid Organ Transplant Recipients	Not Available	Not Available	[88]
		NCT05158140	3	Randomized, Double-blind, Placebo-controlled Study (850 participants)	Booster dose Vaccinated healthy adults (50 Years) or Older aged adults for Pneumococcal Infection	Not Available	Not Available	[89]
		NCT04811664	3	Randomized Controlled Study, Crossover Assignment (1958 participants)	Adults (18–29 years)	Not Available	Not Available	[90]
		NCT04805125	3	Randomized, Parallel Assignment (610 participants)	Immunocompromised patients	Not Available	Not Available	[91]
		NCT05054218		Observational, Cohort (336 participants)	Cancer patients	Not Available	Not Available	[92]
		NCT04405076	2	Randomized, Observer-Blind, Placebo Controlled, Dose-Confirmation Study (660 participants)	Adults (18 Years) and Older	Injection site, headache, and fatigue	Not Available	[93]
		NCT05366322		Cohort, Retrospective (124,879 participants)	Immunocompromised Adults in the United States	It was observed that 2 doses of mRNA-1273 produces lower overall rate of medically-attended COVID-19 as compared to BNT162b2.	Not Available	[94]
		NCT04785144	1	Open-Label, Randomized Study (135 participants)	Naïve and Previously Vaccinated Adults	Well tolerated, safe and acceptable	Not Available	[95]
		NCT04283461	1	Open-Label, Dose-Ranging Study (120 participants)	Healthy participants and Older Adults	Well tolerated, mild or moderate	Not Available	[85,96]

Table 4. *Cont.*

Brand Name	Company	Clinical Trials Gov. Identifier	Phase of Clinical Trials	Study Design	Race of the Participants	Safety Key Results	Efficacy and Key Results	References
Comirnaty® (BNT 162b2)	Pfizer–BioNTech	NCT04816669	3	Randomized, observer-blind study (629 participants)	Healthy adults (18–55 years)	Not Available	Not Available	[97]
		NCT04368728	3	Multinational, placebo-controlled, observer-blinded, pivotal efficacy trial (45,713 participants)	83% were White, 9% were Black or African American, 28% were Hispanic or Latinx	Administration of two doses of BNT162b2 provided 95% protection against COVID-19 in persons 16 years of age or older.	95% effective in preventing COVID-19 Vaccine efficacy (90 to 100%) was observed across subgroups defined by age, sex, race, ethnicity, baseline body-mass index, and the presence of coexisting conditions	[98]
		NCT04887948	3	Randomized, double blind trial, Parallel Assignment (570 participants)	Adults 65 years of age and older	Not Available	Not Available	[99]
		NCT05308680		Case-control, Prospective study (336 participants)	Israeli health care workers	Local pain at injection site, fatigue, myalgia, sore throat etc.	Increase in serum troponin levels was documented after 4th dose of vaccine in among 0.62% of healthy health care workers	[100]
		NCT04949490	2	Open-label, Rollover Trial (137 participants)	BNT162-04 Trial Subjects	Not Available	Not Available	[101]
		NCT04754594	2	Placebo-controlled, randomized, observer-blind study (349 participants)	Healthy pregnant women	Not Available	96% and 97% effective in documented infection and symptomatic infection (7–56 days), respectively	[102]
		NCT04713553	3	Randomized, observer-blind study (1574 participants)	Healthy participants 18 through 50 years of age	Not Available	Not Available	[103]
		NCT04588480	1	Randomized, placebo-controlled, and observer-blind study (160 participants)	Healthy Japanese adults	No serious adverse events	n the younger and older age groups, respectively, SARS-CoV-2 50% serum neutralizing geometric mean titers were 571 and 366, and geometric mean fold increments were 55.8 and 36.6 one month after dose 2	[104]
		NCT04649021	2	Randomized, double-blind, placebo-controlled trial (950 participants)	Han Chinese adults	Mild or moderate	After one month of vaccination, the neutralizing titer was 294.4 and 5.0 in BNT162b2 and placebo, respectively	[105]

After the second dose of the vaccine, local and systemic reactogenicity events increased in frequency and were primarily of moderate severity. The incidence of erythema was found in three participants and lasted for 5 to 7 days. Solicited systemic adverse events such as fever and fatigue occurred in the older subgroup prominently. All these findings suggest that the adverse events solicited or unsolicited were mild to moderately severe. Thus mRNA-1273 was further tested for phase 2/3 trials to assess safety and efficacy in larger populations [95]. Phase 3 clinical trial was a randomized, stratified, observer-blinded, and placebo-controlled study, involving 30,420 volunteers of age 18 years or older, assigned randomly to receive a vaccine (0.5 mL with 100 µg of dose) or placebo. Local reactions for 7 days following immunization, systemic adverse events, unanticipated adverse reactions after 28 days of dose administration, and any significant adverse events were tracked for safety assessment. Solicited adverse effects were predominant in mRNA-1273 in comparison to the placebo group (84.2%, vs. 19.8%). Some of the most observed events were pain at the injection site after vaccination, erythema, tenderness, and induration. These events were cleared up within 4–5 days post-vaccination. After the second dose, the mRNA-1273 group solicited systemic events that became more severe. The presence of hypersensitivity reactions was there in 1.5% and 1.1% of participants in the vaccine and placebo groups, respectively. Other than these complaints, no safety concerns were raised after vaccine administration [106].

A third dose of vaccine was required due to waning protection following two SARS-CoV-2 mRNA injections and the introduction of variations. After administering a third dose of the mRNA vaccine to people who had previously received the mRNA-1273 primary series in the Phase 1 study, their early safety and immunogenicity were assessed. A cross-sectional study performed in Naples (Italy) assessed the preparedness to take the COVID-19 vaccine booster. In this group, the acceptance of the booster dose was nearly 86%. Furthermore, older persons in better health after the main vaccine series, those living with friends or family members who tested positive for COVID-19, and those who had received disease-related information from official public institutions were willing to obtain the booster dose [107].

The bivalent vaccination contained 25 mcg of each mRNA-1273 and mRNA-1273.351, while the booster vaccine formulations contained 100 mcg of mRNA-1273, 50 mcg of mRNA-1273.351, which encodes the Beta variant spike protein. A third dose of the mRNA vaccine showed adequate reactogenicity and safety. When compared to peak responses after the second dosage, vaccination-induced increased in binding and neutralizing antibody titers to D614G, Beta, and Delta variants were similar or larger. It was noticed that neutralizing and binding antibodies reduced constantly. However, detection of antibodies was there at 10–11 months (before third dose) in participants regardless of age and initial primary series dose (e.g., 25, 50, 100, and 250 µg). Injection site pain, weariness, myalgia, and chills were the most often reported adverse effects following the third dosage of the mRNA vaccine, and the frequency of these events was comparable among the three booster vaccine regimens (monovalent prototype, monovalent variant and bivalent groups). With usage of the monovalent or bivalent Beta variant vaccines, no specific advantage or disadvantage was seen in the cellular responses to the epitopes within the Beta-mutated peptides. All of these findings support the current suggestion that a monovalent prototype mRNA-1273 boost be used to provide extensive immunological cross-protection between variants [95].

As per a survey, Heterologous BNT162b2 (BNT) administration in ChAdOx1 (ChAd)-primed participants (ChAd/BNT) demonstrated non-inferior immunogenicity to homologous BNT administration (both prime and booster were BNT vaccines, BNT/BNT), with tolerable reactogenicity and greater T cell responses. In comparison to homologous ChAdOX1 vaccination (ChAd/ChAd), heterologous ChAd/BNT vaccination elicited stronger immunogenicity (ChAd/BNT vs. ChAd/ChAd, antibody titer ratio: 9.2) [108].

A phase 1 trial for BNT162b2 was conducted on 76 participants; they were randomized to receive 10 µg, 30 µg, and 100 µg vaccine doses, and the other group was given the placebo. 58.3% of subjects receiving 10 µg and 100% of 30 µg and 100 µg experienced solicited local reaction pain at the site of the injection after the first dose. The severity of all local reactions was mild to moderate. Fatigue and headache in BNT162b2 were common systemic events. Additionally, chills, muscle pain, and joint pain were also observed. On increasing doses, systemic events were reported more after the second dose was given. A total of 50.0 percent of participants who received either 10 or 30 g of BNT162b1, 58.3 percent of persons who received 100 g of BNT162b1, and 11.1 percent of placebo recipients reported experiencing adverse events. No serious adverse events were reported [109].

In a clinical trial of The Pfizer/BioNTech vaccine (BNT162b2) which was a multinational, placebo-controlled, observer-blinded, randomized, and pivotal efficacy trial, 43,548 participants aged 16 years or older were randomly allocated. A total of 21,720 volunteers were given 30 µg per dose of BNT162b2 and 21,728 with placebo. To determine the safety profile of BNT162b2 characteristics such as pain at the injection site, which is short-term, mild to moderate in case of severity, fatigue, and headache were evaluated. Two injections of BNT162b2 or placebo were given to all the participants, according to randomization 21 days apart, in the deltoid muscle [98]. Local reactions in those who received the BNT162b2 vaccine were reported more as compared to the placebo group. Mild to moderate pain at the site of injection was the most common complaint registered amongst the recipients of BNT162b2 within one week. Severe pain was reported in less than 1% of the population. The pain was observed less in older participants in comparison to that of younger ones. Redness or swelling was less observed. After administration of the second dose, local reactions were less reported [110].

Younger participants who received the vaccine encountered more systemic events than older recipients did. Fatigue and headache (59% and 52%) were the most commonly reported events, and very less vaccinated subjects (<2%) experienced any severe systemic events. After the second dose of the vaccine, 16% of younger groups and 11% of older age reported fever (temperature $\geq$ 38 °C), which increased the use of antipyretic or pain killers. However, post-delivery of the first dose cases of fever were reported very less [110]. Lymphadenopathy was noticed as an adverse event in BNT162b2 receivers in comparison to the placebo group. A shoulder injury related to the vaccination, right axillary lymphadenopathy, paroxysmal ventricular arrhythmia, and right leg paresthesia were among the unfavourable events recorded among BNT162b2 recipients [98]. Rare adverse effects observed are Bell's palsy, acute myocardial infarction, cerebral venous sinus thrombosis, pulmonary embolism, Guillain–Barré syndrome, lymphadenopathy, herpes zoster reactivation, stroke, neurological complications, and thrombosis with thrombocytopenia syndrome, and autoimmunity (e.g., autoimmune peripheral neuropathies and autoimmune hepatitis). Among these certain adverse effects such as anaphylaxis, myocarditis, and appendicitis were common in younger people while Guillain–Barré syndrome and myocardial infarction increased with age. These vaccine-associated adverse effects are less frequent than the additional serious adverse effects that occur after severe COVID-19. A recent study reveals the risk of neurological complications in COVID-19 vaccine receivers. The molecular foundation of these adverse effects is unknown. We hypothesize that, since most of these are also apparent in severe COVID-19, it may be associated with acute inflammation produced by both the vaccine and the virus, as well as in the common SARS-CoV-2 S protein. In the BNT162b2 and mRNA-1273 vaccines encoded antigen (S protein) is stabilized it is therefore probable that, if entering the circulation and systemically distributed throughout the body, it can contribute to these adverse effects in susceptible individuals [111].

7.2. *Efficacy of mRNA Vaccines*

For efficacy assessment of mRNA-1273, the vaccine's primary endpoints were efficacy to prevent symptomatic COVID-19 infection after 14 days of the second dose of vaccine. As a secondary endpoint, prevention of severe COVID-19 infection with persistent symptoms was used. Results after vaccination show that 11 cases of COVID-19 were there in the vaccinated group and 185 cases in the placebo group, indicating 94.1% efficacy of the mRNA-1273 vaccine for treating symptomatic COVID-19. For secondary efficacy endpoints, evaluation of preventing severe COVID-19 was performed. The results indicated 100% efficacy of the vaccine as 30 participants with viral infection were in the placebo group. A study carried out in Qatar showed vaccine efficacy (VE) of mRNA-1273 95.7% against severe, critical, or fatal COVID-19 infection. After $\geq$14 days of the first dose, effectiveness was 88.1% against B.1.1.7 (alpha) variant and was 100% post second dose. 61.3% and 96.4% of VE were reported after the first and second doses of immunization against the B.1.351 (beta) strain. Therefore, the vaccine is quite successful against both the strain, whether symptomatic or asymptomatic and against any COVID-19 hospitalization and death, even after a single dose [112].

BNT162b2 vaccine's efficacy (VE) against confirmed COVID-19 having an onset of at least 7 days after the second dose in individuals who were free from virologic or serologic evidence of SARS-CoV-2 infection was the first primary endpoint. The second primary endpoint measured the effectiveness in participants with and without evidence of prior infection and prevention of severe COVID-19 infection. In a research with a total of 36,523 people, 8 instances of COVID-19 with the beginning at 7 days after the second dosage occurred in the vaccination group, compared to 162 cases in the placebo group. This shows 95% of vaccine efficacy. However, the observed VE against the viral disease was 52% between the first and second doses, and it was 91% in the first 7 days following dose 2, attaining complete efficacy against disease with an onset at least 7 days after dose 2. Only 1 of the 10 severe COVID-19 instances that were seen after the first dosage occurred in the group that received the vaccination. This observation is in line with the excellent overall efficacy against all COVID-19 patients. Two cases of infection were there in vaccine recipients amongst hypertension patients and 44 cases in the placebo group. This case reports 94.6% of vaccine efficacy in hypertension patients. Thus BNT162b2 vaccine meets both primary and secondary efficacy endpoints in vaccinated participants [113]. Apart from SARS-CoV-2 infection, with a single dose of the BNT162b2 vaccine, the predicted vaccination efficacy against symptomatic disease with the delta variant (B.1.617.2) was about 36%. After two doses, VE was about 88 percent [114].

8. Regulatory Challenges

Regulatory science is the foundation on which regulatory decisions are made. Its primary objective is to develop new methods, tools, and standards for evaluating the safety, efficacy, quality, and performance of regulated products at all stages of their life cycle [115]. mRNA vaccines face the same sorts of regulatory hurdles as any other type of vaccine, including the need to show proof of safety and efficacy in pre-clinical studies, clinical trials, and post-marketing surveillance, as well as maintaining a high standard for the raw materials used in production and consistency of manufacture. Vaccine testing relies heavily on the reliability and reproducibility of enzymes, nucleotides, and linear DNA templates [116]. Raw components, such as lipids, should be strictly regulated, and their purity should be proven. Current good manufacturing practices (cGMPs) should be followed when creating the linear DNA template. To ensure the drug substance is of the highest quality, it is essential to keep an eye on the percentage of capped and polyadenylated mRNA, the number of short transcripts, and the presence of double-stranded RNA. Polyadenylation and capping the 5′ end of mRNA ensure stability and effective translation [21]. The translation efficiency is closely linked to poly (A) tail [114]. Quantifying the amount of mRNA encapsulated in the particle and determining the size distribution of the particles is critical for the drug product because it allows the manufacturer to ensure manufacturing uniformity. Monitoring is typically performed on a number of characteristics, including those pertaining to stability, identity, and sterility. One of the issues for vaccine developers, regulators, and users is the thermal stability of mRNA vaccines [115]. Conventional vaccinations are subjected to stress testing, including prolonged exposure to elevated temperatures, in order to determine their stability under a variety of storage circumstances. This must also be conducted for mRNA vaccines, where it is necessary to evaluate not only the stability of the mRNA molecule but also the preservation of the structure of the vaccine particle itself. Integrity testing protocols for individual mRNA components in multi-component mRNA vaccines are still in need of development. A nucleic acid vaccine's identification is determined by its sequence. In general, the sequence of the first DNA plasmid used as a template is sufficient for mRNA vaccinations. This is because DNA is instantly translated into RNA. It is not known that sequencing the mRNA, either directly or by converting it to cDNA and then sequencing that DNA, provides any additional information. Even though the error rates of RNA polymerases are substantially greater than those of DNA polymerases, the stated error rates of 1 error every 104–105 nucleotides would be difficult to detect in RNA due to the random nature of the errors. Based on current research suggesting that mRNA vaccines provide protective immunity in animal models, this error rate does not seem to alter the formation of an immunogenic antigen.

Lipid quantification can be conducted by LC-MS/MS [116]. If the protein is translated too quickly, it may not fold appropriately into a functional antigen, which can have the unintended consequence of lowering vaccine efficacy.

9. Discussion

In 2021, mRNA vaccines gained attention for their critical position in the pharmaceutical industry's reaction to COVID-19. Unlike traditional viral vaccines, which use weakened, non-replicating copies of viruses to display antigens and elicit an immune response, the mRNA strategy uses optimized single-stranded mRNA molecules that can provide biological induction. Once you have the vaccine, the cells will take it in, 'read' the mRNA sequence, and produce the spike protein. Since your body lacks proteins that resemble that spike, your immune system interprets it as harmful and launches an assault against it. In addition, if you are infected with the coronavirus later, the immune system remembers the spike protein and even recognizes it. The remarkable pace at which the first two COVID-19 vaccines were developed and made publicly available in the USA backs the notion that mRNA vaccines from Pfizer and Moderna received emergency use permission from the FDA in December 2020—less than a year after Chinese scientists announced the coronavirus's gene makeup. The major benefit of mRNA-based vaccine technologies is their potential to be quickly modified for various diseases since the processing of the target antigen is 'outsourced' to host cells, which means that only the genetic code of the antigen is used to design a vaccine candidate. The time between the Chinese government exchanging their SARS-CoV-2 genetic structure and Moderna transporting its vaccine candidate to the National Institutes of Health (NIH) in the United States for phase one studies was just 44 days. mRNA vaccine vaccines have not historically gained regulatory clearance for use in humanity due to a perceived lack of clinical trials for this method, as well as technical challenges related to product stability and distribution. With such an increase in mRNA vaccines in the market, more precise advice to help in the development and assessment of new mRNA vaccines is possible. Control is another field where mRNA vaccine science is in its infancy. There are currently no official guidelines from the US Food and Drug Administration or the European Medicines Agency for mRNA vaccines, even though the drugs are safe enough for major clinical trials.

10. Concluding Remarks and Future Prospects

Before 2020, mRNA was not a well-known scientific term in the vaccine world. More than a year since the catastrophic global COVID-19 pandemic began, mRNA-based clinical programs have seen a substantial increase in support, both from the general public and from big pharma. More than 80 million Americans have been vaccinated against SARS-CoV-2-the virus that causes COVID-19, using the game-changing possibilities of mRNA technology. "The vaccine field has been forever transformed and forever advanced because of COVID-19," says Dan Barouch, MD, Ph.D., director of the Centre for Virology and Vaccine Research at Harvard Medical School. Mostly in a situation of the COVID-19 vaccine, the mRNA strand is engineered to produce the unique coronavirus's "spike protein," which produces an immune response that could guard against infection with the actual virus. The vaccines developed by Moderna and Pfizer/BioNTech have been the only mRNA-based vaccines to obtain emergency approval from key regulators, and real-world evidence from the global COVID-19 launch would be critical in vindicating their long-term effectiveness and safety features against the coronavirus and some other viral agents. Exosome-based mRNA delivery will also be the future of mRNA-based therapeutics [117,118]. Mostly with implications of mRNA-based technology becoming apparent as these first-generation vaccines begin to be deployed globally, there is currently a boom in mRNA clinical research for infectious diseases, and industry researchers anticipate an increase in interest in mRNA platforms for other therapeutic fields, especially oncology, but even uncommon autoimmune conditions and neurodegenes.

Author Contributions: V.P.C. prepared the manuscript's backbone and wrote the original draft of the manuscript along with G.J., S.D., B.M.P., L.V.N., K.K. and V.P.C. critically revised the manuscript for important intellectual content. All authors have read and agreed to the published version of the manuscript.

Funding: This research received no external funding.

Institutional Review Board Statement: Not applicable.

Informed Consent Statement: Not applicable.

Data Availability Statement: Not applicable.

Acknowledgments: VPC wants to dedicate this work to L M College of Pharmacy as a part of the 75th year celebration of the college.

Conflicts of Interest: The authors declare no conflict of interest.

References

1. WHO. WHO Coronavirus (COVID-19) Dashboard 2023. Available online: https://covid19.who.int/ (accessed on 17 January 2023).
2. Pal, R.; Yadav, U. COVID-19 Pandemic in India: Present Scenario and a Steep Climb Ahead. *J. Prim. Care Community Health* **2020**, *11*, 2150132720939402. [CrossRef] [PubMed]
3. Keni, R.; Alexander, A.; Nayak, P.G.; Mudgal, J.; Nandakumar, K. COVID-19: Emergence, Spread, Possible Treatments, and Global Burden. *Front. Public Health* **2020**, *8*, 216. [CrossRef] [PubMed]
4. Chavda, V.P.; Ping, F.-F.; Chen, Z.-S. An Impact of COVID-19 on Cancer Care: An Update. *Vaccines* **2022**, *10*, 2072. [CrossRef] [PubMed]
5. Harapan, H.; Itoh, N.; Yufika, A.; Winardi, W.; Keam, S.; Te, H.; Megawati, D.; Hayati, Z.; Wagner, A.L.; Mudatsir, M. Coronavirus Disease 2019 (COVID-19): A Literature Review. *J. Infect. Public Health* **2020**, *13*, 667–673. [CrossRef] [PubMed]
6. Chavda, V.P.; Chhabria, M.T.; Apostolopoulos, V. Aged Population and Immunocompromised Patients: Impact on SARS-CoV-2 Variants and Treatment Outcomes. *Biologics* **2022**, *2*, 165–170. [CrossRef]
7. Chavda, V.P.; Redwan, E.M. SARS-CoV-2: Immunopeptidomics and Other Immunological Studies. *Vaccines* **2022**, *10*, 1975. [CrossRef]
8. Kyriakidis, N.C.; López-Cortés, A.; González, E.V.; Grimaldos, A.B.; Prado, E.O. SARS-CoV-2 Vaccines Strategies: A Comprehensive Review of Phase 3 Candidates. *Npj Vaccines* **2021**, *6*, 28. [CrossRef]
9. Ssentongo, P.; Ssentongo, A.E.; Voleti, N.; Groff, D.; Sun, A.; Ba, D.M.; Nunez, J.; Parent, L.J.; Chinchilli, V.M.; Paules, C.I. SARS-CoV-2 Vaccine Effectiveness against Infection, Symptomatic and Severe COVID-19: A Systematic Review and Meta-Analysis. *BMC Infect. Dis.* **2022**, *22*, 439. [CrossRef]
10. Chavda, V.P.; Vora, L.K.; Vihol, D.R. COVAX-19® Vaccine: Completely Blocks Virus Transmission to Non-Immune Individuals. *Clin. Complement Med. Pharmacol.* **2021**, *1*, 100004. [CrossRef]
11. Chavda, V.P.; Vora, L.K.; Pandya, A.K.; Patravale, V.B. Intranasal Vaccines for SARS-CoV-2: From Challenges to Potential in COVID-19 Management. *Drug Discov. Today* **2021**, *26*, 2619–2636. [CrossRef]
12. Kaur, S.P.; Gupta, V. COVID-19 Vaccine: A Comprehensive Status Report. *Virus Res.* **2020**, *288*, 198114. [CrossRef]
13. Vasireddy, D.; Atluri, P.; Malayala, S.V.; Vanaparthy, R.; Mohan, G. Review of COVID-19 Vaccines Approved in the United States of America for Emergency Use. *J. Clin. Med. Res.* **2021**, *13*, 204. [CrossRef] [PubMed]
14. Zheng, C.; Shao, W.; Chen, X.; Zhang, B.; Wang, G.; Zhang, W. Real-World Effectiveness of COVID-19 Vaccines: A Literature Review and Meta-Analysis. *Int. J. Infect. Dis.* **2022**, *114*, 252–260. [CrossRef]

15. Alagoz, O.; Sethi, A.K.; Patterson, B.W.; Churpek, M.; Alhanaee, G.; Scaria, E.; Safdar, N. The Impact of Vaccination to Control COVID-19 Burden in the United States: A Simulation Modeling Approach. *PLoS ONE* **2021**, *16*, e0254456. [CrossRef]
16. Cromer, D.; Steain, M.; Reynaldi, A.; Schlub, T.E.; Wheatley, A.K.; Juno, J.A.; Kent, S.J.; Triccas, J.A.; Khoury, D.S.; Davenport, M.P. Neutralising Antibody Titres as Predictors of Protection against SARS-CoV-2 Variants and the Impact of Boosting: A Meta-Analysis. *Lancet Microbe* **2022**, *3*, e52–e61. [CrossRef]
17. Zhao, J.; Zhao, S.; Ou, J.; Zhang, J.; Lan, W.; Guan, W.; Wu, X.; Yan, Y.; Zhao, W.; Wu, J.; et al. COVID-19: Coronavirus Vaccine Development Updates. *Front. Immunol.* **2020**, *11*, 2256. [CrossRef] [PubMed]
18. Chung, Y.H.; Beiss, V.; Fiering, S.N.; Steinmetz, N.F. COVID-19 Vaccine Frontrunners and Their Nanotechnology Design. *ACS Nano* **2020**, *14*, 12522–12537. [CrossRef] [PubMed]
19. Jain, S.; Venkataraman, A.; Wechsler, M.E.; Peppas, N.A. Messenger RNA-Based Vaccines: Past, Present, and Future Directions in the Context of the COVID-19 Pandemic. *Adv. Drug Deliv. Rev.* **2021**, *179*, 114000. [CrossRef] [PubMed]
20. Arashkia, A.; Jalilvand, S.; Mohajel, N.; Afchangi, A.; Azadmanesh, K.; Salehi-Vaziri, M.; Fazlalipour, M.; Pouriayevali, M.H.; Jalali, T.; Mousavi Nasab, S.D.; et al. Severe Acute Respiratory Syndrome-Coronavirus-2 Spike (S) Protein Based Vaccine Candidates: State of the Art and Future Prospects. *Rev. Med. Virol.* **2021**, *31*, e2183. [CrossRef]
21. Park, J.W.; Lagniton, P.N.P.; Liu, Y.; Xu, R.H. MRNA Vaccines for COVID-19: What, Why and How. *Int. J. Biol. Sci.* **2021**, *17*, 1446. [CrossRef]
22. Zhu, N.; Zhang, D.; Wang, W.; Li, X.; Yang, B.; Song, J.; Zhao, X.; Huang, B.; Shi, W.; Lu, R.; et al. A Novel Coronavirus from Patients with Pneumonia in China, 2019. *N. Engl. J. Med.* **2020**, *382*, 727–733. [CrossRef] [PubMed]
23. Wang, M.Y.; Zhao, R.; Gao, L.J.; Gao, X.F.; Wang, D.P.; Cao, J.M. SARS-CoV-2: Structure, Biology, and Structure-Based Therapeutics Development. *Front. Cell. Infect. Microbiol.* **2020**, *10*, 7269. [CrossRef] [PubMed]
24. Chavda, V.P.; Hossain, M.K.; Beladiya, J.; Apostolopoulos, V. Nucleic Acid Vaccines for COVID-19: A Paradigm Shift in the Vaccine Development Arena. *Biologics* **2021**, *1*, 337–356. [CrossRef]
25. Chavda, V.P.; Pandya, R.; Apostolopoulos, V. DNA Vaccines for SARS-CoV-2: Toward Third-Generation Vaccination Era. *Expert Rev. Vaccines* **2021**, *20*, 1549–1560. [CrossRef] [PubMed]
26. Yang, H.; Rao, Z. Structural biology of SARS-CoV-2 and implications for therapeutic development. *Nat. Rev. Microbiol.* **2021**, *19*, 685–700. [CrossRef]
27. Kumar, S.; Nyodu, R.; Maurya, V.K.; Saxena, S.K.; Kumar, S.; Nyodu, R.; Maurya, V.K.; Saxena, S.K. Host Immune Response and Immunobiology of Human SARS-CoV-2 Infection. *Coronavirus Dis. 2019 (COVID-19)* **2020**, 43–53. [CrossRef]
28. Asturias, E.J.; Duclos, P.; MacDonald, N.E.; Nohynek, H.; Lambert, P.H. Advanced Vaccinology Education: Landscaping Its Growth and Global Footprint. *Vaccine* **2020**, *38*, 4664–4670. [CrossRef]
29. Kardani, K.; Bolhassani, A.; Shahbazi, S. Prime-Boost Vaccine Strategy against Viral Infections: Mechanisms and Benefits. *Vaccine* **2016**, *34*, 413–423. [CrossRef]
30. Chen, J.M. Should the World Collaborate Imminently to Develop Neglected Live-Attenuated Vaccines for COVID-19? *J. Med. Virol.* **2022**, *94*, 82–87. [CrossRef]
31. Chavda, V.P.; Vihol, D.R.; Solanki, H.K.; Apostolopoulos, V. The Vaccine World of COVID-19: India's Contribution. *Vaccines* **2022**, *10*, 1943. [CrossRef]
32. Ashraf, M.U.; Kim, Y.; Kumar, S.; Seo, D.; Ashraf, M.; Bae, Y.S. COVID-19 Vaccines (Revisited) and Oral-Mucosal Vector System as a Potential Vaccine Platform. *Vaccines* **2021**, *9*, 171. [CrossRef]
33. Lesser, K.; Whittaker, G.R. Vaccination for COVID-19: Benchmarks in Public Health and Virus Transmission. *Public Health* **2021**, *197*, e23. [CrossRef] [PubMed]
34. Chavda, V.P.; Apostolopoulos, V. Is Booster Dose Strategy Sufficient for Omicron Variant of SARS-CoV-2? *Vaccines* **2022**, *10*, 367. [CrossRef] [PubMed]
35. Chavda, V.P.; Bezbaruah, R.; Athalye, M.; Parikh, P.K.; Chhipa, A.S.; Patel, S.; Apostolopoulos, V. Replicating Viral Vector-Based Vaccines for COVID-19: Potential Avenue in Vaccination Arena. *Viruses* **2022**, *14*, 759. [CrossRef]
36. Chavda, V.P.; Apostolopoulos, V. COVID-19 Vaccine Design and Vaccination Strategy for Emerging Variants. *Expert Rev. Vaccines* **2022**, *21*, 1359–1361. [CrossRef] [PubMed]
37. Chavda, V.P.; Vuppu, S.; Mishra, T.; Kamaraj, S.; Patel, A.B.; Sharma, N.; Chen, Z.-S. Recent Review of COVID-19 Management: Diagnosis, Treatment and Vaccination. *Pharmacol. Rep.* **2022**, *74*, 1120–1148. [CrossRef]
38. Chavda, V.P.; Chen, Y.; Dave, J.; Chen, Z.-S.; Chauhan, S.C.; Yallapu, M.M.; Uversky, V.N.; Bezbaruah, R.; Patel, S.; Apostolopoulos, V. COVID-19 and Vaccination: Myths vs Science. *Expert Rev. Vaccines* **2022**, *21*, 1603–1620. [CrossRef]
39. Chavda, V.P.; Bezbaruah, R.; Deka, K.; Nongrang, L.; Kalita, T. The Delta and Omicron Variants of SARS-CoV-2: What We Know So Far. *Vaccines* **2022**, *10*, 1926. [CrossRef]
40. Fioretti, D.; Iurescia, S.; Fazio, V.M.; Rinaldi, M. DNA Vaccines: Developing New Strategies against Cancer. *J. Biomed. Biotechnol.* **2010**, *2010*, 174378. [CrossRef]
41. Zhao, Z.; Deng, Y.; Niu, P.; Song, J.; Wang, W.; Du, Y.; Huang, B.; Wang, W.; Zhang, L.; Zhao, P.; et al. Co-Immunization With CHIKV VLP and DNA Vaccines Induces a Promising Humoral Response in Mice. *Front. Immunol.* **2021**, *12*, 925. [CrossRef]

42. Kalams, S.A.; Parker, S.D.; Elizaga, M.; Metch, B.; Edupuganti, S.; Hural, J.; De Rosa, S.; Carter, D.K.; Rybczyk, K.; Frank, I. Safety and Comparative Immunogenicity of an HIV-1 DNA Vaccine in Combination with Plasmid Interleukin 12 and Impact of Intramuscular Electroporation for Delivery. *J. Infect. Dis.* **2013**, *208*, 818–829. [CrossRef]
43. Bezbaruah, R.; Chavda, V.P.; Nongrang, L.; Alom, S.; Deka, K.; Kalita, T.; Ali, F.; Bhattacharjee, B.; Vora, L. Nanoparticle-Based Delivery Systems for Vaccines. *Vaccines* **2022**, *10*, 1946. [CrossRef] [PubMed]
44. Karam, M.; Daoud, G. MRNA Vaccines: Past, Present, Future. *Asian J. Pharm. Sci.* **2022**, *17*, 491–522. [CrossRef] [PubMed]
45. Dolgin, E. The Tangled History of MRNA Vaccines. *Nature* **2021**, *597*, 318–324. [CrossRef] [PubMed]
46. Hoerr, I.; Obst, R.; Rammensee, H.G.; Jung, G. undefined In Vivo Application of RNA Leads to Induction of Specific Cytotoxic T Lymphocytes and Antibodies. *Eur. J. Immunol.* **2000**, *30*, 1–7. [CrossRef]
47. Kose, N.; Fox, J.M.; Sapparapu, G.; Bombardi, R.; Tennekoon, R.N.; Dharshan De Silva, A.; Elbashir, S.M.; Theisen, M.A.; Humphris-Narayanan, E.; Ciaramella, G.; et al. A Lipid-Encapsulated MRNA Encoding a Potently Neutralizing Human Monoclonal Antibody Protects against Chikungunya Infection. *Sci. Immunol.* **2019**, *4*, eaaw6647. [CrossRef]
48. Sahin, U.; Karikó, K.; Türeci, Ö. MRNA-Based Therapeutics—Developing a New Class of Drugs. *Nat. Rev. Drug Discov.* **2014**, *13*, 759–780. [CrossRef]
49. Moss, P. The T cell immune response against SARS-CoV-2. *Nat. Immunol.* **2022**, *23*, 186–193. [CrossRef] [PubMed]
50. Nance, K.D.; Meier, J.L. Modifications in an Emergency: The Role of N1-Methylpseudouridine in COVID-19 Vaccines. *ACS Cent. Sci.* **2021**, *7*, 748–756. [CrossRef]
51. Kremsner, P.G.; Ahuad Guerrero, R.A.; Arana-Arri, E.; Aroca Martinez, G.J.; Bonten, M.; Chandler, R.; Corral, G.; De Block, E.J.L.; Ecker, L.; Gabor, J.J.; et al. Efficacy and Safety of the CVnCoV SARS-CoV-2 MRNA Vaccine Candidate in Ten Countries in Europe and Latin America (HERALD): A Randomised, Observer-Blinded, Placebo-Controlled, Phase 2b/3 Trial. *Lancet Infect. Dis.* **2022**, *22*, 329–340. [CrossRef]
52. Blakney, A.K.; Ip, S.; Geall, A.J. An Update on Self-Amplifying MRNA Vaccine Development. *Vaccines* **2021**, *9*, 97. [CrossRef] [PubMed]
53. Yılmaz, E. New Hopes in Vaccine Technology: mRNA Vaccines. *Mikrobiyol. Bul.* **2021**, *55*, 265–284. [CrossRef]
54. Jackson, N.A.C.; Kester, K.E.; Casimiro, D.; Gurunathan, S.; DeRosa, F. The Promise of MRNA Vaccines: A Biotech and Industrial Perspective. *Npj Vaccines 2020 51* **2020**, *5*, 11. [CrossRef] [PubMed]
55. Bloom, K.; van den Berg, F.; Arbuthnot, P. Self-amplifying RNA vaccines for infectious diseases. *Gene. Ther.* **2021**, *28*, 117–129. [CrossRef]
56. Kon, E.; Elia, U.; Peer, D. Principles for Designing an Optimal MRNA Lipid Nanoparticle Vaccine. *Curr. Opin. Biotechnol.* **2022**, *73*, 329. [CrossRef] [PubMed]
57. Li, Y.; Teague, B.; Zhang, Y.; Su, Z.; Porter, E.; Dobosh, B.; Wagner, T.; Irvine, D.J.; Weiss, R. In Vitro Evolution of Enhanced RNA Replicons for Immunotherapy. *Sci. Rep.* **2019**, *9*, 6932. [CrossRef] [PubMed]
58. Linares-Fernández, S.; Lacroix, C.; Exposito, J.Y.; Verrier, B. Tailoring MRNA Vaccine to Balance Innate/Adaptive Immune Response. *Trends Mol. Med.* **2020**, *26*, 311–323. [CrossRef]
59. Sample, P.J.; Wang, B.; Reid, D.W.; Presnyak, V.; McFadyen, I.J.; Morris, D.R.; Seelig, G. Human 5′ UTR Design and Variant Effect Prediction from a Massively Parallel Translation Assay. *Nat. Biotechnol.* **2019**, *37*, 803–809. [CrossRef]
60. Kumar, P.; Sweeney, T.R.; Skabkin, M.A.; Skabkina, O.V.; Hellen, C.U.; Pestova, T.V. Inhibition of Translation by IFIT Family Members Is Determined by Their Ability to Interact Selectively with the 5′-Terminal Regions of Cap0-, Cap1-and 5′ Ppp-MRNAs. *Nucleid Acids Res.* **2014**, *42*, 3228–3245. [CrossRef]
61. Strenkowska, M.; Grzela, R.; Majewski, M.; Wnek, K.; Kowalska, J.; Lukaszewicz, M.; Zuberek, J.; Darzynkiewicz, E.; Kuhn, A.N.; Sahin, U.; et al. Cap Analogs Modified with 1,2-Dithiodiphosphate Moiety Protect MRNA from Decapping and Enhance Its Translational Potential. *Nucleic Acids Res.* **2016**, *44*, 9578–9590. [CrossRef]
62. Rydzik, A.M.; Warminski, M.; Sikorski, P.J.; Baranowski, M.R.; Walczak, S.; Kowalska, J.; Zuberek, J.; Lukaszewicz, M.; Nowak, E.; Claridge, T.D.W.; et al. MRNA Cap Analogues Substituted in the Tetraphosphate Chain with CX2: Identification of O-to-CCl2 as the First Bridging Modification That Confers Resistance to Decapping without Impairing Translation. *Nucleic Acids Res.* **2017**, *45*, 8661–8675. [CrossRef] [PubMed]
63. Nicholson, A.L.; Pasquinelli, A.E. Tales of Detailed Poly (A) Tails. *Trends Cell Biol.* **2019**, *29*, 191–200. [CrossRef] [PubMed]
64. Pelletier, J.; Sonenberg, N. The Organizing Principles of Eukaryotic Ribosome Recruitment. *Annu. Rev. Chem.* **2019**, *88*, 307–335. [CrossRef]
65. Pascolo, S. The Messenger's Great Message for Vaccination. *Expert Rev. Vaccines* **2014**, *14*, 153–156. [CrossRef]
66. Rosa, S.S.; Prazeres, D.M.F.; Azevedo, A.M.; Marques, M.P.C. MRNA Vaccines Manufacturing: Challenges and Bottlenecks. *Vaccine* **2021**, *39*, 2190. [CrossRef] [PubMed]
67. Pascolo, S. Messenger RNA: The Inexpensive Biopharmaceutical. *J. Multidiscip. Eng. Sci. Technol. JMEST* **2017**, *4*, 2458–9403.
68. Thanh Le, T.; Andreadakis, Z.; Kumar, A.; Gómez Román, R.; Tollefsen, S.; Saville, M.; Mayhew, S. The COVID-19 Vaccine Development Landscape. *Nat. Rev. Drug Discov.* **2020**, *19*, 305–306. [CrossRef]
69. Maruggi, G.; Zhang, C.; Li, J.; Ulmer, J.B.; Yu, D. MRNA as a Transformative Technology for Vaccine Development to Control Infectious Diseases. *Mol. Ther.* **2019**, *27*, 757–772. [CrossRef]

70. Jeeva, S.; Kim, K.H.; Shin, C.H.; Wang, B.Z.; Kang, S.M. An Update on MRNA-Based Viral Vaccines. *Vaccines* **2021**, *9*, 965. [CrossRef]
71. Liu, T.; Liang, Y.; Huang, L. Development and Delivery Systems of MRNA Vaccines. *Front. Bioeng. Biotechnol.* **2021**, *9*, 8753. [CrossRef]
72. Reichmuth, A.M.; Oberli, M.A.; Jeklenec, A.; Langer, R.; Blankschtein, D. MRNA Vaccine Delivery Using Lipid Nanoparticles. *Ther. Deliv.* **2016**, *7*, 319–334. [CrossRef]
73. Schoenmaker, L.; Witzigmann, D.; Kulkarni, J.A.; Verbeke, R.; Kersten, G.; Jiskoot, W.; Crommelin, D.J.A. MRNA-Lipid Nanoparticle COVID-19 Vaccines: Structure and Stability. *Int. J. Pharm.* **2021**, *601*, 120586. [CrossRef] [PubMed]
74. Pilkington, E.H.; Suys, E.J.A.; Trevaskis, N.L.; Wheatley, A.K.; Zukancic, D.; Algarni, A.; Al-Wassiti, H.; Davis, T.P.; Pouton, C.W.; Kent, S.J.; et al. From influenza to COVID-19: Lipid nanoparticle mRNA vaccines at the frontiers of infectious diseases. *Acta Biomater* **2021**, *131*, 16–40. [CrossRef]
75. Tenchov, R.; Bird, R.; Curtze, A.E.; Zhou, Q. Lipid Nanoparticles from Liposomes to MRNA Vaccine Delivery, a Landscape of Research Diversity and Advancement. *ACS Nano* **2021**, *15*, 16982–17015. [CrossRef] [PubMed]
76. Ramachandran, S.; Satapathy, S.R.; Dutta, T. Delivery Strategies for MRNA Vaccines. *Pharm. Med.* **2022**, *36*, 11–20. [CrossRef] [PubMed]
77. Pardi, N.; Hogan, M.J.; Porter, F.W.; Weissman, D. MRNA Vaccines-a New Era in Vaccinology. *Nat. Rev. Drug Discov.* **2018**, *17*, 261–279. [CrossRef] [PubMed]
78. Zhang, R.; Tang, L.; Tian, Y.; Ji, X.; Hu, Q.; Zhou, B.; Ding, Z.; Xu, H.; Yang, L. DP7-C-Modified Liposomes Enhance Immune Responses and the Antitumor Effect of a Neoantigen-Based MRNA Vaccine. *J. Control. Release* **2020**, *328*, 210–221. [CrossRef]
79. Alfagih, I.M.; Aldosari, B.; AlQuadeib, B.; Almurshedi, A.; Alfagih, M.M. Nanoparticles as Adjuvants and Nanodelivery Systems for MRNA-Based Vaccines. *Pharmaceutics* **2020**, *13*, 45. [CrossRef]
80. Qin, S.; Tang, X.; Chen, Y.; Chen, K.; Fan, N.; Xiao, W.; Zheng, Q.; Li, G.; Teng, Y.; Wu, M.; et al. MRNA-Based Therapeutics: Powerful and Versatile Tools to Combat Diseases. *Signal Transduct. Target. Ther.* **2022**, *7*, 166. [CrossRef]
81. Damase, T.R.; Sukhovershin, R.; Boada, C.; Taraballi, F.; Pettigrew, R.I.; Cooke, J.P. The Limitless Future of RNA Therapeutics. *Front. Bioeng. Biotechnol.* **2021**, *9*, 161. [CrossRef]
82. Brito, L.A.; Chan, M.; Shaw, C.A.; Hekele, A.; Carsillo, T.; Schaefer, M.; Archer, J.; Seubert, A.; Otten, G.R.; Beard, C.W.; et al. A Cationic Nanoemulsion for the Delivery of Next-Generation RNA Vaccines. *Mol. Ther. J. Am. Soc. Gene Ther.* **2014**, *22*, 2118–2129. [CrossRef] [PubMed]
83. Adam, A.; Shi, Q.; Wang, B.; Zou, J.; Mai, J.; Osman, S.R.; Wu, W.; Xie, X.; Aguilar, P.V.; Bao, X.; et al. A Modified Porous Silicon Microparticle Potentiates Protective Systemic and Mucosal Immunity for SARS-CoV-2 Subunit Vaccine. *Transl. Res.* **2022**, *249*, 13–27. [CrossRef] [PubMed]
84. Uddin, M.N.; Roni, M.A. Challenges of Storage and Stability of Mrna-Based COVID-19 Vaccines. *Vaccines* **2021**, *9*, 1033. [CrossRef] [PubMed]
85. Anderson, E.J.; Rouphael, N.G.; Widge, A.T.; Jackson, L.A.; Roberts, P.C.; Makhene, M.; Chappell, J.D.; Denison, M.R.; Stevens, L.J.; Pruijssers, A.J.; et al. Safety and Immunogenicity of SARS-CoV-2 MRNA-1273 Vaccine in Older Adults. *N. Engl. J. Med.* **2020**, *383*, 2427–2438. [CrossRef]
86. El Sahly, H.M.; Baden, L.R.; Essink, B.; Doblecki-Lewis, S.; Martin, J.M.; Anderson, E.J.; Campbell, T.B.; Clark, J.; Jackson, L.A.; Fichtenbaum, C.J.; et al. Efficacy of the MRNA-1273 SARS-CoV-2 Vaccine at Completion of Blinded Phase. *N. Engl. J. Med.* **2021**, *385*, 1774–1785. [CrossRef]
87. Ali, K.; Berman, G.; Zhou, H.; Deng, W.; Faughnan, V.; Coronado-Voges, M.; Ding, B.; Dooley, J.; Girard, B.; Hillebrand, W.; et al. Evaluation of MRNA-1273 SARS-CoV-2 Vaccine in Adolescents. *N. Engl. J. Med.* **2021**, *385*, 2241–2251. [CrossRef]
88. A Study to Evaluate Safety and Immunogenicity of MRNA-1273 Vaccine to Prevent COVID-19 in Adult Organ Transplant Recipients and in Healthy Adult Participants—Full Text View—ClinicalTrials.Gov. Available online: https://clinicaltrials.gov/ct2/show/NCT04860297 (accessed on 10 January 2023).
89. Safety, Tolerability, and Immunogenicity of V110 or V114 Co-Administered With a Booster Dose of MRNA-1273 in Healthy Adults (V110-911)—Full Text View—ClinicalTrials.Gov. Available online: https://clinicaltrials.gov/ct2/show/NCT05158140 (accessed on 10 January 2023).
90. A Study of SARS-CoV-2 Infection and Potential Transmission in Individuals Immunized With Moderna COVID-19 Vaccine—Full Text View—ClinicalTrials.Gov. Available online: https://www.clinicaltrials.gov/ct2/show/NCT04811664 (accessed on 10 January 2023).
91. Kusejko, K.; Chammartin, F.; Smith, D.; Odermatt, M.; Schuhmacher, J.; Koller, M.; Günthard, H.F.; Briel, M.; Bucher, H.C.; Speich, B.; et al. Developing and Testing a Corona VaccinE TRiAL PLatform (COVERALL) to Study COVID-19 Vaccine Response in Immunocompromised Patients. *BMC Infect. Dis.* **2022**, *22*, 654. [CrossRef]
92. COVID-19 Immunogenicity of a Third Dose of MRNA-1273 Vaccine Among Cancer Patients—Full Text View—ClinicalTrials.Gov. Available online: https://clinicaltrials.gov/ct2/show/NCT05054218 (accessed on 10 January 2023).
93. Chu, L.; McPhee, R.; Huang, W.; Bennett, H.; Pajon, R.; Nestorova, B.; Leav, B. A Preliminary Report of a Randomized Controlled Phase 2 Trial of the Safety and Immunogenicity of MRNA-1273 SARS-CoV-2 Vaccine. *Vaccine* **2021**, *39*, 2791–2799. [CrossRef]

94. Mues, K.E.; Kirk, B.; Patel, D.A.; Gelman, A.; Chavers, L.S.; Talarico, C.A.; Esposito, D.B.; Martin, D.; Mansi, J.; Chen, X.; et al. Real-World Comparative Effectiveness of MRNA-1273 and BNT162b2 Vaccines among Immunocompromised Adults Identified in Administrative Claims Data in the United States. *Vaccine* **2022**, *40*, 6730–6739. [CrossRef]
95. Choi, A.; Koch, M.; Wu, K.; Chu, L.; Ma, L.; Hill, A.; Nunna, N.; Huang, W.; Oestreicher, J.; Colpitts, T.; et al. Safety and Immunogenicity of a Third Dose of SARS-CoV-2 MRNA Vaccine—An Interim Analysis. *Res. Sq.* 2022; *preprint*. [CrossRef]
96. Jochum, S.; Kirste, I.; Hortsch, S.; Grunert, V.P.; Legault, H.; Eichenlaub, U.; Kashlan, B.; Pajon, R. Clinical Utility of Elecsys Anti-SARS-CoV-2 S Assay in COVID-19 Vaccination: An Exploratory Analysis of the MRNA-1273 Phase 1 Trial. *Front. Immunol.* **2022**, *12*, 8117. [CrossRef] [PubMed]
97. A Study to Evaluate Safety, Tolerability & Immunogenicity of Multiple Formulations of BNT162b2 Against COVID-19 in Healthy Adults—Full Text View—ClinicalTrials.Gov. Available online: https://clinicaltrials.gov/ct2/show/NCT04816669 (accessed on 10 January 2023).
98. Polack, F.P.; Thomas, S.J.; Kitchin, N.; Absalon, J.; Gurtman, A.; Lockhart, S.; Perez, J.L.; Pérez Marc, G.; Moreira, E.D.; Zerbini, C.; et al. Safety and Efficacy of the BNT162b2 MRNA COVID-19 Vaccine. *N. Engl. J. Med.* **2020**, *383*, 2603–2615. [CrossRef]
99. Safety and Immunogenicity Study of 20vPnC When Coadministered With a Booster Dose of BNT162b2—Study Results—ClinicalTrials.Gov. Available online: https://clinicaltrials.gov/ct2/show/NCT04887948 (accessed on 10 January 2023).
100. Levi, N.; Moravsky, G.; Weitsman, T.; Amsalem, I.; Bar-Sheshet Itach, S.; Algur, N.; Lapidus, I.; Mitz, O.; Glikson, M.; Wiener-Well, Y.; et al. A Prospective Study on Myocardial Injury after BNT162b2 MRNA COVID-19 Fourth Dose Vaccination in Healthy Persons. *Eur. J. Heart Fail.* 2022; *online*. [CrossRef] [PubMed]
101. Quandt, J.; Muik, A.; Salisch, N.; Lui, B.G.; Lutz, S.; Krüger, K.; Wallisch, A.K.; Adams-Quack, P.; Bacher, M.; Finlayson, A.; et al. Omicron BA.1 Breakthrough Infection Drives Cross-Variant Neutralization and Memory B Cell Formation against Conserved Epitopes. *Sci. Immunol.* **2022**, *7*, eabq2427. [CrossRef]
102. Mohapatra, S.; Ananda, P.; Tripathy, S. Pharmacological Consideration of COVID-19 Infection and Vaccines in Pregnancy. *J. Chin. Med. Assoc. JCMA* **2022**, *85*, 537–542. [CrossRef] [PubMed]
103. A Phase 3 Study to Evaluate the Safety, Tolerability, and Immunogenicity of Multiple Production Lots and Dose Levels of BNT162b2 RNA-Based COVID-19 Vaccines Against COVID-19 in Healthy Participants—Full Text View—ClinicalTrials.Gov. Available online: https://clinicaltrials.gov/ct2/show/NCT04713553 (accessed on 10 January 2023).
104. Haranaka, M.; Baber, J.; Ogama, Y.; Yamaji, M.; Aizawa, M.; Kogawara, O.; Scully, I.; Lagkadinou, E.; Türeci, Ö.; Şahin, U.; et al. A Randomized Study to Evaluate Safety and Immunogenicity of the BNT162b2 COVID-19 Vaccine in Healthy Japanese Adults. *Nat. Commun.* **2021**, *12*, 7105. [CrossRef]
105. Hui, A.M.; Li, J.; Zhu, L.; Tang, R.; Ye, H.; Lin, M.; Ge, L.; Wang, X.; Peng, F.; Wu, Z.; et al. Immunogenicity and Safety of BNT162b2 MRNA Vaccine in Chinese Adults: A Phase 2 Randomised Clinical Trial. *Lancet Reg. Health West. Pac.* **2022**, *29*, 100586. [CrossRef] [PubMed]
106. Baden, L.R.; El Sahly, H.M.; Essink, B.; Kotloff, K.; Frey, S.; Novak, R.; Diemert, D.; Spector, S.A.; Rouphael, N.; Creech, C.B.; et al. Efficacy and Safety of the MRNA-1273 SARS-CoV-2 Vaccine. *N. Engl. J. Med.* **2021**, *384*, 403–416. [CrossRef]
107. Al Bawab, W.; Hammad, A.Q.; Ling, A.; Alasmari, J.; Al-Qerem, W.; Al Bawab, A.Q.; Hammad, A.; Ling, J.; Alasmari, F. Willingness of the Jordanian Population to Receive a COVID-19 Booster Dose: A Cross-Sectional Study. *Vaccines* **2022**, *10*, 410. [CrossRef]
108. Chiu, N.C.; Chi, H.; Tu, Y.K.; Huang, Y.N.; Tai, Y.L.; Weng, S.L.; Chang, L.; Huang, D.T.N.; Huang, F.Y.; Lin, C.Y. To Mix or Not to Mix? A Rapid Systematic Review of Heterologous Prime–Boost COVID-19 Vaccination. *Expert Rev. Vaccines* **2021**, *20*, 1211–1220. [CrossRef]
109. Preparation, V.; Information, G.; Indications, A.; Schedule, V.; Vaccine, T.F. *Pfizer-BioNTech COVID-19 Vaccine Pfizer-BioNTech COVID-19 Vaccine*; CDC: Atlanta, GA, USA, 2022; pp. 4–6.
110. Thomas, S.J.; Moreira, E.D.; Kitchin, N.; Absalon, J.; Gurtman, A.; Lockhart, S.; Perez, J.L.; Pérez Marc, G.; Polack, F.P.; Zerbini, C.; et al. Safety and Efficacy of the BNT162b2 MRNA COVID-19 Vaccine through 6 Months. *N. Engl. J. Med.* **2021**, *385*, 1761–1773. [CrossRef] [PubMed]
111. Trougakos, I.P.; Terpos, E.; Alexopoulos, H.; Politou, M.; Paraskevis, D.; Scorilas, A.; Kastritis, E.; Andreakos, E.; Dimopoulos, M.A. Adverse Effects of COVID-19 MRNA Vaccines: The Spike Hypothesis. *Trends Mol. Med.* **2022**, *28*, 542–554. [CrossRef]
112. Naik, R.; Peden, K. *Regulatory Considerations on the Development of MRNA Vaccines*; Part of the Current Topics in Microbiology and Immunology book series (CT MICROBIOLOGY, Volume 440); Springer: Cham, Switzerland, 2020. [CrossRef]
113. Lopez Bernal, J.; Andrews, N.; Gower, C.; Gallagher, E.; Simmons, R.; Thelwall, S.; Stowe, J.; Tessier, E.; Groves, N.; Dabrera, G.; et al. Effectiveness of COVID-19 Vaccines against the B.1.617.2 (Delta) Variant. *N. Engl. J. Med.* **2021**, *385*, 585–594. [CrossRef] [PubMed]
114. Park, J.; Yi, H.; Kim, Y.; Chang, H.; Cell, V.K.-M. Regulation of Poly (A) Tail and Translation during the Somatic Cell Cycle. *Mol. Cell.* **2016**, *62*, 462–471. [CrossRef] [PubMed]
115. Knezevic, I.; Liu, M.; Peden, K.; Zhou, T.; Kang, H.-N. Development of MRNA Vaccines: Scientific and Regulatory Issues. *Vaccines* **2021**, *9*, 81. [CrossRef] [PubMed]

116. Hassett, K.J.; Benenato, K.E.; Jacquinet, E.; Lee, A.; Woods, A.; Yuzhakov, O.; Himansu, S.; Deterling, J.; Geilich, B.M.; Ketova, T.; et al. Optimization of Lipid Nanoparticles for Intramuscular Administration of MRNA Vaccines. *Mol. Ther. Nucleic Acids* **2019**, *15*, 1–11. [CrossRef] [PubMed]
117. Krishnan, A.; Gangadaran, P.; Chavda, V.P.; Jogalekar, M.P.; Muthusamy, R.; Valu, D.; Vadivalagan, C.; Ramani, P.; Laishevtcev, A.; Katari, N.K.; et al. Convalescent Serum-Derived Exosomes: Attractive Niche as COVID-19 Diagnostic Tool and Vehicle for MRNA Delivery. *Exp. Biol. Med. Maywood* **2022**, *247*, 1244–1252. [CrossRef] [PubMed]
118. Chavda, V.P.; Soni, S.; Vora, L.K.; Soni, S.; Khadela, A.; Ajabiya, J. MRNA-Based Vaccines and Therapeutics for COVID-19 and Future Pandemics. *Vaccines* **2022**, *10*, 2150. [CrossRef] [PubMed]

vaccines

MDPI

Review

An Overview of the Strategies to Boost SARS-CoV-2-Specific Immunity in People with Inborn Errors of Immunity

Emma Chang-Rabley [1], Menno C. van Zelm [2,3,4], Emily E. Ricotta [1,5,*] and Emily S. J. Edwards [2,3,*]

1 The Laboratory of Clinical Immunology and Microbiology, National Institute of Allergy and Infectious Diseases, National Institutes of Health, Bethesda, MD 20892, USA
2 Allergy and Clinical Immunology Laboratory, Department of Immunology, Central Clinical School, Monash University, Melbourne, VIC 3800, Australia
3 The Jeffrey Modell Diagnostic and Research Centre for Primary Immunodeficiencies in Melbourne, Melbourne, VIC 3000, Australia
4 Department of Immunology, Erasmus MC, University Medical Center, 3015 GD Rotterdam, The Netherlands
5 Department of Preventive Medicine and Biostatistics, Uniform Services University of the Health Sciences, Bethesda, MD 20814, USA
* Correspondence: emily.ricotta@usuhs.edu (E.E.R.); emily.edwards@monash.edu (E.S.J.E.); Tel.: +1-301-7617784 (E.E.R.); +61-3-9903-0197 (E.S.J.E.)

Abstract: The SARS-CoV-2 pandemic has heightened concerns about immunological protection, especially for individuals with inborn errors of immunity (IEI). While COVID-19 vaccines elicit strong immune responses in healthy individuals, their effectiveness in IEI patients remains unclear, particularly against new viral variants and vaccine formulations. This uncertainty has led to anxiety, prolonged self-isolation, and repeated vaccinations with uncertain benefits among IEI patients. Despite some level of immune response from vaccination, the definition of protective immunity in IEI individuals is still unknown. Given their susceptibility to severe COVID-19, strategies such as immunoglobulin replacement therapy (IgRT) and monoclonal antibodies have been employed to provide passive immunity, and protection against both current and emerging variants. This review examines the efficacy of COVID-19 vaccines and antibody-based therapies in IEI patients, their capacity to recognize viral variants, and the necessary advances required for the ongoing protection of people with IEIs.

Keywords: COVID-19 vaccination; SARS-CoV-2-specific antibody therapies; immune memory; inborn errors of immunity; breakthrough infections

1. Introduction

Since its emergence in November 2019, severe acute respiratory coronavirus-2 (SARS-CoV-2) has caused over 775 million confirmed cases of coronavirus disease 2019 (COVID-19) and over 7 million deaths worldwide [1]. The global fatality rates range across countries and age groups, from <1% in those aged <50 years to ~4–25% in healthy individuals 60–80 years of age [2,3].

SARS-CoV-2 is an enveloped virus with a linear RNA genome belonging to the *Coronaviridae* family [4]. The infectious nature of SARS-CoV-2 potentiated the quick establishment of a pandemic, rather than the epidemic (SARS-CoV, MERS-CoV) or endemic (seasonal coronaviruses) outbreaks of its predecessors [5,6].

Infection is established when the spike receptor binding domain (RBD) of the SARS-CoV-2 virus engages the angiotensin-converting enzyme 2 (ACE2) receptor on the surface of host T-cells, especially lung, heart, and kidney cells [7,8]. While, in most healthy individuals, SARS-CoV-2 infection causes asymptomatic or mild respiratory disease including fever, cough, and lethargy, a subset of individuals mount an inappropriately strong inflammatory response to high viral loads, resulting in severe illness, hospitalization, respiratory support, and in some cases death [9,10]. This leads to overwhelming concern that people with defective immunity, particularly those with rare inherited immunodeficiencies (approximately 1 in 10,000 people) [11] or more common acquired immunodeficiencies (approximately 1 in 1200 people) [12], may be at increased risk of severe COVID-19 disease.

Whilst public health measures, such as mask wearing, hand washing, social distancing, and shielding, have undoubtedly helped to protect people with inborn errors of immunity (IEIs), this has posed other issues, including feelings of isolation and adverse impacts on quality of life [13,14]. As such, the medical and scientific community rapidly pivoted to combat the global pandemic by providing novel and innovative solutions for SARS-CoV-2 testing, vaccination, and therapies to treat disease and help cover the gap in immunity in an effort to reduce virus transmission and COVID-19 disease severity. Here, we provide an in-depth overview of the current understanding of COVID-19 vaccine efficacy in people with IEI, the efficacy of SARS-CoV-2-specific antibody products, and new insights and technological advances that can enhance protection for people with IEI or other immunocompromised conditions in the changing SARS-CoV-2 landscape [15].

1.1. Inborn Errors of Immunity (IEI)

At present, genetic variants in more than 485 genes are known to cause IEIs. Patients with IEIs can be broadly classified into nine groups capturing the diversity of clinical, genetic, and immunological phenotypes of disease, plus an additional tenth category covering IEI phenocopies. Groups are defined by the nature of the rare genetic defect identified, the immune cell(s) affected, and infections to which individuals exhibit increased susceptibility [16]. Of these nine categories, the most prevalent is predominantly antibody deficiency (PAD) [17,18], including patients with Common Variable Immunodeficiency (CVID) and agammaglobulinemia. Other categories include combined immunodeficiencies (CID) and diseases of immune dysregulation known to have defects in multiple immune cell lineages. A common presenting feature in PAD is profound antibody deficiency, poor responses to vaccination, and increased susceptibility to sinopulmonary infections underpinned by defects in B-cell development, differentiation, and function [17,19,20]. It is generally accepted that many of these diseases are accompanied by defects in other immune cells involved in innate and adaptive responses. These include T-cells, which are integral for robust generation of imunity to infectious agents and may have a key role in vaccine efficacy for some pathogens, particularly those of viral origin. As a result, in people with PAD and other IEIs, reduced vaccine efficacy can result in increased susceptibility to vaccine-preventable disease. For these individuals, preventative therapy centers around tackling antibody deficiency, including lifelong immunoglobulin replacement therapy (IgRT), annual vaccinations (e.g., for influenza), and prophylactic antibiotics, in a complicated attempt to reduce the infectious burden [21,22]. Thus, the emergence of the novel SARS-CoV-2 virus presents unprecedented challenges for protecting and treating those with IEIs [17,20].

1.2. COVID-19 Infection in People with IEI

While, in healthy individuals, SARS-CoV-2 infection generates functional memory B- (Bmem), memory $CD4^+$ T- ($CD4^+$ Tmem), and $CD8^+$ T-cell ($CD8^+$ Tmem) responses, as well as neutralizing antibodies [5,6,23], some of these responses are perturbed in people with IEI, resulting in more severe disease outcomes [3]. These have been extensively reviewed elsewhere and will not be described in depth here. Briefly, Tangye et al. recently reported that ~1330 infections with SARS-CoV-2 in IEI had been published to date, with 60% of reported individuals diagnosed with antibody deficiency [3]. Among these, a case fatality rate of 8.5% was documented in people with IEIs as compared to ~1.1% in the general population. It was noted that the case fatality rate for children 0–19 years old with IEIs was up to 100 times higher than that observed for those of the same age in the general population [3,24].

Within the IEI population, individuals with defects in genes including *AIRE* (autoimmune regulator), *IRF7* (interferon regulatory factor 7), and *IFNAR1/2* (interferon-α/β receptor) had significantly higher COVID-19 case fatality rates, clearly demonstrating that genetics can adversely impact patient outcomes to SARS-CoV-2 infection [3]. In particular, individuals with biallelic variants in *AIRE* experienced the most severe COVID-19 disease as a consequence of the production of neutralizing antibodies to cytokines, including type I interferon (IFN). These anti-IFN antibodies prevent binding of IFN-α or β to its receptor (IFNAR), thereby inhibiting the pivotal role of IFNs in mediating a host response to viruses [25]. Furthermore, SARS-CoV-2 has unmasked undiagnosed IEI in otherwise asymptomatic individuals, with these individuals presenting with life-threatening COVID-19. The first identified genetic cause of severe COVID-19 disease was published in 2020 by van der Made et al. Here, rare X-linked (XL) loss-of-function (LOF) variants in the gene encoding Toll-like receptor 7 (*TLR7*) were identified in four young males with critical COVID-19 disease [26]. These variants were shown to cause impaired type I and II IFN responses, known to be crucial for immune responses against viruses. Later studies have additionally revealed novel, rare XL LOF variants in *TLR7* in young males critically ill with COVID-19, with these defects being shown to underlie severe COVID-19 disease in 1–2% of men under 60 years of age [26–29]. Additionally, *TLR7* genetic variants in the *TLR3* gene have been found to compromise local type I IFN-mediated innate immune responses. Together, variants in these genes are estimated to be the cause of severe COVID-19 in up to 5% of people under 70 years of age [26,27,30].

Additional studies have identified additional loci where enrichment of rare autosomal recessive (AR) or autosomal dominant (AD) variants in *IFNAR1* (AR/AD), *IFNAR2* (AD), *IRF3* (AD), *IRF7* (AR/AD), *TBK1* (AD), *TICAM1* (AD), *TLR3* (AD), and *UNC931* (AD), predispose ~3.5% of individuals with severe SARS-CoV-2 infection to critical COVID-19 pneumonia [31]. These genes are known to control TLR3 and IRF7-dependent induction and enhancement of type I IFN signaling, showing the important role of these pathways in the control of SARS-CoV-2 infection. Thus, this suggests that type I IFN administration might reduce disease severity if administered early in the course of the disease [31]. These findings were subsequently followed by the discovery of additional rare variants in *IFNAR1* (AR) [32,33], *TNFRSF13B* (AD), and *TBK1* (AD) underlying severe COVID-19 [34].

Strikingly, although only a few individuals have been identified with rare AR *IFNAR1* or *IFNAR2* variants, COVID-19 lethality rates are 57% in these individuals [31–33,35]. *IFNAR1* and *IFNAR2* encode the α and β chain of the type I interferon (IFN)-α/β receptor (IFNAR), respectively, which, along with IFN-I, form the IFNAR receptor. Upon binding of IFN-α or β to the IFNAR receptor, the IFNAR1 chain binds tyrosine kinase-2 (TYK2) and IFNAR2 interacts with Janus Kinase-1 (JAK1) and signal transduction and transcription activation (STAT), mediating downstream JAK/STAT (primarily STAT1 and STAT2) signal transduction and resulting in the IFN-I induced cellular response [36].

Further, an international study has identified recessive defects, including XL *TLR7* and AR *IFNAR1*, *STAT2*, and *TYK2*, in 10% of pediatric patients hospitalized with COVID-19 pneumonia [37]. Together, the predisposition of individuals with variants in the aforementioned genes to severe COVID-19 disease demonstrates the critical role of type I IFN in host defense against SARS-CoV-2, whilst this pathway is redundant for other infectious agents. Interestingly, a more recent retrospective cohort study by Ngyuen et al. found that many studies of infection outcomes in IEI did not control for factors classified as social determinants of health, such as race/ethnicity [38]. In their cohort of various combined, humoral, or innate immunodeficiencies and ages (2 months to 69 years), they identified an association between an increased risk of hospitalization and race, ethnicity, obesity, and neurological disease. The authors posit that these findings have important implications for current treatment and COVID-19 disease management guidelines for IEI populations, which center around cellular and genetic mechanisms of severe disease risk.

1.3. SARS-CoV-2 Variants

Over the pandemic, multiple SARS-CoV-2 variants have evolved, with the first, Alpha, detected in September 2020 (Table S1). Viral variants contain mutations that are advantageous for viral spread, e.g., increased infectivity, viral fitness, or escape from immune responses [39]. Multiple predisposing factors, including geographical location, environmental and economic conditions, and access to vaccination, favor viral diversification, thus leading to the emergence of variants in the general population [40]. Indeed, this concern extends to the unvaccinated, and inequitable global vaccine access may play a role in the ongoing development of SARS-CoV-2 variants. There is also evidence that the delayed viral clearance observed in people with immune disorders contributes to the emergence of viral variants [41–44].

Whilst over 30 different SARS-CoV-2 genetic clades have been identified to date, not all have been cause for heightened concern or attention. Therefore, the World Health Organization (WHO) monitored variants with increased viral transmissibility or virulence or escape from the host antibody. For example, the Omicron BA.1 variant, which emerged in November 2021, has 37 spike protein mutations, resulting in increased ACE2 binding affinity and decreased humoral immune recognition [45]. To date, the Omicron lineage is the most divergent variant due to the high number of mutations it harbors, with all sublineages maintaining properties of increased immune evasion and preference for binding to ACE2 compared to earlier SARS-CoV-2 variants [46,47] (Table S1).

Due to the ongoing evolution of SARS-CoV-2 variants, there was a shift in variant predominance from Omicron XBB.1.5 and XBB.1.6. in July 2023 to Omicron E.G.5.1 in December 2023, with the epidemiology differing by geographical location (Figure 1). The current dominant variants have an immune evasion advantage, but result in less severe infections in the general population [39,48]. Here, more observation is needed to determine how variant transmission impacts the IEI community in terms of infection rates and severity of illness.

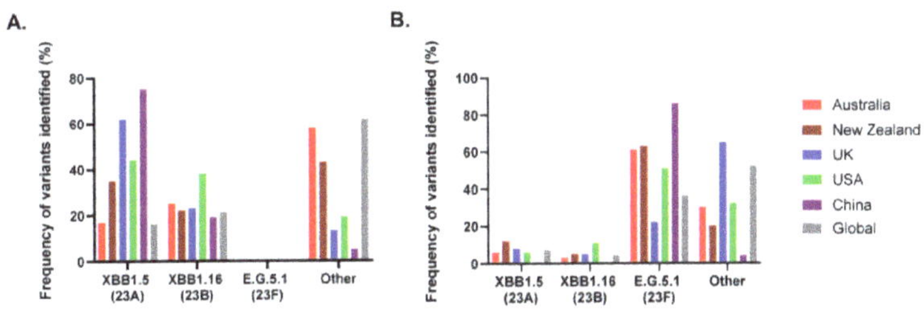

Figure 1. Shifting predominance of SARS-CoV-2 variants over time and in different geographical locations worldwide. SARS-CoV-2 variant predominance in different countries and globally (**A**) as at 10 July 2023 and (**B**) 18 December 2023. Global data from [49] and individual country data from [50].

2. COVID-19 Vaccines and Vaccine-Induced Responses in Healthy Individuals

The emergence of SARS-CoV-2 and the rapid roll-out of new vaccine formulations have provided a unique opportunity to examine vaccine responses in infection- or vaccine-naïve individuals with or without IEI. This has the capacity to provide novel insights into the immunological defects in individual IEI patients [19], as well as to provide crucial information to direct future vaccination programs.

2.1. Vaccine Formulations for COVID-19

During the pandemic, the WHO evaluated and provided Emergency Use Authorization (EUA) qualification for COVID-19 vaccines in July 2020, with the initial aim to provide protection from viral transmission, severe disease, hospitalization, and death [51,52]. As viral transmissibility increased (September 2020), the focus switched to the latter aspects of vaccine efficacy, as well as the predominance of breakthrough infections [2,53]. To date, more than 13.6 billion doses of COVID-19 vaccine have been administered in the ongoing fight against SARS-CoV-2. This includes receipt of at least one dose of COVID-19 vaccine by 70.6% of the world's population and 32.9% of people in low-income countries [1]. This, in isolation, shows the disparity in vaccine access between low and middle/high income countries. Granular data are not available in many regions to assess the extent to which this disparity impacts people with IEI.

The vaccine formulations used for primary dosing in Australia, the UK, and the USA included mRNA vaccines (Comirnaty (BNT162b2, Pfizer BioNTech)), SpikeVax (mRNA-1273, Moderna), viral vector vaccines (Ad26.COV2.S (Johnson & Johnson, Janssen), adenoviral vector based ChAdOx1 nCoV-19 (Oxford/AstraZeneca)), and one protein subunit vaccine (Novavax, Nuvaxovid). All vaccines are generally safe and highly effective at preventing hospitalization in healthy populations. Notable exceptions included the increased incidence of thrombosis with thrombocytopenia syndrome or severe anaphylactic reactions to polyethylene glycol in certain individuals with specific vaccine formulations [54,55]. Importantly, these five authorized COVID-19 vaccines induce a robust humoral response in healthy individuals, with some variation in antibody levels identified between different formulations as well as based on timings between doses [53,54,56]. For example, it has been shown that spike RBD-specific IgG antibody levels are higher in healthy individuals who received two primary doses of the Comirnaty mRNA vaccine compared to those who received two primary doses of the ChAdOx1 nCOV-19 adenoviral vaccine [5,6,57,58]. The development and rollout of the primary immunization series, and any subsequent boosters, are now an indispensable cornerstone of the global response against COVID-19.

In comparison, other authorized vaccination regimens, including Coronavac (Sinovac Biotech), Sputnik-V (Gam-COVID-Vac), and BBIBP-CorV (SinoPharm, Beijing Institute Biological Products), produce a substantially reduced antibody response with seropositivity rates of 36.9–50%, known to be substantially lower than those seen in convalescence. This explains the reduced efficacy of these vaccines with respect to both protection from symptomatic infection and severe infection and hospitalization [59–61].

Despite the emergence of SARS-CoV-2 variants as early as May 2021, most COVID-19 vaccine formulations until late 2022/early 2023 exclusively contained the spike protein of the ancestral WH1 strain. To combat ongoing viral evolution, bivalent mRNA vaccines were developed and released to further boost immunity to emerging Omicron variants, with the aim of providing protection from severe disease, hospitalization, and death. To date, four bivalent vaccines have emerged: the Pfizer bivalent vaccine containing equal amounts of WH-1 and Omicron BA.1 (Comirnaty Original/Omicron BA.1) or Omicron BA.4/BA.5 spike (Comirnaty Original/Omicron BA.4-5) [62] and the Moderna bivalent vaccine containing equal amounts of WH-1 and Omicron BA.1 (Spikevax Bivalent Original/Omicron BA.1) or Omicron BA.4/BA.5 spike (Spikevax Bivalent Original/Omicron BA.4-5). In May 2023, due to the increased prevalence of Omicron XBB.1 lineages, the WHO recommended use of the monovalent XBB.1.5 as the antigen for ongoing COVID-19 vaccination. Since then, two monovalent Omicron XBB.1.5 vaccines, Pfizer (Comirnaty) Omicron XBB.1.5. and Moderna (Spikevax) Omicron XBB.1.5, have been approved for use by the U.S. Food and Drug Administration (FDA), Australian Technical Advisory Group on Immunization (ATAGI), and the UK medicines regulator [15,63,64].

Due to the sparsity of information regarding the efficacy of bivalent vaccinations in IEI populations, this review summarizes the information to date on the healthy individual and IEI patient response to the original monovalent vaccination formulations.

2.2. The COVID-19 Vaccine-Induced Response in Immunocompetent Individuals

In immunocompetent individuals, COVID-19 vaccination generates neutralizing antibodies, as well as functional SARS-CoV-2-specific B-cell memory (Bmem) and $CD4^+$ and $CD8^+$ T memory (Tmem) responses, namely towards the RBD known to directly bind the ACE2 receptor. These correlates define a protective immune response emerging 1–2 weeks following vaccination. Whilst specific antibody and neutralizing titers have been shown to wane 1–3 months post-vaccination, protection against severe infection has been shown to persist for at least 4–6 months. Importantly, vaccine-induced Bmem and Tmem responses are known to persist longer-term, and likely represent a more durable marker of immune protection than antibodies [5,6].

Moreover, it has been shown that booster vaccination can significantly boost Bmem responses specific for ancestral virus and are cross-protective against Omicron subvariant RBD [56–58]. It is important to note that vaccine formulation can have a dramatic impact on the magnitude of response, such that individuals who received a two-dose primary regimen of Pfizer BNT162b2 generated a significantly higher magnitude of ancestral WH1 RBD-specific plasma IgG and Bmem compared to those receiving the two-dose adenoviral ChAdOx1 vaccine [56,58]. However, upon boosting with a third dose of mRNA vaccine, both groups demonstrated a significant increase in ancestral WH1 RBD-specific plasma IgG and Bmem numbers, with the magnitude of response being similar between both groups. Furthermore, the mRNA third-dose booster increased recognition of the Omicron BA.2 and BA.5 variants by both antibodies and Bmem [56]. This further exemplifies the need to assess these attributes of the immune response in COVID-19-vaccinated IEI patients and to determine whether the boosters have the same benefit in this population.

3. The COVID-19 Vaccination Response in IEI Patients

Globally, it has been acknowledged that immunocompromised individuals, including those with IEIs, may benefit from extra doses of COVID-19 vaccines to generate responses equivalent to those observed in healthy individuals [65–68]. First, it was recommended by the U.S. FDA, ATAGI, and UK medicines regulator that an additional (third) dose be added to the primary regimen. This differs from the two-dose regimen (except for Ad26.CoV2.S, which comprised a 1-dose regimen) for the general population [55,67,69]. Vaccines approved by the aforementioned regulatory bodies showed evidence of a high efficacy for protection from infection, as well as protection from severe disease, hospitalization, and death [54,70]. Whilst breakthrough infections with SARS-CoV-2 variants have been documented in patients with IEIs, those who have been vaccinated experience lower disease severity [71].

In contrast to the general population, individuals with IEI have variable immunological responses to vaccination, with responses being impaired in some patients [72–77] (Figure 2). This section will review the humoral response reported in the literature in a variety of IEIs. For the purposes of this review, we refer to doses 1–3 as the "primary" series for people with IEIs and any additional doses as "boosters". This differs from healthy individuals, where the "primary" series refers to doses one and two, with doses three and onwards qualifying as boosters.

3.1. Humoral Response—Antibodies

People with antibody deficiencies generate a particularly poor antibody response to vaccination; indeed, "diagnostic vaccination" is used to clinically evaluate individuals for the presence of humoral IEI [78]. It was, therefore, an early concern whether these populations would develop any meaningful protection from COVID-19 vaccines, especially those using novel mRNA vaccine platforms. Here, we review 58 papers evaluating the humoral immune response generated by individuals with different IEIs to COVID-19 primary vaccines and/or booster doses (Table S2, Figure 2). In many cases [72,79–86], studies age-matched IEI patients to healthy controls to compare the robustness and quality of their antibody responses to those of the general population. This is important because otherwise, known age-related changes in the immune system would confound the results of each study. The published study designs varied from observational [74,80,86–100] to interventional studies and clinical trials [83,85,86,101,102]. Furthermore, humoral responses were reported according to seroconversion, antibody concentration/titers, and, in some cases, virus neutralization/pseudo-neutralization capacity (Figure 3 and Table 1). Samples were generally collected between approximately two weeks to one month post-vaccination, with a smaller portion of studies collecting samples at two, three, or six months post-vaccination [91,92,103]. These differences in sampling time post-vaccination can have dramatic effects on the status of the immune response. For these reasons, care should be taken when comparing studies, as variations in sample collection time points and experimental methodology affect the quantitative ranges, etc. (Figure 3 and Table 1).

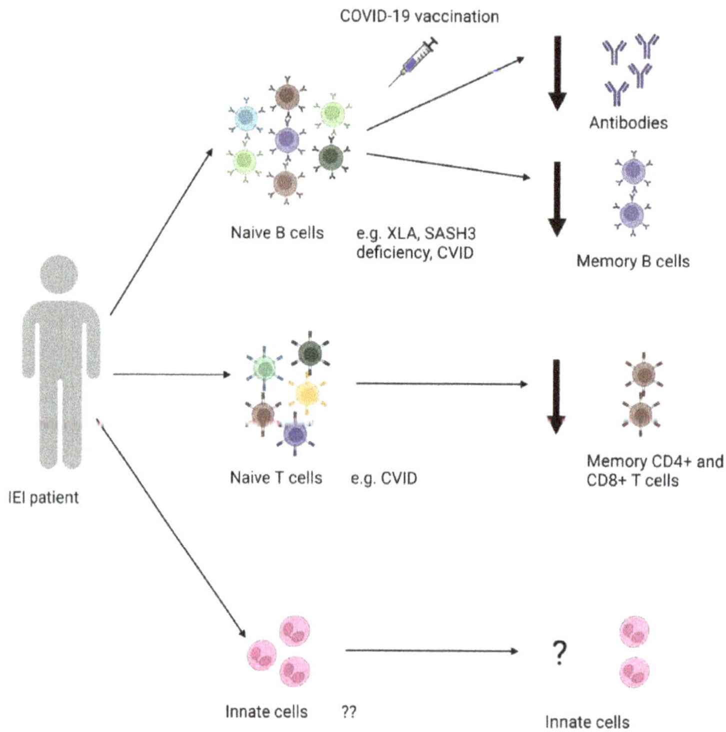

Figure 2. Generation of SARS-CoV-2-specific immunity in responses to COVID-19 vaccination in IEI patients. In healthy individuals, after administration of the COVID-19 vaccination, naive B- and T-cells are primed and expand to generate long-lived memory specific for the SARS-CoV-2 spike protein contained in the vaccine. This includes spike-specific antibodies, memory B cells, and memory T-cells that are ready for action upon re-exposure to antigen because of either booster vaccination or natural infection. In contrast, IEI patients are reported to generate a variable and, in some cases, poor response to COVID-19 vaccination which is dependent upon the genetic defect they possess. In most studies, COVID-19 vaccination of IEI patients can result in reduced COVID-19-specific antibody, memory B-cell, and/or memory T-cell responses, dependent upon the nature of the genetic lesion and the arm of the immune system affected. Above, we indicate IEIs for which perturbed COVID-19 vaccination responses have been reported in the literature. Additionally, innate cells play a pivotal role in the first line of defense against viruses. However, the responses of these cells to vaccination are currently unknown. ? depict unknown response and downwards depicts known reduced response. Figure generated with BioRender.

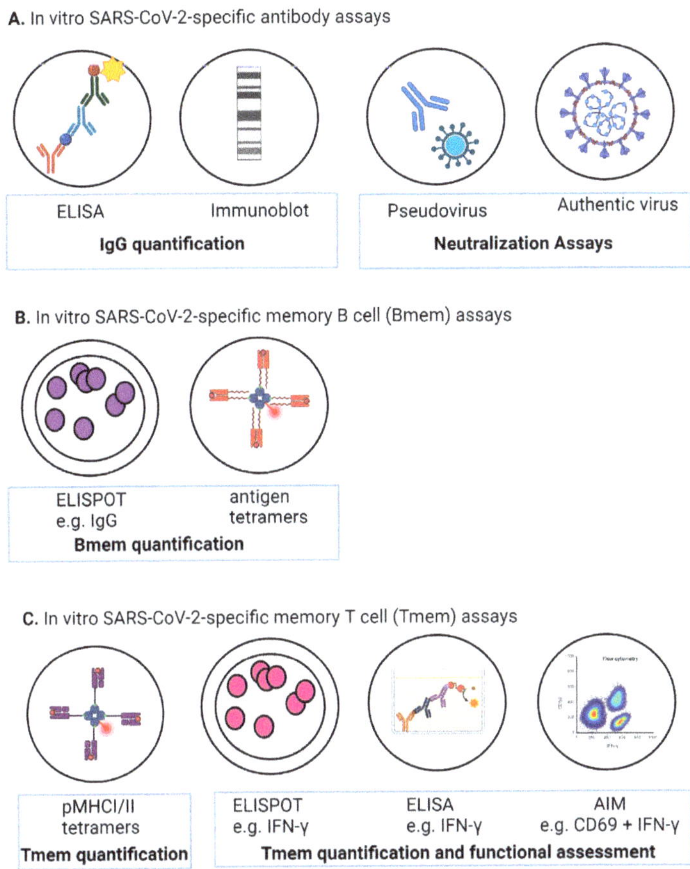

Figure 3. Main methods for the in vitro detection of SARS-CoV-2-specific humoral and cellular immunity in the peripheral blood of humans. (**A**) SARS-CoV-2-specific antibodies can be detected by ELISA or immunoblot, whilst SARS-CoV-2 virus neutralization is most frequently quantified using pseudovirus or authentic virus neutralization assays. (**B**) SARS-CoV-2-specific memory B cells (Bmem) can be identified either by the capture of IgG after antigenic stimulation in an ELISPOT or using fluorescently labeled SARS-CoV-2 antigen containing fluorochromes. (**C**) SARS-CoV-2-specific memory T-cells (Tmem) can be identified either by binding to fluorescently tagged peptide loaded MHC tetramers or after stimulation with whole protein or overlapping peptide pools. Here, SARS-CoV-2-specific Tmem are enumerated by either the production of cytokines such as IFN-γ in ELISPOTs or ELISAs or intracellular detection of cytokines coupled with cell surface expression of activation-induced markers (AIM) such as CD69, CD134, and CD137. Together, multiple methods have been used to assess immune responses to vaccination, preventing a robust comparison between various published reports (Table 2). Figure generated with BioRender.

Table 1. Methods used for the evaluation of cellular and humoral immune responses.

Assay	References	
	Studies Investigating	
	IEI Patient Responses to COVID-19 Vaccination	**Quantity and Quality of IgG Antibodies in IgRT**
SARS-CoV-2-binding IgG antibodies		
SARS-CoV-2 IgG II Quant Assay	[87]	-
Luciferase immunoprecipitation	[100]	-
ELISA	[82–84,86,92,94,97,103–117]	[118–125]
Abbott/Phadia ELiA SARS-CoV-2-Sp1 IgG assay	-	[126,127]
Roche Elecsys immunoassay	[80,82,83,104,128,129]	[130]
DiaSorin IgG immunoassay	[80,81,88,103,129,131]	-
Microblot assay	[112]	-
Abbot nucleoprotein assay	[81]	-
His-tagged spike and RBD binding probes	[90]	-
Abbott IgG assay	[85,91]	-
Luminex Ab binding	[98,124]	-
Extracted cell-free DNA sequenced by DNBSEQ	[92]	-
Abbott Quant chemiluminescent microparticle immunoassay	-	[132]
Abbot AdviseDx SARS-CoV-2 IgG II assay	-	
V-PLEX SARS-CoV-2 10-plex IgG		[133]
SARS-CoV-2-neutralizing antibodies		
SARS-CoV-2 Neutralization Antibody Detection Kit	[110,124,134]	-
Pseudovirus neutralization assay	[74,82,86,90,92,95,117,131,135]	[120,125,132,136–139]
ELISA	[72,73,89,96]	-
Live neutralization assays using Vero cells	[76,102,128]	[126]
B-cell measurement	[84]	-
Luminex based assays	[98]	[130]
SARS-CoV-2-specific B cells		
SARS-CoV-2-specific tetramers	[73,84,90,101,140]	-
SARS-CoV-2-specific T-cells		
AIMS (cell surface + intracellular cytokines)	[79,86,94,110,134,141]	-
Intracellular cytokine staining	[92,96,135,142]	-
Interferon-y ELISA	[88,89,102,103,143]	-
Interferon-y ELISPOT	[73,76,79,84,86,92,101,128,131,144]	-
Whole blood IGRA	[74,99,112]	-
Tetramers/multimers		
pMHCI	[142]	
pMHCII	[90]	

AIMS, activation-induced markers; DNBSEQ, DNA nanoballs sequencing; EliA, Enzyme fluoroimmunoassay; ELISA, enzyme-linked immunosorbent assay; ELISPOT, enzyme-linked immunosorbent spot; IgG, Immunoglobulin G; IGRA, IFN-γ release assay; pMHCI, peptide major histocompatibility complex I; pMHCII, peptide major histocompatibility complex II; SARS-CoV-2, Severe Acute Respiratory Syndrome Coronavirus-2.

Overall, seroconversion in populations with IEIs was much more variable and occurred at a lower magnitude compared to healthy controls across the primary series and additional doses [77,79–81,86,97,100,103–108,134,145–147], regardless of different methods of measurement. This is due to the heterogenous genetic and immunologic phenotype of disease in these individuals. In one study, individuals with IEI overwhelmingly displayed poorer seroconversion rates (ranging from 16.6–61.4%) compared to healthy controls (90–100%), after two doses of the mRNA vaccine (Comirnaty, SpikeVax) [76]. Despite the lower seroconversion rate at post-dose 2, it is clear that booster doses increased seropositivity (76–100%) in IEI patients after 3 vaccine doses [76,77,80].

As described in Section 1.1, the immune defects in patients with IEIs are highly diverse and likely impact the outcomes of COVID-19 vaccination. Most patients examined in the literature had PAD, in line with this group of diseases being the most prevalent IEI group (42% worldwide IEI diagnoses) [18]. In those receiving an mRNA vaccine, 20.6%

to 90.0% of individuals with PAD seroconverted after two doses [74,77,84]. In contrast, in a cohort of individuals with primary or secondary antibody deficiencies vaccinated with either Comirnaty or ChAdOx1 nCoV-19, the overall seroprevalence rose from 61.4% to 76.0% after a third dose [76]. Tandon et al., 2023, assessed the differences between an adult (n = 62) and relatively smaller pediatric (n = 13) PADs cohort, finding that antibody levels were higher in the pediatric cohort after a primary series (Comirnaty), as well as after a monovalent booster, but only for those classified as having mild PADs [109]. Otherwise, there was limited research on pediatric PAD cohorts. A study by Shin et al. specifically investigated the clinical and/or immunological factors in a group of mixed PADs that might predict their COVID-19 vaccination response [110]. They found a lower seroconversion rate and neutralizing antibody levels to vaccination in CVID patients compared to other PAD categories (e.g., IgG deficiency, IgG2 subclass deficiency, and specific antibody deficiency (SpAD)). This was associated with a number of factors, including lower baseline IgG, IgA, and proportion of Bmem cells; a higher proportion of $CD8^+$ Tmem cells; and a co-diagnosis of an autoimmune disorder [110]. Mizera et al. also found that, in their cohort study of various PADs, all patients in their CVID subgroup had around fivefold lower titers than other subgroups [108]. Thus, as stated by Quinti et al., with the high immunological and clinical diversity within CVID, each patient should be assessed individually for their capacity to mount a protective vaccination response [111].

In contrast, several studies have reported on smaller groups of patients with specific IEI diagnoses. For example, one report of individuals with STAT1-GOF (n = 7) found that 57% seroconverted after two doses of the vaccine [112]. Another case report on one individual with XMEN/MAGT1 deficiency reported a reactive spike-specific total antibody response after two doses of the mRNA vaccine [93]. In addition, Timothy et al. also completed a retrospective chart review of eight patients with CTLA-4 deficiency (two children and six adults). Of those who had their SARS-CoV-2-specific IgG levels tested (n = 2), antibody titers were lower (<6.25%) than those of the healthy unvaccinated controls [113]. Multiple studies evaluated antibody responses in individuals with XLA. In all studies, patients had nearly nonexistent antibody responses after two doses with either ChAdOx1 nCoV-19 or Comirnaty [84,102]. In fact, in one case study of three people with XLA, only one was able to mount a measurable antibody response post-vaccination [114] (Figure 2). This is consistent with the inherent B-cell defects in these individuals, whereby peripheral B cells are low or absent, resulting in an absence of serum immunoglobulins and an inadequacy in terms of generating a B-cell response to vaccination [16,17]. In this case, the observed post-vaccination antibody response is likely due to the IgRT received by the patient to treat their underlying antibody deficiency (See Section 3.1).

In several studies with more diverse cohorts of IEI, seroconversion differed by subgroup. Van Leeuwen et al. found significantly lower seroconversion rates in those with CVID, XLA, and CID compared to SpAD, undefined antibody deficiency, and phagocytic defects [74]. In studies which evaluated possible predictors of antibody responses in IEI populations, certain factors, such as condition severity [81,83], previous history of autoimmunity [72], underlying immunosuppressive treatment [81,83], and low numbers of Bmem cells pre-vaccination [84], were associated with poor responses (Figure 2).

This is important, as previous studies have established a connection between the humoral and cellular response to infection outcomes in healthy individuals [115].

Interestingly, in some studies which compared both COVID-19-naïve individuals and those with a history of previous SARS-CoV-2 infection, recovery from natural SARS-CoV-2 infection corresponded with a more efficacious antibody response to the vaccination series (i.e., "hybrid immunity"). This includes a more robust seroconversion rate [101,102], higher neutralization capacity [79], and better protection against the Delta variant [116]. Additionally, Abella et al. found that, even in the cohort with plasma cell diseases, those with multiple myeloma who had hybrid immunity had a higher plasma neutralization capacity than infection-naïve individuals 3 months post-vaccination [117]. This provides insights into whether hybrid immunity provides a more robust immune response than vaccination alone, in addition to the capacity of natural infection to shape immunity.

Recently, Abo-Helo et al. found that antibody levels remained poor in people with more severe disorders of humoral immunity 5–6 months after vaccination, suggesting the need for additional doses to preserve sufficient protection [85]. Van Leeuwen et al. conducted a large multicenter study of patients with PADs, following them up to 6 months past the primary vaccine series and a through a third dose for smaller subset of 50 CVID patients. Their cohort all received mRNA-1273 for their primary series, and either BNT16b2 or an unspecified vaccine formulation for a third dose, if applicable. At 6 months past the primary series, the decline in antibodies ranged from 5.9- to 11.2-fold, measured in GMT of S-specific IgG. However, seropositivity rates at 6 months ranged from 73% to 98%, with those in the XLA subgroup maintaining a relatively low rate of 24% [148]. Another study of a mixed cohort of more than 50 patients who received at least one dose of any mRNA-based OR inactivated vaccine, or a combination of both, found no significant difference in antibody levels across formulations [149].

There remains limited knowledge about the efficacy and durability of responses to different COVID-19 vaccine formulations in people with IEIs. Leung et al. studied the humoral response to both Comirnaty and CoronaVac ("Sinovac") formulations in their cohort of mixed IEIs and found that 73% of individuals were seropositive after a full series of either formulation [96]. Some studies found that a full Comirnaty vaccination series was more efficacious than ChAdOx1 nCoV-19 [131], and this superior protection was maintained for about 6 months after the second dose [76]. Overall, most individuals had increased neutralizing activity after a partial or full vaccine series [72–74,76,86,96,102,116,131]. Furthermore, a follow-up from the COV-AD study using a live virus neutralization assay with Vero cells found that 99.8% of their study subjects had neutralization activity after a booster dose [102]. However, whether this was a bona fide response to vaccination or a consequence of receiving SARS-CoV-2-specific antibody-containing IgRT was not evident, although in at least one study, IgRT did not appear to be significantly associated with either titer or neutralization activity [77]. It is also important to note the sparsity of data surrounding SARS-CoV-2-specific Bmem generation in individuals with IEIs in response both to natural infection and SARS-CoV-2 infection, which is necessary to provide information about the generation and durability of the Bmem cells in these populations and their ongoing ability to produce antibodies.

Furthermore, to date, some IEI patients may have received five or more vaccine doses; however, information on the efficacy of these later doses is limited. This is likely due to lack of available participants with sufficient time elapsed since their most recent dose [102], and also insufficient time elapsed to enable sample analysis and reliable reporting of findings.

3.2. *Memory T-Cells*

Like humoral immunity, cellular immunity in people with IEIs is more variable than it is in healthy populations. Recent research has focused attention specifically on the mechanisms of Bmem, Tmem, and innate immune cells following COVID-19 vaccination in IEI populations.

As such, we reviewed 43 papers investigating the overall cellular response and its relationship with the humoral response of IEI populations after receiving COVID-19 vaccination (Table S3). As with antibody production, IEI patients demonstrated suboptimal $CD4^+$ and/or $CD8^+$ T-cell responses compared to the general population, ranging from ~30 to 80% of that of healthy controls [73,80,96,102,142,150]. A number of studies found that individuals with IEI could mount measurable $CD4^+$ and/or $CD8^+$ T-cell responses [89,106,107,143], measured as the percentage of IFN-γ-positive T-cells via IFN-γ release assay (IGRA), ELISpot assay, or flow cytometry (Figure 2, Table 1).

Studies evaluating both cellular and humoral post-vaccination immunity have found varying levels of correlation between these two responses, making it difficult to draw definitive conclusions about their relationship [96,99,101]. Sauerwein et al. found an association between intact spike-specific CD4$^+$ T-cell responses and normal IgG responses, defined as a titer of spike protein 3x the limit or more, in individuals with CVID or milder antibody deficiency [134]. Oyaert et al. found a positive and significant correlation between anti-spike IgG and IFN-γ levels in IEI and chronic kidney disease (CKD) subgroups [103]. Notably, Gao et al. were able to confirm a positive correlation between antibodies and spike-specific CD4$^+$ T-cells in all their study groups, both healthy and immunocompromised [141].

Other studies found that a negative humoral response was associated with a poor cellular response. Bergman et al. found that low levels of naïve CD4$^+$ T-cells correlated with a poor antibody response in the CVID participants of their prospective clinical trial [79]. Similarly, Antoli et al. established that low CD4$^+$ and CD8$^+$ T-cell counts were a predictor of poor antibody response specifically in CVID patients [88]. Barmettler et al. also observed a correlation between low CD4$^+$ T-helper cells and low specific antibody responses in their mixed cohort of individuals with secondary and severe primary PADs, including complicated CVID/SpAD, activated P13K-syndrome, TACI deficiency, NFKB1 deficiency, HGG, and IgG subclass deficiency. This observation was evident for both mRNA and the Ad26.CoV.S vaccines [82].

In contrast, several studies reported no association or a discordant relationship between the humoral and cellular responses [96,99,101]. For example, Pulvirenti et al. found nearly no T-cell response in their vaccinated cohort of people with CVID, despite this cohort presenting a positive (albeit suboptimal) IgG response [101]. Findings from a subsequent paper by Pulvirenti et al. demonstrate that T-cell abnormalities resulting from CVID may play a role in the lack of specific antibody responses after vaccination [94]. Interestingly, in a separate cohort followed by Goschl et al. had a robust specific CD4$^+$ and CD8$^+$ T-cell response to vaccination; they found no significant correlation between that response and antibody levels [128]. Similarly, a case study of five individuals with PAD by Steiner et al. found a robust cellular response, yet no humoral response in their entire cohort [151]. Mizera et al., in their study on a cohort of individuals with primary antibody deficiencies receiving 2–4 doses, found that anti-SARS-CoV-2 IgG did not correlate with either CD4$^+$ or CD8$^+$ levels, but rather NK cells [108]. This underscores the suggestion made by previous papers to measure both the cellular and humoral response in order to develop a more complete post-vaccination immune profile in each individual [152,153].

Importantly, some studies evaluated the spectrum of T-cell responses by IEI patients to identify specific characteristics or factors that may predict poor or robust responses. Shin et al. found a correlation between baseline immune profiles as well as comorbidities, where poor vaccine responders among their mixed cohort of PADs had autoimmune diseases, low levels of baseline IgG, low naïve CD8$^+$ T-cells, and higher levels of effector CD8$^+$ Tmem [110]. Gao et al., who looked extensively at T-cell profiles between subgroups of immunocompromised individuals, found that overall, specific CD8$^+$ T-cells were generated at a higher rate than CD4$^+$ T-cells. These frequencies were comparable at 35 days after dose 2 between healthy controls, IEI, HIV, and HSCT, but lower in SOT and CLL [141]. This study found that individuals enrolled in the trial generated higher levels of higher frequencies of SARS-CoV-2-specific CD4$^+$ T-cells after two vaccine doses [141]. Similarly, van Leeuwen et al. conducted a multicenter study of different subgroups of IEI compared to healthy controls. Only the CVID subgroup had significantly lower IFN-γ response rates compared to healthy controls. Within this subgroup, lower responses were associated with age and lymphoproliferative diseases [74].

Similarly, we identified case reports of vaccination among less researched IEIs, including STAT1-GOF and X-linked *SASH3* deficiency, which found that nearly all studied individuals were able to mount both a cellular response and a humoral response despite a suboptimal baseline immune profile due to their inborn immune disorders [112,154] (Figure 2). Notably, Bloomfield et al. found that 85% of their STAT1-GOF cohort, including two individuals on the JAK inhibitor ruxolitinib, produced cellular responses comparable to healthy controls [112].

Like with post-vaccination antibody levels, exogenous factors such as natural SARS-CoV-2 infection and vaccine formulation appear to impact T-cell responses in certain settings. Some studies found that SARS-CoV-2 infection increased T-cell activity in antibody-deficient individuals [155], while another found poor $CD4^+$ and $CD8^+$ T-cell responses after both previous infection and subsequent vaccination [101]. Other studies have reported that prior SARS-CoV-2 infection results in improved immune response after the first [156] and second [102] vaccine doses. Additionally, other studies have reported the phenomena of pre-existing cross-reactive $CD4^+$ T-cells that can recognize SARS-CoV-2 [157]. The COV-AD study follow-up found that receipt of heterologous vaccines by infection-naïve IEI individuals was associated with a significantly higher likelihood of T-cell response generation compared to homogenous boosting [76]. Lin et al. found that a third dose increased the amount of SARS-CoV-2-specific $CD4^+$ and $CD8^+$ T-cells generated [90], and Goda et al. were able to demonstrate a 30% increase in T-cell activity after a third dose of Comirnaty following two ChAdOx1 n CoV-19 in individuals with CVID [131].

The rise of viral variants has sparked questions about the durability of T-cells, as well as whether strain-specific T-cells are broadly protective against variants in the IEI population. While few studies have been published to date in either healthy populations or individuals with IEI, there is some evidence of sustained reactivity.

In terms of longevity, Hurme et al. conducted a longitudinal cohort study over 22 months in a mixed cohort of primary and secondary antibody deficiencies, finding a robust cellular response. Specifically, across 1–4 doses of either mRNA-1273, BNT162b2, or ChAdOx1, 95% of their cohort had detectable T-cell responses after the primary series as measured by flow cytometry, dropping down to 78% at 3 months following a fourth dose. In a smaller subset of individuals, they observed that CD4+ cell responses were higher than $CD8^+$ at the same timepoints when stimulated with wildtype SARS-CoV-2 strain [105].

Van Leeuwen et al. extended their investigations to observe cellular responses at 6 months post-primary vaccination in their mixed IEI cohort, finding that while IFN levels decreased significantly in most of their subgroups (XLA, CVID, IgG/SPAD), these responses were still detectable at varying levels [148]. Barouch et al. found that the Ad26.CoV2.S vaccine induces durable cellular immunity, with minimal decreases over the course of 8 months in a healthy population [135]. In another healthy individual cohort, Liu et al. found that both the Ad26.CoV2.S and Comirnaty vaccines induced durable spike-specific $CD4^+$ and $CD8^+$ T-cell responses. Here, 82–84% $CD8^+$ T-cell responses were cross-reactive to the Omicron B.1.1.529 variant [150]. Sanchez et al. recently demonstrated that people with XLA had increased T-cell responses to variants compared to healthy controls, while individuals with CVID had reduced responses [144]. More evidence is needed to understand the post-vaccine T-cell response in general, as well as its ability to provide protection in the face of future SARS-CoV-2 variants. This, coupled with correlation between generation and durability of Tmem and Bmem responses, will provide crucial information about whether, for example, the generation of Tmem responses in the absence of Bmem is sufficient for protection from disease.

3.3. Memory B Cells and Innate Cells

Very few studies have evaluated the post-vaccination production of Bmem or the innate immune response (Table S4). Those that have tended to concentrate on the correlation between the presence of these cells and SARS-CoV-2-specific antibody levels. Most studies reviewed found an association between measures of Bmem and humoral responses. In three studies following individuals with antibody deficiencies, their reduced antibody responses correlated with reduced Bmem count [79,88,110]. However, other studies found little to no correlation between B-cell measurements and humoral responses [101,154], likely due to patients receiving IgRT, where antibodies from the product are indistinguishable from vaccine-induced antibodies. As with the T-cell response, Lin et al. found a similar effect of a third vaccine dose, which increased SARS-CoV-2-specific B-cell responses [90]. The previously mentioned individual with SASH3 deficiency had marked B-cell lymphopenia and reduced switched Bmem cells [154]. Pulvirenti et al. found that SARS-CoV-2 infection produced a more classical Bmem cell response in unvaccinated individuals with CVID, whilst vaccine recipients with CVID had more atypical [$CD19^{+}CD27^{-}CD24^{-}CD38^{-}$] Bmem responses [101].

At the time of this review, there was limited literature regarding specific innate cell responses to SARS-CoV-2 primary vaccination in individuals with IEIs. Notably, Cuapio et al. recently conducted a clinical trial observing natural killer (NK) cells in IEI/SID individuals during COVID-19 vaccination. They found a positive correlation between the frequency of NK cells at baseline and antibody titers taken about a month after vaccination (2.1 T-cell section). Therefore, further elucidation of the innate cell response to vaccination will be important in terms of fully understanding the efficacy of COVID-19 vaccines in these populations [158]. Mortari et al., 2023, conducted a longitudinal study on their cohort of only CVID patients who received 1–4 doses of BNT162b2 and identified four functional groups of B cell phenotypes and clinical characteristics. With respect specifically to Bmem cells, they classified their cohort into those with both low- and high-affinity Bmem cells, those who only had low-affinity Bmem cells, those with neither low- nor high-affinity Bmem cells, and non-responders (neither Bmem cells nor specific antibodies). Overall, their CVID group had significantly lower levels of low- and high-affinity Bmem cells compared to healthy volunteers [145]. Steiner et al., 2023, in their smaller cohort of only CVID patients, found that after a primary vaccine series, those who did seroconvert had significantly lower levels of class-switched Bmem cells [107]. Finally, Yam-Puc et al. conducted interesting analyses of the role of age-associated B cells (ABC) in the vaccine responses of those with IEIs or cancer, finding that a higher baseline level of ABC is associated with lower levels of specific memory B cells and less neutralizing activity [147].

The reviewed literature highlights the important finding that, for certain IEI conditions, solely relying on measurements of antibody response as a proxy for overall immunity may be underestimating the durability and efficacy of COVID-19 vaccines [79]. Given the potential confounding factors of disease, IgRT, and other adjunctive therapies (see below), it will be important to devote future research initiatives to specifically evaluating the SARS-CoV-2-specific Tmem, Bmem, and innate immune cell responses to COVID-19 vaccination in IEIs to further clarify their efficacy in these populations. Furthermore, it is evident that there is a paucity of information defining what response level of each individual immune correlate is required to confer protection against SARS-CoV-2. This information is urgently needed to accurately discern whether COVID-19 vaccines generate protective responses in people with IEIs.

4. Impact of Adjunctive Antibody Therapies on COVID-19 Immunity

Antibodies that are generated against commonly encountered pathogens and vaccine antigens are readily present in IgRT, which reduces the infectious burden in the recipient of this therapy [22,25]. Considering the ongoing pandemic, the presence of SARS-CoV-2-specific antibodies in IgRT and its capacity to protect people with IEIs from infection and/or severe COVID-19 has been of great interest to patients, clinicians, and the scientific community. Furthermore, the development and rollout of monoclonal SARS-CoV-2 antibody (mAb)-based therapeutics as preventatives and treatment options for COVID-19 has been extremely pertinent (Table 2), particularly considering the known lag between infection (and, once available, vaccination) of the general population and emergence of these antibodies in IgRT. Here, we review our current understanding regarding the content and functional capacity of SARS-CoV-2 antibody-containing products and their ability to protect against circulating SARS-CoV-2 variants.

Table 2. Adjunctive therapies for prophylaxis or treatment of SARS-CoV-2 infection.

	Monoclonal		**Polyclonal**
Example	Evusheld (AZD7442)	Xevudy (sotrovimab)	IgRT (IVIg or SCIg)
Company	AstraZeneca	VUR Biotechnology GlaxoSmithKline	Various
Pre or Post Exposure Prophylaxis	Pre	Post	N/A
Antibody Isotype	Hu IgG1κ	Hu IgG1κ	Various
SARS-CoV-2 Target	RBD	RBD	Broad range including NCP and RBD
Origin/Platform	Isolated from B cells of convalescent patients	Natural antibody from convalescent patient with SARS-CoV-2	Purified antibodies from plasma of >1000 donors/product batch
Half-life	~6 months	LS mutation of Fc increases half life	~28 days
Doses required	1 *	1	ongoing
Dosage	150 mg of tixagevimab + 150 mg cilgavimab	500 mg	Dependent on factors including weight and IgG trough levels
Frequency of redosing	Every 6 months	N/A	Every week to every month depending on IgG trough levels
Route of administration	IM	IV	IV or SC
Approved recipients Age COVID-19 exposure Clinical disease	 >12 years weighing at least 40 kg Not infected and no recent exposure Moderate to severe immunocompromised state	 >12 years weighing at least 40 kg COVID-19$^+$ PCR Moderate to severe immunocompromised state	Dependent on established clinical guidelines
Neutralization Omicron BA.1 BA.2	 344-fold decrease 9-fold decrease	 Unknown Unknown	 Unknown Unknown
Emergency Authorization US FDA Australian TGA	 12/21–1/23 11/21–1/22	 05/21–3/22 08/21–3/22	N/A
Emergency approval for use in	Australia, UK, and USA	Australia, UK, and EU	N/A
References	[159–161]	[55,160,162,163]	[164]

COVID-19, coronavirus 19; FDA, Food and Drugs Administration; Hu, human; IgRT, immunoglobulin replacement therapy; IM, intramuscular; IVIg, intravenous immunoglobulin; subcutaneous immunoglobulin, SCIg; N/A, not applicable; nucleoprotein, NCP; receptor-binding domain, RBD; severe acute respiratory coronavirus-2, SARS-CoV-2; TGA, therapeutic goods administration (* Dose increased to 300 mg each antibody in 12/22 due to emergence of Omicron BA.1 and BA.1.1 [165]).

4.1. Immunoglobulin Replacement Therapy (IgRT)

IgRT is the cornerstone of treatment for antibody-deficient individuals. For over 25 years, prophylactic administration, either intravenously (IVIg) or subcutaneously (SCIg), has been shown to be safe and tolerable, reducing the incidence and severity of infection [21,22,164]. IgRT is a polyclonal IgG product purified from pooled human plasma (>1000 donors) containing a broad range of antibody specificities directed against commonly encountered pathogens, either because of natural infection or vaccination in the general population (Table S5) [164]. However, when SARS-CoV-2 first emerged, there was a period of multiple months before IgRT products contained IgG against SARS-CoV-2. This gap in protection was problematic due to the reliance of antibody-deficient individuals on the protection this product provides against a variety of infections. It was believed that this gap in protection would compound the immune defects already predisposing immune-deficient individuals to severe COVID-19 disease.

However, even when SARS-CoV-2-specific antibodies from natural infection and, later, vaccination in plasma donors emerged in IgRT, it was unclear whether they would neutralize the virus in recipients. Moreover, early insights into the protective capacity and persistence of SARS-CoV-2-specific neutralizing antibodies (nAbs) in plasma from convalescent COVID-19 patients showed that these antibodies could protect from viral transmission and remained stable in plasma from 15 months post-infection while retaining their capacity to protect from infection [5,6,23]. This provided an avenue for treatment for at-risk individuals who contracted the virus, including those with IEIs, to both limit infection and protect from severe disease. This also provided promise that, when antibodies emerged in IgRT, they would provide some protection against SARS-CoV-2 [23,118,119]. Despite this, it was necessary to obtain data to prove the retention of antibody function after the IgRT manufacturing process.

We reviewed 21 papers (Table S4) documenting the occurrence of SARS-CoV-2-specific antibodies in products derived from plasma donations mainly from Europe and the USA. At the time of printing, information regarding SARS-CoV-2-specific antibody content in other countries, including Australia, was not available. Observational studies showed that products generated from pre-pandemic plasma contained antibodies which were cross-reactive to seasonal coronaviruses and SARS-CoV; however, none demonstrated the capacity to neutralize the SARS-CoV-2 virus [120–123,136]. A study by Farcet et al. first detected SARS-CoV-2-specific antibodies in products generated from USA-donated plasma in September 2020 [137], and Romero et al. documented the first positive pools from donations in Spain and the USA in July through September of the same year [138]. A later update by Farcet et al. showed that neutralization towards the ancestral WH1 strain plateaued in products between May 2021 and April 2022, with the drop in titers in European plasma being slower compared to the USA [139], likely due to changes in infections rates in these locations. Importantly, antibody titers in IgRT products steadily increased longitudinally with increasing incidence of SARS-CoV-2 infection, with 93% of IgRT lots containing SARS-CoV-2-specific antibodies by January 2021 [126,137]. A later study by Raphael et al. documented a twofold increase in SARS-CoV-2-spike-specific IgG antibodies in products between February and March 2021. Importantly, this paper associated products with high antibody titers with donations from countries with high rates of COVID-19 infection and products with low titers with countries with low infection rates [166]. Additionally, while the published studies clearly document the emergence of anti-spike SARS-CoV-2 IgG levels [119–127,137–139,167], in a few cases, nucleocapsid-specific IgG was also observed, resulting from natural infection of the donors prior to plasma donation [124,139,167]. This clearly demonstrates the association between geographical location, timing of plasma donations and natural infection, vaccination rates at the time of donation, and the subsequent emergence and levels of SARS-CoV-2 antibody in commercial IgRT.

Additionally, ongoing assessment of IgRT demonstrated that, while the recognition of ancestral WH1 remained high, cross-reactivity towards variants decreased incrementally with continued mutation of the RBD of SARS-CoV-2. Here, the cross-recognition levels of the Omicron variant were lowest [130,133,168], mirrored by a decreased neutralization capacity and reduced inhibition of ACE2 receptor binding [133,168]. This is in line with observations from healthy donor plasma post-vaccination [56–58].

Neutralization capacity of antibody in IgRT to the ancestral SARS-CoV-2 strain was assessed in 11 publications, although multiple assays (Table 1) were utilized, making definitive comparisons between the neutralizing capacity of products between studies difficult [118–120,123–126,132,136,137,139]. Despite the continuing emergence of SARS-CoV-2 variants, few of these studies assessed the presence or neutralization capacity of antibodies to these variants. In one study in April 2022, all lots derived from US plasma could neutralize Omicron B.1.1.529, albeit at a 12-fold lower level compared to the ancestral strain and a 22-fold lower level in donated plasma from Europe [139]. A second study showed 32-fold lower Omicron neutralization compared to the ancestral strain [126]. A third study demonstrated neutralization of Omicron BA.1, BA.4/5, BQ.1.1, and XBB, with these antibodies retaining neutralization capacity in the plasma of patients receiving these products [130]. Notably, the latter study is the only one to date that tested the product administered to each patient alongside their plasma both pre- and post-infusion. This enabled the dissection of whether detected antibodies were endogenously produced in response to vaccination or were due to antibodies contained in IgRT. Importantly, this tracks the IgRT products' capacity to retain its function within recipients and infers that these products play a role in limiting severe COVID-19 disease. Additionally, neutralization of ancestral and omicron variants was boosted after receipt of the product, further supporting the importance of this treatment for protection against SARS-CoV-2 infection. This, again, reflects the dynamics of the timing and levels of natural infection and vaccination in different geographical locations where plasma is donated. It also shows the decreased antibody recognition of variants, which has also been documented in studies examining antibodies induced by COVID-19 vaccination [57,58]. This observed reduction in RBD-specific antibody binding to the Omicron B.1.1.529 variant was also observed in serum from convalescent COVID-19 patients and COVID-19-vaccinated individuals [169]. These observations led to concerns regarding the ongoing efficacy of antibody-based therapies in the treatment of COVID-19.

The progressive loss of variant recognition and reduced neutralization potency is indicative of viral evasion from antibodies. These variables make it difficult to infer the level of protection IgRT confers towards breakthrough infection, much less the clinical dose that is efficacious in preventing severe disease. These facets will require further examination to provide valuable information to clinicians regarding clinical dosing with IgRT and the clinical need for other supportive treatments, including mAbs and antivirals, for the treatment of COVID-19.

4.2. *Prophylactic Monoclonal Antibody (mAb) Therapies to Prevent Severe COVID-19 in IEI*

Monoclonal antibodies were developed as a treatment option for immunocompromised individuals who were deemed highly susceptible to severe COVID-19, including individuals with IEIs and those who had received solid organ or hematopoietic stem cell transplants. Up to April 2022, a dozen mAbs targeting the RBD spike protein were rapidly developed and deployed for clinical use as a preventative against SARS-CoV-2 infection, or for treating those infected or recently exposed to SARS-CoV-2 to reduce the chance of severe disease, hospitalization, and death [170].

mAbs consisted of either single (e.g., sotrovimab or bebtelovimab) or combination therapies (e.g., Evusheld) aimed at reducing or limiting infection by preventing spike protein binding to the ACE2 receptor and targeting the virus for elimination either by direct neutralization, antibody-dependent-cellular phagocytosis, antibody-dependent T-cell-mediated cytotoxicity, or complement activation. While antibodies targeting other domains of the spike protein or other viral proteins are in development, here, we will review the literature surrounding the efficacy of sotrovimab and Evusheld (Table S5), the mAb modalities most prominently used as preventatives or therapeutics for SARS-CoV-2 in Australia, the UK, and the USA. We discuss their efficacy towards the ancestral WH-1 virus and VOC (Table S6), as well as future iterations currently in development to combat the ongoing emergence of VOC.

4.2.1. Sotrovimab

Sotrovimab (Xevudy, VUR Biotechnology GlaxoSmith Kline) is a single-dose mAb administered intravenously for the treatment of SARS-CoV-2, and was first authorized for emergency use by the FDA in May 2021 (Table 2) [171]. In people treated with sotrovimab, antibody titers of the drug have been proven to be high at three months post-infusion [172]. This mAb has proven efficacy to the ancestral WH-1 strain of SARS-CoV-2 and the strains preceding Omicron, as evidenced by reduced COVID-19 hospitalization rates in individuals receiving treatment [173,174]. Separately, modeling studies have shown that sotrovimab's efficacy could be predicted by the clinical stage of the disease at treatment, with treatment during early disease yielding better therapeutic efficacy [175]. However, the emergence of Omicron sublineages has been suggested to reduce mAb efficacy. Sotrovimab has been shown to maintain its efficacy in reducing the progression of breakthrough infection with Omicron BA.1 and BA.2, as evidenced by reduced hospitalization and/or death rates within 28–30 days of mAb administration [173,176–180]. Importantly, both subvariants showed a similar risk of hospital admission [179,181]. In contrast, a separate study showed no protective effect of sotrovimab against BA.2 [182]. Here, measurement of sotrovimab-treated individuals showed that neutralization of BA.1 was 4-fold lower than for BA.2, demonstrating a dramatic loss in spike protein recognition [181]. Furthermore, in murine models, sotrovimab administration to mice expressing the ACE2 receptor showed reduced lung infection with either Omicron BA.1 and BA.2. This illustrates that, despite reduced in vitro neutralization capacity, this mAb retained protective capacity against severe lung disease [183].

Continuous evolution of Omicron has been associated with ongoing immune evasion [5,6]. Here, the progressive loss of the neutralization efficacy of sotrovimab has been observed starting with the Omicron BA.1 lineage, with a full loss of efficacy predicted from BA.4.6 [183–189]. To date, Omicron BQ.1.1.10, BA.4.6.3, XBB.1.1, XBB.1.5, and CH.1.1 are the most antibody-evasive strains, with sotrovimab exhibiting reduced neutralization and binding to ACE2, resulting in increased viral transmissibility [190–192]. This demonstrated loss in efficacy resulted in a retraction of the authorization of sotrovimab use for the treatment of COVID-19 [193]. It is important to note that cell lines used for neutralization varied in their expression of ACE2, making the comparison of neutralization data between studies difficult (Figure 3, Table 2).

4.2.2. Evusheld

Evusheld (AZD7442) is a mAb combination of cilgavimab and tixagevimab, which both bind to non-overlapping epitopes on the SARS-CoV-2 RBD, causing direct neutralization of the virus [194]. These antibodies, initially isolated from previously infected individuals, were engineered to extend their half-life (Table 2). Phase I trials showed that intramuscular administration of 300 mg Evusheld resulted in 10-fold higher levels of neutralization 3 months post-administration, with levels remaining above those of convalescent serum at 9 months. Furthermore, antibodies were detectable in nasal mucosa, a SARS-CoV-2 infection site, which might help to limit infection [194]. Furthermore, non-human primate models of SARS-CoV-2 showed that infection was prevented by prophylactic administration of Evusheld, while accelerated viral clearance was achieved by therapeutic administration [194]. Therefore, while this mAb combination was the only approved pre-exposure prophylaxis for COVID-19 in some countries [172,189,195], other countries, including Europe and Japan, approved Evusheld solely as a treatment of COVID-19. This demonstrates regulators' dogmatic focus on not licensing COVID-19 mAbs for simultaneous prophylactic and treatment purposes [189].

Antibody levels in individuals receiving Evusheld were high 3 months post-administration, with breakthrough infections rare in recipients [172]. As of the Delta surge, increased serum antibody levels and efficient neutralization of the Delta variant were observed in all individuals receiving Evusheld [196]. In comparison, neutralization was decreased 344-fold in Omicron BA.1 and 9-fold in BA.2, with 13.8% of Evusheld recipients exhibiting breakthrough infections with these subvariants [196]. This was confirmed in vitro, where neutralization capacity was shown to be significantly reduced in Omicron BA.1, with a high rate of BA.1 breakthrough infections observed in kidney transplant recipients treated with Evusheld [195,197]. In comparison, Evusheld retained strong neutralization capacity against BA.2 in vitro for at least 8 weeks post-administration [172,195]. This shows the importance of ongoing testing of mAb therapeutics for emerging variants.

What was evident for Evusheld is that cilgavimab demonstrated better efficacy against both BA.1 and BA.2 than tixagevimab, accounting for Evusheld's retained efficacy [185,196]. The ongoing evolution of variants has resulted in a progressive loss of variant recognition by Evusheld, reducing its capacity to neutralize the SARS-CoV-2 virus and protect from infection. As of January 2023, the FDA has rescinded authorization for emergency use of Evusheld as a pre-exposure prophylaxis for COVID-19 in the US [198]. In response to the ongoing threat from variants, AstraZeneca has now registered and is recruiting for a Phase I/III study to test a new pre-exposure prophylaxis in the SUPERNOVA (Study Understanding Pre-Exposure pRophylaxis of NOVel Antibodies; NCT05648110) trial. It is noted that Phase I will investigate this therapy in healthy adults, with extension in to immunocompromised adults and adolescents in phase III [199,200].

Altogether, this highlights the importance of ongoing assessment of mAb recognition of emerging viral variants to determine neutralization capacity, as well as, thus, the efficacy of these therapeutics.

5. Discussion and Future Directions

The SARS-CoV-2 pandemic has shed light on the role that cellular and humoral immunity play in the control of SARS-CoV-2 infection and elicitation of robust vaccination responses. Importantly, it has shown that solely assessing antibody responses to natural infection and/or COVID-19 vaccination is insufficient for monitoring the efficacy and longevity of SARS-CoV-2-specific immunity, especially in people with IEIs [100], particularly as spike-specific antibody levels wane over time [5,6,23,57,58]. Additionally, IgRT and other antibody-based therapeutics confound the measurement of endogenous infection- or vaccination-induced antibodies. This highlights the urgent need for strategies to easily detect antigen-specific Bmem and Tmem responses, particularly as the assessment of antibody responses traditionally used to measure vaccine responses is confounded by IgRT administration. These facets of immunity work in concert to provide robust protection against infection, severe disease, and death. Thus, measurement of their quantity, quality and longevity is paramount for assessing vaccine efficacy and their potential to protect from severe disease in both healthy individuals and those with conditions impacting immune function [179,180].

At present, assays examining these compartments vary and are only available in the research setting, making it difficult to compare findings between individual studies. Translating these assays to the diagnostic setting requires the dedication of resources, including funding and further refinement and testing of methodology, to ensure they are robust, standardized, and high-throughput. The availability of these assays is particularly important for IEI, as the genetic and immunological complexity of these diseases make it difficult to draw clear conclusions for immune-deficient individuals collectively. As such, individualized assessment is urgently needed to uncover the depth of the defect, the role of the cellular response in the absence of humoral immunity, and the level of protection that may be afforded by each correlate of immune function, thus imparting information regarding the efficacy of COVID-19 vaccination. A prime example of this is in XLA, where T-cell responses play a more prominent role due to the absence of both antibodies and B cells. Comparatively, in disorders with both a T-cell and a B-cell defect (e.g., CVID) it is crucial for immunity to be generated by both compartments to account for defects in both arms of the immune system. Future studies should focus on more than one facet of the immune system in order to understand and correlate responses generated in different compartments and to provide a more holistic picture of each individual patient's response to vaccination. Additionally, analyses such as those from Ngyuen et al. bring attention to the importance of population-level factors such as social determinants of health in determining patient outcome and disease risk. Future investigations should consider adding these key factors into the assessment of the IEI population's response to COVID-19 infection and vaccination in order to provide a more wholistic understanding of what drives disease and protection in these populations.

There is currently a paucity of information regarding the number, function, and phenotype of Bmem and Tmem generated in response to COVID-19 vaccination in people with IEIs, as well as the capacity of these cells to bind and neutralize SARS-CoV-2 variants. This is important in the ever-evolving landscape of viral mutation, where even in healthy individuals, antibodies and Bmem cells exhibit reduced recognition of variants. In the context of IEI, reduced efficacy could render these populations more susceptible to severe disease and possibly death.

Finally, to date, assessments of vaccine responses in IEI patients have only been published for up to 3–4 doses of COVID-19 vaccines [76,82,87,90,94,96,131]. While this has provided critical information on early post-vaccination immune responses, immune-deficient individuals are recommended to receive boosters every 3–6 months. Thus, at present, some IEI patients have received six or more doses of the vaccine compared to 4–5 in the general population. Therefore, information regarding the efficacy of these later doses, especially those with the bivalent formulations, and protein-based vaccines (e.g., NovaVax) is required in order to determine whether certain vaccine platforms elicit a superior immune response and whether individuals with humoral deficiencies may benefit from a formulation such as NovaVax that specifically induces a T-cell response. This information is urgently needed to ascertain the benefit of continued vaccination and novel formulations in IEI populations. Together, this knowledge will inform future COVID-19 vaccine recommendations for people with IEI, and more widely, other immunodeficient populations. Additionally, these insights might also have implications for the regimens for other currently administered vaccines (e.g., influenza) and for pathogenic threats that may emerge in the future.

In summation, there is much that is left to understand about COVID-19 vaccinations in people with IEIs. These complex issues require intensive research to provide robust recommendations concerning timing between doses, vaccine formulations for individual disorders, and whether vaccines provide sufficient protection to allay the anxiety brought by increased transmission of SARS-CoV-2. In addition, it is important to generate continued evidence of the capacity of IgRT and mAb treatments to bind and neutralize emerging variants to inform the clinical care of people with IEIs as both prophylactic and treatment options for COVID-19. This ongoing pandemic is known to affect those with IEIs physically, mentally, and socioeconomically. We hope the information in this review and that of ongoing and future studies will benefit individuals with IEI, ultimately improving their quality-of-life post-pandemic.

Final Thoughts

This review shows that COVID-19 vaccine responses in people with IEIs are highly variable after a primary vaccine regimen of three doses (compared to two in the general population). Whilst there is limited information on the responses of people with IEIs to booster doses of the vaccine, it is clear that this variability still exists. Furthermore, there is limited research on the capacity of cross-recognition of SARS-CoV-2 variants by immune cells in people with IEIs. Despite this, we can infer from information in the general population that repeated vaccination is required to boost immunity to Omicron variants [56], which is presumed to enable ongoing protection from severe disease.

However, in order to make specific recommendations for this population, further research is needed to accurately determine whether these same patterns are observed in people with IEIs, as well as to standardize the methodology for measuring antigen-specific immunity in peripheral blood. Research in three main areas is required. These are: 1. IEI patient responses to three or more doses of COVID-19 vaccine to provide evidence of protective immunity and to ascertain the requirement for continued administration of booster vaccine doses and their frequency. 2. The capacity of antibodies in IgRT products to recognize and neutralize circulating Omicron variants; this will demonstrate that these products provide some protection against severe disease in people with IEIs. 3. Further information on the severity and duration of COVID-19 disease upon infection and incidence of long COVID in IEI people to ascertain the vulnerability of this population to circulating Omicron variants, the efficacy of methods to limit disease, and the ongoing measures required to protect this population.

Once more of this information is available, then these data will prove crucial in drafting guidelines for vaccination of this population, not only for COVID-19, but also for other viral pathogens.

Supplementary Materials: The following supporting information can be downloaded at: https://www.mdpi.com/article/10.3390/vaccines12060675/s1, Table S1: Current and previous SARS-CoV-2 variants and their characteristics; Table S2: Antibody responses; Table S3: Memory T-cell responses, Table S4: Bmem and Innate responses; Table S5: IgRT; Table S6: Therapeutic mAbs. References [39,201–227] are cited in the Supplementary Materials.

Author Contributions: Conceptualization E.S.J.E. and E.E.R.; writing—original draft, E.E.R., E.C.-R., and E.S.J.E.; writing—review and editing, all authors. All authors have read and agreed to the published version of the manuscript.

Funding: This work was funded in part by the Division of Intramural Research, National Institute of Allergy and Infectious Diseases, National Institutes of Health, USA (E.E.R, E.C.-R.), an Allergy and Immunology Foundation of Australasia (AIFA) Primary Immunodeficiency Clinical Research Grant (supported by CSL Behring (Australia), E.S.J.E), an Australasian Government Medical Research Future Fund (MRFF, Project no. 2016108, M.C.v.Z), and the Jeffrey Modell Foundation (M.C.v.Z).

Acknowledgments: The authors would like to acknowledge the ongoing support and mentorship of Robyn E. O'Hehir, Luigi D. Notarangelo, Michail S. Lionakis, and Steven M. Holland.

Conflicts of Interest: The authors declare no conflicts of interest. Neither the authors nor their family members have financial interest in any commercial product, service, or organization providing financial support for this research. The opinions and assertions expressed herein are those of the author(s) and do not reflect the official policy or position of the Uniformed Services University of the Health Sciences, the National Institutes of Health, the US Department of Health and Human Services, or the US Department of Defense. References to non-Federal entities or products do not constitute or imply a Department of Defense or Uniformed Services University of the Health Sciences endorsement. This work was prepared by a military or civilian employee of the US Government as part of the individual's official duties and therefore is in the public domain and does not possess copyright protection (public domain information may be freely distributed and copied; however, as a courtesy it is requested that the Uniformed Services University and the author be given an appropriate acknowledgement).

References

1. World Health Organization. *WHO Coronavirus (COVID-19) Dashboard*; World Health Organization: Geneva, Switzerland, 2023.
2. COVID-19 Data Explorer—Our World in Data. Available online: https://ourworldindata.org/explorers/coronavirus-data-explorer?zoomToSelection=true&time=2020-03-01..latest&facet=none&pickerSort=asc&pickerMetric=location&Metric=Case+fatality+rate&Interval=7-day+rolling+average&Relative+to+Population=true&Color+by+test+positivity=false&country=JPN~USA~GBR~ITA~DEU~FRA~CAN (accessed on 5 January 2023).
3. Tangye, S.G. COVID Human Genetic Effort consortium Impact of SARS-CoV-2 infection and COVID-19 on patients with inborn errors of immunity. *J. Allergy Clin. Immunol.* **2023**, *151*, 818–831. [CrossRef] [PubMed]
4. Chiu, S.S.; Hung Chan, K.; Wing Chu, K.; Kwan, S.W.; Guan, Y.; Man Poon, L.L.; Peiris, J.S.M. Human Coronavirus NL63 Infection and Other Coronavirus Infections in Children Hospitalized with Acute Respiratory Disease in Hong Kong, China. *Clin. Infect. Dis.* **2005**, *40*, 1721–1729. [CrossRef] [PubMed]
5. Hartley, G.E.; Edwards, E.S.J.; O'Hehir, R.E.; van Zelm, M.C. New insights into human immune memory from SARS-CoV-2 infection and vaccination. *Allergy* **2022**, *77*, 3553–3566. [CrossRef] [PubMed]
6. Fryer, H.A.; Hartley, G.E.; Edwards, E.S.J.; O'Hehir, R.E.; van Zelm, M.C. Humoral immunity and B-cell memory in response to SARS-CoV-2 infection and vaccination. *Biochem. Soc. Trans.* **2022**, *50*, 1643–1658. [CrossRef] [PubMed]
7. Yi, C.; Sun, X.; Ye, J.; Ding, L.; Liu, M.; Yang, Z.; Lu, X.; Zhang, Y.; Ma, L.; Gu, W.; et al. Key residues of the receptor binding motif in the spike protein of SARS-CoV-2 that interact with ACE2 and neutralizing antibodies. *Cell. Mol. Immunol.* **2020**, *17*, 621–630. [CrossRef] [PubMed]

8. Jiang, S.; Hillyer, C.; Du, L. Neutralizing Antibodies against SARS-CoV-2 and Other Human Coronaviruses. *Trends Immunol.* **2020**, *41*, 355–359. [CrossRef] [PubMed]
9. Folegatti, P.M.; Ewer, K.J.; Aley, P.K.; Angus, B.; Becker, S.; Belij-Rammerstorfer, S.; Bellamy, D.; Bibi, S.; Bittaye, M.; Clutterbuck, E.A.; et al. Safety and immunogenicity of the ChAdOx1 nCoV-19 vaccine against SARS-CoV-2: A preliminary report of a phase 1/2, single-blind, randomised controlled trial. *Lancet* **2020**, *396*, 467–478. [CrossRef]
10. Polack, F.P.; Thomas, S.J.; Kitchin, N.; Absalon, J.; Gurtman, A.; Lockhart, S.; Perez, J.L.; Pérez Marc, G.; Moreira, E.D.; Zerbini, C.; et al. Safety and Efficacy of the BNT162b2 mRNA Covid-19 Vaccine. *N. Engl. J. Med.* **2020**, *383*, 2603–2615. [CrossRef]
11. Meyts, I.; Bousfiha, A.; Duff, C.; Singh, S.; Lau, Y.L.; Condino-Neto, A.; Bezrodnik, L.; Ali, A.; Adeli, M.; Drabwell, J. Primary Immunodeficiencies: A Decade of Progress and a Promising Future. *Front. Immunol.* **2021**, *11*, 625753. [CrossRef]
12. Szepanowski, F.; Warnke, C.; Meyer Zu Hörste, G.; Mausberg, A.K.; Hartung, H.-P.; Kleinschnitz, C.; Stettner, M. Secondary Immunodeficiency and Risk of Infection Following Immune Therapies in Neurology. *CNS Drugs* **2021**, *35*, 1173–1188. [CrossRef]
13. Pulvirenti, F.; Cinetto, F.; Milito, C.; Bonanni, L.; Pesce, A.M.; Leodori, G.; Garzi, G.; Miglionico, M.; Tabolli, S.; Quinti, I. Health-Related Quality of Life in Common Variable Immunodeficiency Italian Patients Switched to Remote Assistance During the COVID-19 Pandemic. *J. Allergy Clin. Immunol. Pract.* **2020**, *8*, 1894–1899.e2. [CrossRef]
14. Sowers, K.L.; Galantino, M.L. Living with primary immunodeficiency disease during the Covid-19 pandemic. *J. Public Health* **2022**, *30*, 2753–2760. [CrossRef]
15. About Coronavirus (COVID-19). Available online: https://www.health.gov.au/topics/covid-19/about (accessed on 2 January 2024).
16. Tangye, S.G.; Al-Herz, W.; Bousfiha, A.; Cunningham-Rundles, C.; Franco, J.L.; Holland, S.M.; Klein, C.; Morio, T.; Oksenhendler, E.; Picard, C.; et al. Human Inborn Errors of Immunity: 2022 Update on the Classification from the International Union of Immunological Societies Expert Committee. *J. Clin. Immunol.* **2022**, *42*, 1473–1507. [CrossRef]
17. Edwards, E.S.J.; Bosco, J.J.; Ojaimi, S.; O'Hehir, R.E.; van Zelm, M.C. Beyond monogenetic rare variants: Tackling the low rate of genetic diagnoses in predominantly antibody deficiency. *Cell. Mol. Immunol.* **2021**, *18*, 588–603. [CrossRef]
18. Quinn, J.; Modell, V.; Orange, J.S.; Modell, F. Growth in diagnosis and treatment of primary immunodeficiency within the global Jeffrey Modell Centers Network. *Allergy Asthma Clin. Immunol.* **2022**, *18*, 19. [CrossRef] [PubMed]
19. Hartley, G.E.; Edwards, E.S.J.; Bosco, J.J.; Ojaimi, S.; Stirling, R.G.; Cameron, P.U.; Flanagan, K.; Plebanski, M.; Hogarth, P.M.; O'Hehir, R.E.; et al. Influenza-specific IgG1$^+$ memory B-cell numbers increase upon booster vaccination in healthy adults but not in patients with predominantly antibody deficiency. *Clin. Transl. Immunol.* **2020**, *9*, e1199. [CrossRef] [PubMed]
20. Edwards, E.S.J.; Bosco, J.J.; Aui, P.M.; Stirling, R.G.; Cameron, P.U.; Chatelier, J.; Hore-Lacy, F.; O'Hehir, R.E.; van Zelm, M.C. Predominantly Antibody-Deficient Patients With Non-infectious Complications Have Reduced Naive B, Treg, Th17, and Tfh17 Cells. *Front. Immunol.* **2019**, *10*, 2593. [CrossRef]
21. Durandy, A.; Kracker, S.; Fischer, A. Primary antibody deficiencies. *Nat. Rev. Immunol.* **2013**, *13*, 519–533. [CrossRef] [PubMed]
22. Lucas, M.; Lee, M.; Lortan, J.; Lopez-Granados, E.; Misbah, S.; Chapel, H. Infection outcomes in patients with common variable immunodeficiency disorders: Relationship to immunoglobulin therapy over 22 years. *J. Allergy Clin. Immunol.* **2010**, *125*, 1354–1360.e4. [CrossRef]
23. Hartley, G.E.; Edwards, E.S.J.; Aui, P.M.; Varese, N.; Stojanovic, S.; McMahon, J.; Peleg, A.Y.; Boo, I.; Drummer, H.E.; Hogarth, P.M.; et al. Rapid generation of durable B cell memory to SARS-CoV-2 spike and nucleocapsid proteins in COVID-19 and convalescence. *Sci. Immunol.* **2020**, *5*, eabf8891. [CrossRef]
24. Giardino, G.; Milito, C.; Lougaris, V.; Punziano, A.; Carrabba, M.; Cinetto, F.; Scarpa, R.; Dellepiane, R.M.; Ricci, S.; Rivalta, B.; et al. The Impact of SARS-CoV-2 Infection in Patients with Inborn Errors of Immunity: The Experience of the Italian Primary Immunodeficiencies Network (IPINet). *J. Clin. Immunol.* **2022**, *42*, 935–946. [CrossRef]
25. Puel, A.; Bastard, P.; Bustamante, J.; Casanova, J.-L. Human autoantibodies underlying infectious diseases. *J. Exp. Med.* **2022**, *219*, e20211387. [CrossRef]
26. Asano, T.; Boisson, B.; Onodi, F.; Matuozzo, D.; Moncada-Velez, M.; Maglorius Renkilaraj, M.R.L.; Zhang, P.; Meertens, L.; Bolze, A.; Materna, M.; et al. X-linked recessive TLR7 deficiency in ~1% of men under 60 years old with life-threatening COVID-19. *Sci. Immunol.* **2021**, *6*, eabl4348. [CrossRef] [PubMed]
27. Mantovani, S.; Daga, S.; Fallerini, C.; Baldassarri, M.; Benetti, E.; Picchiotti, N.; Fava, F.; Gallì, A.; Zibellini, S.; Bruttini, M.; et al. Rare variants in Toll-like receptor 7 results in functional impairment and downregulation of cytokine-mediated signaling in COVID-19 patients. *Genes Immun.* **2022**, *23*, 51–56. [CrossRef] [PubMed]
28. Fallerini, C.; Daga, S.; Mantovani, S.; Benetti, E.; Picchiotti, N.; Francisci, D.; Paciosi, F.; Schiaroli, E.; Baldassarri, M.; Fava, F.; et al. Association of Toll-like receptor 7 variants with life-threatening COVID-19 disease in males: Findings from a nested case-control study. *eLife* **2021**, *10*, e67569. [CrossRef] [PubMed]
29. Solanich, X.; Vargas-Parra, G.; Van Der Made, C.I.; Simons, A.; Schuurs-Hoeijmakers, J.; Antolí, A.; Del Valle, J.; Rocamora-Blanch, G.; Setién, F.; Esteller, M.; et al. Genetic Screening for TLR7 Variants in Young and Previously Healthy Men With Severe COVID-19. *Front. Immunol.* **2021**, *12*, 719115. [CrossRef] [PubMed]
30. Van Der Made, C.I.; Simons, A.; Schuurs-Hoeijmakers, J.; Van Den Heuvel, G.; Mantere, T.; Kersten, S.; Van Deuren, R.C.; Steehouwer, M.; Van Reijmersdal, S.V.; Jaeger, M.; et al. Presence of Genetic Variants Among Young Men With Severe COVID-19. *JAMA* **2020**, *324*, 663–673. [CrossRef] [PubMed]

31. Zhang, Q.; Bastard, P.; Liu, Z.; Le Pen, J.; Moncada-Velez, M.; Chen, J.; Ogishi, M.; Sabli, I.K.D.; Hodeib, S.; Korol, C.; et al. Inborn errors of type I IFN immunity in patients with life-threatening COVID-19. *Science* **2020**, *370*, eabd4570. [CrossRef] [PubMed]
32. Abolhassani, H.; Landegren, N.; Bastard, P.; Materna, M.; Modaresi, M.; Du, L.; Aranda Guillén, M.; Sardh, F.; Zuo, F.; Zhang, P.; et al. Inherited IFNAR1 Deficiency in a Child with Both Critical COVID-19 Pneumonia and Multisystem Inflammatory Syndrome. *J. Clin. Immunol.* **2022**, *42*, 471–483. [CrossRef] [PubMed]
33. Khanmohammadi, S.; Rezaei, N.; Khazaei, M.; Shirkani, A. A Case of Autosomal Recessive Interferon Alpha/Beta Receptor Alpha Chain (IFNAR1) Deficiency with Severe COVID-19. *J. Clin. Immunol.* **2022**, *42*, 19–24. [CrossRef]
34. Schmidt, A.; Peters, S.; Knaus, A.; Sabir, H.; Hamsen, F.; Maj, C.; Fazaal, J.; Sivalingam, S.; Savchenko, O.; Mantri, A.; et al. TBK1 and TNFRSF13B mutations and an autoinflammatory disease in a child with lethal COVID-19. *npj Genomic Med.* **2021**, *6*, 55. [CrossRef]
35. Duncan, C.J.A.; Skouboe, M.K.; Howarth, S.; Hollensen, A.K.; Chen, R.; Børresen, M.L.; Thompson, B.J.; Stremenova Spegarova, J.; Hatton, C.F.; Stæger, F.F.; et al. Life-threatening viral disease in a novel form of autosomal recessive *IFNAR2* deficiency in the Arctic. *J. Exp. Med.* **2022**, *219*, e20212427. [CrossRef] [PubMed]
36. Platanias, L.C. Mechanisms of type-I- and type-II-interferon-mediated signalling. *Nat. Rev. Immunol.* **2005**, *5*, 375–386. [CrossRef] [PubMed]
37. Zhang, Q.; Matuozzo, D.; Le Pen, J.; Lee, D.; Moens, L.; Asano, T.; Bohlen, J.; Liu, Z.; Moncada-Velez, M.; Kendir-Demirkol, Y.; et al. Recessive inborn errors of type I IFN immunity in children with COVID-19 pneumonia. *J. Exp. Med.* **2022**, *219*, e20220131. [CrossRef] [PubMed]
38. Nguyen, A.A.; Habiballah, S.B.; LaBere, B.; Day-Lewis, M.; Elkins, M.; Al-Musa, A.; Chu, A.; Jones, J.; Fried, A.J.; McDonald, D.; et al. Rethinking Immunological Risk: A Retrospective Cohort Study of Severe SARS-Cov-2 Infections in Individuals With Congenital Immunodeficiencies. *J. Allergy Clin. Immunol. Pract.* **2023**, *11*, 3391–3399.e3. [CrossRef] [PubMed]
39. World Health Organization Tracking SARS-CoV-2 Variants. Available online: https://www.who.int/activities/tracking-SARS-CoV-2-variants (accessed on 24 January 2023).
40. Parra-Lucares, A.; Segura, P.; Rojas, V.; Pumarino, C.; Saint-Pierre, G.; Toro, L. Emergence of SARS-CoV-2 Variants in the World: How Could This Happen? *Life* **2022**, *12*, 194. [CrossRef] [PubMed]
41. Van Egeren, D.; Novokhodko, A.; Stoddard, M.; Tran, U.; Zetter, B.; Rogers, M.S.; Joseph-McCarthy, D.; Chakravarty, A. Controlling long-term SARS-CoV-2 infections can slow viral evolution and reduce the risk of treatment failure. *Sci. Rep.* **2021**, *11*, 22630. [CrossRef] [PubMed]
42. Wilkinson, S.A.J.; Richter, A.; Casey, A.; Osman, H.; Mirza, J.D.; Stockton, J.; Quick, J.; Ratcliffe, L.; Sparks, N.; Cumley, N.; et al. Recurrent SARS-CoV-2 mutations in immunodeficient patients. *Virus Evol.* **2022**, *8*, veac050. [CrossRef] [PubMed]
43. Halfmann, P.J.; Minor, N.R.; Haddock, L.A.; Maddox, R.; Moreno, G.K.; Braun, K.M.; Baker, D.A.; Riemersa, K.K.; Prasad, A.; Alman, K.J.; et al. Evolution of a globally unique SARS-CoV-2 Spike E484T monoclonal antibody escape mutation in a persistently infected, immunocompromised individual. *Virus Evol.* **2023**, *9*, veac104. [CrossRef] [PubMed]
44. Scherer, E.M.; Babiker, A.; Adelman, M.W.; Allman, B.; Key, A.; Kleinhenz, J.M.; Langsjoen, R.M.; Nguyen, P.-V.; Onyechi, I.; Sherman, J.D.; et al. SARS-CoV-2 Evolution and Immune Escape in Immunocompromised Patients. *N. Engl. J. Med.* **2022**, *386*, 2436–2438. [CrossRef]
45. McCallum, M.; Czudnochowski, N.; Rosen, L.E.; Zepeda, S.K.; Bowen, J.E.; Walls, A.C.; Hauser, K.; Joshi, A.; Stewart, C.; Dillen, J.R.; et al. Structural basis of SARS-CoV-2 Omicron immune evasion and receptor engagement. *Science* **2022**, *375*, 864–868. [CrossRef]
46. Enhancing Response to Omicron SARS-CoV-2 Variant. Available online: https://www.who.int/publications/m/item/enhancing-readiness-for-omicron-(b.1.1.529)-technical-brief-and-priority-actions-for-member-states (accessed on 3 July 2023).
47. Panja, A.; Roy, J.; Mazumder, A.; Choudhury, S.M. Divergent mutations of Delta and Omicron variants: Key players behind differential viral attributes across the COVID-19 waves. *Virus Dis.* **2023**, *34*, 307–320. [CrossRef] [PubMed]
48. Ao, D.; He, X.; Hong, W.; Wei, X. The rapid rise of SARS-CoV-2 Omicron subvariants with immune evasion properties: XBB.1.5 and BQ.1.1 subvariants. *MedComm* **2023**, *4*, e239. [CrossRef] [PubMed]
49. Food and Drug Administration. FDA Takes Key Action in Fight against COVID-19 by Issuing Emergency Use Authorization for First COVID-19 Vaccine. Available online: https://www.fda.gov/news-events/press-announcements/fda-takes-key-action-fight-against-covid-19-issuing-emergency-use-authorization-first-covid-19 (accessed on 31 January 2024).
50. CoVariants: Per Country. Available online: https://covariants.org/per-country (accessed on 10 July 2023).
51. Coronavirus Disease (COVID-19) Situation Reports. Available online: https://www.who.int/emergencies/diseases/novel-coronavirus-2019/situation-reports (accessed on 10 July 2023).
52. Food and Drug Administration. FDA Approves First COVID-19 Vaccine. Available online: https://www.fda.gov/news-events/press-announcements/fda-approves-first-covid-19-vaccine (accessed on 31 January 2024).
53. McIntyre, P.B.; Aggarwal, R.; Jani, I.; Jawad, J.; Kochhar, S.; MacDonald, N.; Madhi, S.A.; Mohsni, E.; Mulholland, K.; Neuzil, K.M.; et al. COVID-19 vaccine strategies must focus on severe disease and global equity. *Lancet* **2022**, *399*, 406–410. [CrossRef]

54. Chirico, F.; Teixeira Da Silva, J.; Tsigaris, P.; Sharun, K. Safety & effectiveness of COVID-19 vaccines: A narrative review. *Indian J. Med. Res.* **2022**, *155*, 91–104. [CrossRef] [PubMed]
55. Food and Drug Administration. Coronavirus (COVID-19) Update: FDA Limits Use of Janssen COVID-19 Vaccine to Certain Individuals. Available online: https://www.fda.gov/vaccines-blood-biologics/coronavirus-covid-19-cber-regulated-biologics/janssen-covid-19-vaccine (accessed on 15 February 2023).
56. Hartley, G.E.; Fryer, H.A.; Gill, P.A.; Boo, I.; Bornheimer, S.J.; Hogarth, P.M.; Drummer, H.E.; O'Hehir, R.E.; Edwards, E.S.J.; Van Zelm, M.C. Third dose COVID-19 mRNA vaccine enhances IgG4 isotype switching and recognition of Omicron subvariants by memory B cells after mRNA but not adenovirus priming. *bioRxiv* **2023**. [CrossRef]
57. Hartley, G.E.; Edwards, E.S.J.; Varese, N.; Boo, I.; Aui, P.M.; Bornheimer, S.J.; Hogarth, P.M.; Drummer, H.E.; O'Hehir, R.E.; van Zelm, M.C. The second COVID-19 mRNA vaccine dose enhances the capacity of Spike-specific memory B cells to bind Omicron BA.2. *Allergy* **2022**, *78*, 855–858. [CrossRef]
58. Fryer, H.A.; Hartley, G.E.; Edwards, E.S.J.; Varese, N.; Boo, I.; Bornheimer, S.J.; Hogarth, P.M.; Drummer, H.E.; O'Hehir, R.E.; Van Zelm, M.C. COVID-19 Adenoviral Vector Vaccination Elicits a Robust Memory B Cell Response with the Capacity to Recognize Omicron BA.2 and BA.5 Variants. *J. Clin. Immunol.* **2023**, *43*, 1506–1518. [CrossRef]
59. Ikegame, S.; Siddiquey, M.N.A.; Hung, C.-T.; Haas, G.; Brambilla, L.; Oguntuyo, K.Y.; Kowdle, S.; Chiu, H.-P.; Stevens, C.S.; Vilardo, A.E.; et al. Neutralizing activity of Sputnik V vaccine sera against SARS-CoV-2 variants. *Nat. Commun.* **2021**, *12*, 4598. [CrossRef]
60. Khoury, D.S.; Cromer, D.; Reynaldi, A.; Schlub, T.E.; Wheatley, A.K.; Juno, J.A.; Subbarao, K.; Kent, S.J.; Triccas, J.A.; Davenport, M.P. Neutralizing antibody levels are highly predictive of immune protection from symptomatic SARS-CoV-2 infection. *Nat. Med.* **2021**, *27*, 1205–1211. [CrossRef]
61. Marta, R.A.; Nakamura, G.E.K.; De Matos Aquino, B.; Bignardi, P.R. COVID-19 vaccines: Update of the vaccines in use and under development. *Vacunas* **2022**, *23*, S88–S102. [CrossRef]
62. Comirnaty® COVID-19 Vaccines (COVID-19 Vaccines) | Pfizer Medical Information—Australia. Available online: https://www.pfizermedicalinformation.com.au/en-au/pfizer-biontech-covid-19-vaccine (accessed on 3 July 2023).
63. Statement on the Antigen Composition of COVID-19 Vaccines. Available online: https://www.who.int/news/item/13-12-2023-statement-on-the-antigen-composition-of-covid-19-vaccines (accessed on 31 January 2024).
64. Department of Health and Aged Care of Australia Government. ATAGI Recommendations on Use of the Moderna and Pfizer Monovalent Omicron XBB.1.5 COVID-19 Vaccines. Available online: https://www.health.gov.au/news/atagi-recommendations-on-use-of-the-moderna-and-pfizer-monovalent-omicron-xbb15-covid-19-vaccines (accessed on 31 January 2024).
65. Edwards, E.; Quinn, K. Why Is a Third COVID-19 Vaccine Dose Important for People Who Are Immunocompromised? Available online: https://theconversation.com/why-is-a-third-covid-19-vaccine-dose-important-for-people-who-are-immunocompromised-166569 (accessed on 3 July 2023).
66. Gernez, Y.; Murugesan, K.; Cortales, C.R.; Banaei, N.; Hoyte, L.; Pinsky, B.A.; Lewis, D.B.; Pham, M.N. Immunogenicity of a third COVID-19 messenger RNA vaccine dose in primary immunodeficiency disorder patients with functional B-cell defects. *J. Allergy Clin. Immunol. Pract.* **2022**, *10*, 1385–1388.e2. [CrossRef]
67. Department of Health and Aged Care of Australia Government. ATAGI Recommendations on the Use of a Third Primary Dose of COVID-19 Vaccine in Individuals Who Are Severely Immunocompromised. Available online: https://www.health.gov.au/resources/publications/atagi-recommendations-on-the-use-of-a-third-primary-dose-of-covid-19-vaccine-in-individuals-who-are-severely-immunocompromised?language=en (accessed on 3 July 2023).
68. Food and Drug Administration. Coronavirus (COVID-19) Update: FDA Authorizes Additional Vaccine Dose for Certain Immunocompromised Individuals. Available online: https://www.fda.gov/news-events/press-announcements/coronavirus-covid-19-update-fda-authorizes-additional-vaccine-dose-certain-immunocompromised (accessed on 4 July 2023).
69. Joint Committee on Vaccination and Immunisation (JCVI) Advice on Third Primary Dose Vaccination. Available online: https://www.gov.uk/government/publications/third-primary-covid-19-vaccine-dose-for-people-who-are-immunosuppressed-jcvi-advice/joint-committee-on-vaccination-and-immunisation-jcvi-advice-on-third-primary-dose-vaccination (accessed on 3 July 2023).
70. Mohammed, I.; Nauman, A.; Paul, P.; Ganesan, S.; Chen, K.-H.; Jalil, S.M.S.; Jaouni, S.H.; Kawas, H.; Khan, W.A.; Vattoth, A.L.; et al. The efficacy and effectiveness of the COVID-19 vaccines in reducing infection, severity, hospitalization, and mortality: A systematic review. *Hum. Vaccines Immunother.* **2022**, *18*, 2027160. [CrossRef]
71. DeSantis, S.M.; Yaseen, A.; Hao, T.; León-Novelo, L.; Talebi, Y.; Valerio-Shewmaker, M.A.; Pinzon Gomez, C.L.; Messiah, S.E.; Kohl, H.W.; Kelder, S.H.; et al. Incidence and Predictors of Breakthrough and Severe Breakthrough Infections of SARS-CoV-2 After Primary Series Vaccination in Adults: A Population-Based Survey of 22 575 Participants. *J. Infect. Dis.* **2023**, *227*, 1164–1172. [CrossRef]
72. Arroyo-Sánchez, D.; Cabrera-Marante, O.; Laguna-Goya, R.; Almendro-Vázquez, P.; Carretero, O.; Gil-Etayo, F.J.; Suàrez-Fernández, P.; Pérez-Romero, P.; Rodríguez de Frías, E.; Serrano, A.; et al. Immunogenicity of Anti-SARS-CoV-2 Vaccines in Common Variable Immunodeficiency. *J. Clin. Immunol.* **2022**, *42*, 240–252. [CrossRef] [PubMed]

73. Hagin, D.; Freund, T.; Navon, M.; Halperin, T.; Adir, D.; Marom, R.; Levi, I.; Benor, S.; Alcalay, Y.; Freund, N.T. Immunogenicity of Pfizer-BioNTech COVID-19 vaccine in patients with inborn errors of immunity. *J. Allergy Clin. Immunol.* **2021**, *148*, 739–749. [CrossRef]
74. van Leeuwen, L.P.M.; GeurtsvanKessel, C.H.; Ellerbroek, P.M.; de Bree, G.J.; Potjewijd, J.; Rutgers, A.; Jolink, H.; van de Veerdonk, F.; van Gorp, E.C.M.; de Wilt, F.; et al. Immunogenicity of the mRNA-1273 COVID-19 vaccine in adult patients with inborn errors of immunity. *J. Allergy Clin. Immunol.* **2022**, *149*, 1949–1957. [CrossRef] [PubMed]
75. Fernandez Salinas, A.; Piano Mortari, E.; Terreri, S.; Milito, C.; Zaffina, S.; Perno, C.F.; Locatelli, F.; Quinti, I.; Carsetti, R. Impaired memory B-cell response to the Pfizer-BioNTech COVID-19 vaccine in patients with common variable immunodeficiency. *J. Allergy Clin. Immunol.* **2022**, *149*, 76–77. [CrossRef] [PubMed]
76. Shields, A.M.; Faustini, S.E.; Hill, H.J.; Al-Taei, S.; Tanner, C.; Ashford, F.; Workman, S.; Moreira, F.; Verma, N.; Wagg, H.; et al. Increased Seroprevalence and Improved Antibody Responses Following Third Primary SARS-CoV-2 Immunisation: An Update From the COV-AD Study. *Front. Immunol.* **2022**, *13*, 912571. [CrossRef]
77. Zendt, M.; Bustos Carrillo, F.A.; Kelly, S.; Saturday, T.; DeGrange, M.; Ginigeme, A.; Wu, L.; Callier, V.; Ortega-Villa, A.; Faust, M.; et al. Characterization of the antispike IgG immune response to COVID-19 vaccines in people with a wide variety of immunodeficiencies. *Sci. Adv.* **2023**, *9*, eadh3150. [CrossRef]
78. Hlongwa, L.; Peter, J.; Mayne, E. Value of diagnostic vaccination in diagnosis of humoral inborn errors of immunity. *Hum. Immunol.* **2023**, *84*, 337–341. [CrossRef]
79. Bergman, P.; Wullimann, D.; Gao, Y.; Wahren Borgström, E.; Norlin, A.-C.; Lind Enoksson, S.; Aleman, S.; Ljunggren, H.-G.; Buggert, M.; Smith, C.I.E. Elevated CD21low B Cell Frequency Is a Marker of Poor Immunity to Pfizer-BioNTech BNT162b2 mRNA Vaccine Against SARS-CoV-2 in Patients with Common Variable Immunodeficiency. *J. Clin. Immunol.* **2022**, *42*, 716–727. [CrossRef] [PubMed]
80. Amodio, D.; Ruggiero, A.; Sgrulletti, M.; Pighi, C.; Cotugno, N.; Medri, C.; Morrocchi, E.; Colagrossi, L.; Russo, C.; Zaffina, S.; et al. Humoral and Cellular Response Following Vaccination With the BNT162b2 mRNA COVID-19 Vaccine in Patients Affected by Primary Immunodeficiencies. *Front. Immunol.* **2021**, *12*, 727850. [CrossRef]
81. Bitzenhofer, M.; Suter-Riniker, F.; Moor, M.B.; Sidler, D.; Horn, M.P.; Gschwend, A.; Staehelin, C.; Rauch, A.; Helbling, A.; Jörg, L. Humoral response to mRNA vaccines against SARS-CoV-2 in patients with humoral immunodeficiency disease. *PLoS ONE* **2022**, *17*, e0268780. [CrossRef] [PubMed]
82. Barmettler, S.; DiGiacomo, D.V.; Yang, N.J.; Lam, T.; Naranbhai, V.; Dighe, A.S.; Burke, K.E.; Blumenthal, K.G.; Ling, M.; Hesterberg, P.E.; et al. Response to Severe Acute Respiratory Syndrome Coronavirus 2 Initial Series and Additional Dose Vaccine in Patients With Predominant Antibody Deficiency. *J. Allergy Clin. Immunol. Pract.* **2022**, *10*, 1622–1634.e4. [CrossRef]
83. Bergman, P.; Blennow, O.; Hansson, L.; Mielke, S.; Nowak, P.; Chen, P.; Söderdahl, G.; Österborg, A.; Smith, C.I.E.; Wullimann, D.; et al. Safety and efficacy of the mRNA BNT162b2 vaccine against SARS-CoV-2 in five groups of immunocompromised patients and healthy controls in a prospective open-label clinical trial. *eBioMedicine* **2021**, *74*, 103705. [CrossRef]
84. Salinas, A.F.; Mortari, E.P.; Terreri, S.; Quintarelli, C.; Pulvirenti, F.; Di Cecca, S.; Guercio, M.; Milito, C.; Bonanni, L.; Auria, S.; et al. SARS-CoV-2 Vaccine Induced Atypical Immune Responses in Antibody Defects: Everybody Does their Best. *J. Clin. Immunol.* **2021**, *41*, 1709–1722. [CrossRef] [PubMed]
85. Abo-Helo, N.; Muhammad, E.; Ghaben-Amara, S.; Cohen, S. Specific antibody response of 14 patients with common variable immunodeficiency to 3 BNT162b2 messenger RNA coronavirus disease 2019 vaccinations. *Ann. Allergy Asthma Immunol.* **2022**, *129*, 108–109. [CrossRef]
86. Erra, L.; Uriarte, I.; Colado, A.; Paolini, M.V.; Seminario, G.; Fernández, J.B.; Tau, L.; Bernatowiez, J.; Moreira, I.; Vishnopolska, S.; et al. COVID-19 Vaccination Responses with Different Vaccine Platforms in Patients with Inborn Errors of Immunity. *J. Clin. Immunol.* **2022**, *43*, 271–285. [CrossRef]
87. Nielsen, B.U.; Drabe, C.H.; Barnkob, M.B.; Johansen, I.S.; Hansen, A.K.K.; Nilsson, A.C.; Rasmussen, L.D. Antibody response following the third and fourth SARS-CoV-2 vaccine dose in individuals with common variable immunodeficiency. *Front. Immunol.* **2022**, *13*, 934476. [CrossRef]
88. Antolí, A.; Rocamora-Blanch, G.; Framil, M.; Mas-Bosch, V.; Navarro, S.; Bermudez, C.; Martinez-Yelamos, S.; Dopico, E.; Calatayud, L.; Garcia-Muñoz, N.; et al. Evaluation of Humoral and Cellular Immune Responses to the SARS-CoV-2 Vaccine in Patients With Common Variable Immunodeficiency Phenotype and Patient Receiving B-Cell Depletion Therapy. *Front. Immunol.* **2022**, *13*, 895209. [CrossRef]
89. Pham, M.N.; Murugesan, K.; Banaei, N.; Pinsky, B.A.; Tang, M.; Hoyte, E.; Lewis, D.B.; Gernez, Y. Immunogenicity and tolerability of COVID-19 messenger RNA vaccines in primary immunodeficiency patients with functional B-cell defects. *J. Allergy Clin. Immunol.* **2022**, *149*, 907–911.e3. [CrossRef] [PubMed]
90. Lin, F.J.; Doss, A.M.A.; Davis-Adams, H.G.; Adams, L.J.; Hanson, C.H.; VanBlargan, L.A.; Liang, C.-Y.; Chen, R.E.; Monroy, J.M.; Wedner, H.J.; et al. SARS-CoV-2 booster vaccination rescues attenuated IgG1 memory B cell response in primary antibody deficiency patients. *Front. Immunol.* **2022**, *13*, 1033770. [CrossRef] [PubMed]
91. Abo-Helo, N.; Muhammad, E.; Ghaben-Amara, S.; Panasoff, J.; Cohen, S. Specific antibody response of patients with common variable immunodeficiency to BNT162b2 coronavirus disease 2019 vaccination. *Ann. Allergy Asthma Immunol.* **2021**, *127*, 501–503. [CrossRef]

92. Liu, L.; Iketani, S.; Guo, Y.; Chan, J.F.-W.; Wang, M.; Liu, L.; Luo, Y.; Chu, H.; Huang, Y.; Nair, M.S.; et al. Striking antibody evasion manifested by the Omicron variant of SARS-CoV-2. *Nature* **2022**, *602*, 676–681. [CrossRef]
93. Jalil, M.; Rowane, M.; Rajan, J.; Hostoffer, R. Successful Anti-SARS-CoV-2 Spike Protein Antibody Response to Vaccination in *MAGT1* Deficiency. *Allergy Rhinol.* **2021**, *12*, 1–4. [CrossRef]
94. Pulvirenti, F.; Di Cecca, S.; Sinibaldi, M.; Piano Mortari, E.; Terreri, S.; Albano, C.; Guercio, M.; Sculco, E.; Milito, C.; Ferrari, S.; et al. T-Cell Defects Associated to Lack of Spike-Specific Antibodies after BNT162b2 Full Immunization Followed by a Booster Dose in Patients with Common Variable Immune Deficiencies. *Cells* **2022**, *11*, 1918. [CrossRef]
95. Sheward, D.J.; Kim, C.; Ehling, R.A.; Pankow, A.; Dopico, X.C.; Martin, D.; Reddy, S.; Dillner, J.; Karlsson Hedestam, G.B.; Albert, J.; et al. Variable loss of antibody potency against SARS-CoV-2 B.1.1.529 (Omicron). *bioRxiv* **2021**. [CrossRef]
96. Leung, D.; Mu, X.; Duque, J.S.R.; Cheng, S.M.S.; Wang, M.; Zhang, W.; Zhang, Y.; Tam, I.Y.S.; Lee, T.S.S.; Lam, J.H.Y.; et al. Safety and immunogenicity of 3 doses of BNT162b2 and CoronaVac in children and adults with inborn errors of immunity. *Front. Immunol.* **2022**, *13*, 982155. [CrossRef] [PubMed]
97. Illes, P.; Csomos, K.; Ujhazi, B.; Dasso, J.; Nagy, B.; Alas, E.; Gordon, S.; Timothy, P.; Miranda, M.A.; Sullivan, S.; et al. The Humoral Immune Response To SARS-CoV-2 Infection and/or Immunization in Immunocompromised Versus Immunocompetent Individuals. *J. Allergy Clin. Immunol.* **2022**, *149*, AB21. [CrossRef]
98. Obeid, M.; Suffiotti, M.; Pellaton, C.; Bouchaab, H.; Cairoli, A.; Salvadé, V.; Stevenel, C.; Hottinger, R.; Pythoud, C.; Coutechier, L.; et al. Humoral Responses Against Variants of Concern by COVID-19 mRNA Vaccines in Immunocompromised Patients. *JAMA Oncol.* **2022**, *8*, e220446. [CrossRef]
99. Lucane, Z.; Slisere, B.; Ozola, L.; Rots, D.; Papirte, S.; Vilne, B.; Gailite, L.; Kurjane, N. Long-Term Immunological Memory of SARS-CoV-2 Is Present in Patients with Primary Antibody Deficiencies for up to a Year after Vaccination. *Vaccines* **2023**, *11*, 354. [CrossRef] [PubMed]
100. Delmonte, O.M.; Bergerson, J.R.E.; Burbelo, P.D.; Durkee-Shock, J.R.; Dobbs, K.; Bosticardo, M.; Keller, M.D.; McDermott, D.H.; Rao, V.K.; Dimitrova, D.; et al. Antibody Responses to the SARS-CoV-2 Vaccine in Individuals with Various Inborn Errors of Immunity. *J. Allergy Clin. Immunol.* **2021**, *148*, 1192–1197. [CrossRef]
101. Pulvirenti, F.; Fernandez Salinas, A.; Milito, C.; Terreri, S.; Piano Mortari, E.; Quintarelli, C.; Di Cecca, S.; Lagnese, G.; Punziano, A.; Guercio, M.; et al. B Cell Response Induced by SARS-CoV-2 Infection Is Boosted by the BNT162b2 Vaccine in Primary Antibody Deficiencies. *Cells* **2021**, *10*, 2915. [CrossRef] [PubMed]
102. Shields, A.M.; Faustini, S.E.; Hill, H.J.; Al-Taei, S.; Tanner, C.; Ashford, F.; Workman, S.; Moreira, F.; Verma, N.; Wagg, H.; et al. SARS-CoV-2 Vaccine Responses in Individuals with Antibody Deficiency: Findings from the COV-AD Study. *J. Clin. Immunol.* **2022**, *42*, 923–934. [CrossRef] [PubMed]
103. Oyaert, M.; De Scheerder, M.-A.; Van Herrewege, S.; Laureys, G.; Van Assche, S.; Cambron, M.; Naesens, L.; Hoste, L.; Claes, K.; Haerynck, F.; et al. Evaluation of Humoral and Cellular Responses in SARS-CoV-2 mRNA Vaccinated Immunocompromised Patients. *Front. Immunol.* **2022**, *13*, 858399. [CrossRef]
104. Murray, C.E.; O'Brien, C.; Alamin, S.; Phelan, S.H.; Argue, R.; Kiersey, R.; Gardiner, M.; Naughton, A.; Keogh, E.; Holmes, P.; et al. Cellular and humoral immunogenicity of the COVID-19 vaccine and COVID-19 disease severity in individuals with immunodeficiency. *Front. Immunol.* **2023**, *14*, 1131604. [CrossRef] [PubMed]
105. Hurme, A.; Jalkanen, P.; Marttila-Vaara, M.; Heroum, J.; Jokinen, H.; Vara, S.; Liedes, O.; Lempainen, J.; Melin, M.; Julkunen, I.; et al. T cell immunity following COVID-19 vaccination in adult patients with primary antibody deficiency—A 22-month follow-up. *Front. Immunol.* **2023**, *14*, 1146500. [CrossRef]
106. La Civita, E.; Zannella, C.; Brusa, S.; Romano, P.; Schettino, E.; Salemi, F.; Carrano, R.; Gentile, L.; Punziano, A.; Lagnese, G.; et al. BNT162b2 Elicited an Efficient Cell-Mediated Response against SARS-CoV-2 in Kidney Transplant Recipients and Common Variable Immunodeficiency Patients. *Viruses* **2023**, *15*, 1659. [CrossRef]
107. Steiner, S.; Schwarz, T.; Corman, V.M.; Jeworowski, L.M.; Bauer, S.; Drosten, C.; Scheibenbogen, C.; Hanitsch, L.G. Impaired B Cell Recall Memory and Reduced Antibody Avidity but Robust T Cell Response in CVID Patients After COVID-19 Vaccination. *J. Clin. Immunol.* **2023**, *43*, 869–881. [CrossRef]
108. Mizera, D.; Dziedzic, R.; Drynda, A.; Gradzikiewicz, A.; Jakieła, B.; Celińska-Löwenhoff, M.; Padjas, A.; Matyja-Bednarczyk, A.; Zaręba, L.; Bazan-Socha, S. Cellular immune response to SARS-CoV-2 in patients with primary antibody deficiencies. *Front. Immunol.* **2023**, *14*, 1275892. [CrossRef]
109. Tandon, M.; DiGiacomo, D.V.; Zhou, B.; Hesterberg, P.; Rosenberg, C.E.; Barmettler, S.; Farmer, J.R. Response to SARS-CoV-2 initial series and additional dose vaccine in pediatric patients with predominantly antibody deficiency. *Front. Immunol.* **2023**, *14*, 1217718. [CrossRef] [PubMed]
110. Shin, J.J.; Par-Young, J.; Unlu, S.; McNamara, A.; Park, H.-J.; Shin, M.S.; Gee, R.J.; Doyle, H.; Afinogenova, Y.; Zidan, E.; et al. Defining Clinical and Immunological Predictors of Poor Immune Responses to COVID-19 mRNA Vaccines in Patients with Primary Antibody Deficiency. *J. Clin. Immunol.* **2022**, *42*, 1137–1150. [CrossRef]
111. Quinti, I.; Locatelli, F.; Carsetti, R. The Immune Response to SARS-CoV-2 Vaccination: Insights Learned From Adult Patients With Common Variable Immune Deficiency. *Front. Immunol.* **2021**, *12*, 815404. [CrossRef]
112. Bloomfield, M.; Parackova, Z.; Hanzlikova, J.; Lastovicka, J.; Sediva, A. Immunogenicity and Safety of COVID-19 mRNA Vaccine in STAT1 GOF Patients. *J. Clin. Immunol.* **2022**, *42*, 266–269. [CrossRef]

113. Timothy, P.; Illes, P.; Ujhazi, B.; Gordon, S.; Nagy, B.; Alas, E.; Sullivan, S.; Miranda, M.A.; Duff, C.; Farmer, J.; et al. Effects Of The COVID-19 Pandemic On A Group Of Patients With Pathogenic Variant of Cytotoxic T-Lymphocyte Associated Protein 4 (CTLA-4) in a Tertiary Center in Florida. *J. Allergy Clin. Immunol.* **2022**, *149*, AB28. [CrossRef]
114. Squire, J.D.; Joshi, A.Y. Response to mRNA COVID-19 vaccination in three XLA patients. *Vaccine* **2022**, *40*, 5299–5301. [CrossRef]
115. Sette, A.; Crotty, S. Adaptive immunity to SARS-CoV-2 and COVID-19. *Cell* **2021**, *184*, 861–880. [CrossRef]
116. Zimmerman, O.; Altman Doss, A.M.; Kaplonek, P.; Liang, C.-Y.; VanBlargan, L.A.; Chen, R.E.; Monroy, J.M.; Wedner, H.J.; Kulczycki, A.; Mantia, T.L.; et al. mRNA vaccine boosting enhances antibody responses against SARS-CoV-2 Omicron variant in individuals with antibody deficiency syndromes. *Cell Rep. Med.* **2022**, *3*, 100653. [CrossRef]
117. Abella, E.; Trigueros, M.; Pradenas, E.; Muñoz-Lopez, F.; Garcia-Pallarols, F.; Ben Azaiz Ben Lahsen, R.; Trinité, B.; Urrea, V.; Marfil, S.; Rovirosa, C.; et al. Efficacy of SARS-CoV-2 vaccination in patients with monoclonal gammopathies: A cross sectional study. *Life Sci. Alliance* **2022**, *5*, e202201479. [CrossRef]
118. Romero, C.; Díez, J.M.; Gajardo, R. Anti-SARS-CoV-2 antibodies in healthy donor plasma pools and IVIG products. *Lancet Infect. Dis.* **2021**, *21*, 765–766. [CrossRef]
119. Volk, A.; Covini-Souris, C.; Kuehnel, D.; De Mey, C.; Römisch, J.; Schmidt, T. SARS-CoV-2 Neutralization in Convalescent Plasma and Commercial Lots of Plasma-Derived Immunoglobulin. *BioDrugs* **2022**, *36*, 41–53. [CrossRef]
120. Ahn, T.S.; Han, B.; Krogstad, P.; Bun, C.; Kohn, L.A.; Garcia-Lloret, M.I.; Damoiseaux, R.; Butte, M.J. Commercial immunoglobulin products contain cross-reactive but not neutralizing antibodies against SARS-CoV-2. *J. Allergy Clin. Immunol.* **2021**, *147*, 876–877. [CrossRef]
121. Dalakas, M.C.; Bitzogli, K.; Alexopoulos, H. Anti-SARS-CoV-2 Antibodies Within IVIg Preparations: Cross-Reactivities With Seasonal Coronaviruses, Natural Autoimmunity, and Therapeutic Implications. *Front. Immunol.* **2021**, *12*, 627285. [CrossRef]
122. Díez, J.-M.; Romero, C.; Gajardo, R. Currently available intravenous immunoglobulin contains antibodies reacting against severe acute respiratory syndrome coronavirus 2 antigens. *Immunotherapy* **2020**, *12*, 571–576. [CrossRef]
123. Manian, D.V.; Jensen, C.; Theel, E.S.; Mills, J.R.; Joshi, A. Non-neutralizing antibodies and limitations of serologic testing for severe acute respiratory syndrome coronavirus 2 in patients receiving immunoglobulin replacement products. *Ann. Allergy Asthma Immunol.* **2021**, *126*, 206–207. [CrossRef]
124. Hirsiger, J.R.; Weigang, S.; Walz, A.-C.; Fuchs, J.; Daly, M.-L.; Eggimann, S.; Hausmann, O.; Schwemmle, M.; Kochs, G.; Panning, M.; et al. Passive immunization against COVID-19 by anti-SARS-CoV-2 spike IgG in commercially available immunoglobulin preparations in severe antibody deficiency. *J. Allergy Clin. Immunol. Pract.* **2022**, *10*, 2452–2455.e3. [CrossRef]
125. Miller, A.L.; Rider, N.L.; Pyles, R.B.; Judy, B.; Xie, X.; Shi, P.-Y.; Ksiazek, T.G. The arrival of SARS-CoV-2–neutralizing antibodies in a currently available commercial immunoglobulin. *J. Allergy Clin. Immunol.* **2022**, *149*, 1958–1959. [CrossRef]
126. Lindahl, H.; Klingström, J.; Da Silva Rodrigues, R.; Christ, W.; Chen, P.; Ljunggren, H.-G.; Buggert, M.; Aleman, S.; Smith, C.I.E.; Bergman, P. Neutralizing SARS-CoV-2 Antibodies in Commercial Immunoglobulin Products Give Patients with X-Linked Agammaglobulinemia Limited Passive Immunity to the Omicron Variant. *J. Clin. Immunol.* **2022**, *42*, 1130–1136. [CrossRef]
127. Stinca, S.; Barnes, T.W.; Vogel, P.; Meyers, W.; Schulte-Pelkum, J.; Filchtinski, D.; Steller, L.; Hauser, T.; Manni, S.; Gardiner, D.F.; et al. Modelling the concentration of anti-SARS-CoV-2 immunoglobulin G in intravenous immunoglobulin product batches. *PLoS ONE* **2021**, *16*, e0259731. [CrossRef]
128. Göschl, L.; Mrak, D.; Grabmeier-Pfistershammer, K.; Stiasny, K.; Haslacher, H.; Schneider, L.; Deimel, T.; Kartnig, F.; Tobudic, S.; Aletaha, D.; et al. Reactogenicity and immunogenicity of the second COVID-19 vaccination in patients with inborn errors of immunity or mannan-binding lectin deficiency. *Front. Immunol.* **2022**, *13*, 974987. [CrossRef]
129. Schulz, E.; Hodl, I.; Forstner, P.; Hatzl, S.; Sareban, N.; Moritz, M.; Fessler, J.; Dreo, B.; Uhl, B.; Url, C.; et al. CD19+IgD+CD27- Naïve B Cells as Predictors of Humoral Response to COVID 19 mRNA Vaccination in Immunocompromised Patients. *Front. Immunol.* **2021**, *12*, 803742. [CrossRef]
130. Upasani, V.; Townsend, K.; Wu, M.Y.; Carr, E.J.; Hobbs, A.; Dowgier, G.; Ragno, M.; Herman, L.S.; Sharma, S.; Shah, D.; et al. Commercial Immunoglobulin Products Contain Neutralizing Antibodies Against Severe Acute Respiratory Syndrome Coronavirus 2 Spike Protein. *Clin. Infect. Dis.* **2023**, *77*, 950–960. [CrossRef]
131. Goda, V.; Kriván, G.; Kulcsár, A.; Gönczi, M.; Tasnády, S.; Matula, Z.; Nagy, G.; Bekő, G.; Horváth, M.; Uher, F.; et al. Specific Antibody and the T-Cell Response Elicited by BNT162b2 Boosting After Two ChAdOx1 nCoV-19 in Common Variable Immunodeficiency. *Front. Immunol.* **2022**, *13*, 907125. [CrossRef]
132. Karbiener, M.; Farcet, M.R.; Schwaiger, J.; Powers, N.; Lenart, J.; Stewart, J.M.; Tallman, H.; Kreil, T.R. Highly Potent SARS-CoV-2 Neutralization by Intravenous Immunoglobulins manufactured from Post-COVID-19 and COVID-19-Vaccinated Plasma Donations. *J. Infect. Dis.* **2021**, *224*, jiab482. [CrossRef]
133. Lindahl, H.; Chen, P.; Åberg, M.; Ljunggren, H.-G.; Buggert, M.; Aleman, S.; Smith, C.I.E.; Bergman, P. SARS-CoV-2 Antibodies in Commercial Immunoglobulin Products Show Markedly Reduced Cross-reactivities Against Omicron Variants. *J. Clin. Immunol.* **2023**, *43*, 1075–1082. [CrossRef]
134. Sauerwein, K.M.T.; Geier, C.B.; Stemberger, R.F.; Akyaman, H.; Illes, P.; Fischer, M.B.; Eibl, M.M.; Walter, J.E.; Wolf, H.M. Antigen-Specific $CD4^{+}$ T-Cell Activation in Primary Antibody Deficiency After BNT162b2 mRNA COVID-19 Vaccination. *Front. Immunol.* **2022**, *13*, 827048. [CrossRef] [PubMed]

135. Barouch, D.H.; Stephenson, K.E.; Sadoff, J.; Yu, J.; Chang, A.; Gebre, M.; McMahan, K.; Liu, J.; Chandrashekar, A.; Patel, S.; et al. Durable Humoral and Cellular Immune Responses 8 Months after Ad26.COV2.S Vaccination. *N. Engl. J. Med.* **2021**, *385*, 951–953. [CrossRef]
136. Schwaiger, J.; Karbiener, M.; Aberham, C.; Farcet, M.R.; Kreil, T.R. No SARS-CoV-2 Neutralization by Intravenous Immunoglobulins Produced From Plasma Collected Before the 2020 Pandemic. *J. Infect. Dis.* **2020**, *222*, 1960–1964. [CrossRef]
137. Farcet, M.R.; Karbiener, M.; Schwaiger, J.; Ilk, R.; Kreil, T.R. Rapidly Increasing Severe Acute Respiratory Syndrome Coronavirus 2 Neutralization by Intravenous Immunoglobulins Produced From Plasma Collected During the 2020 Pandemic. *J. Infect. Dis.* **2022**, *226*, 1357–1361. [CrossRef]
138. Romero, C.; Díez, J.-M.; Gajardo, R. Anti-SARS-CoV-2 antibodies in healthy donor plasma pools and IVIG products—An update. *Lancet Infect. Dis.* **2022**, *22*, 19. [CrossRef]
139. Farcet, M.R.; Karbiener, M.; Knotzer, S.; Schwaiger, J.; Kreil, T.R. Omicron Severe Acute Respiratory Syndrome Coronavirus 2 Neutralization by Immunoglobulin Preparations Manufactured From Plasma Collected in the United States and Europe. *J. Infect. Dis.* **2022**, *226*, 1396–1400. [CrossRef]
140. Sokal, A.; Bastard, P.; Chappert, P.; Barba-Spaeth, G.; Fourati, S.; Vanderberghe, A.; Lagouge-Roussey, P.; Meyts, I.; Gervais, A.; Bouvier-Alias, M.; et al. Human type I IFN deficiency does not impair B cell response to SARS-CoV-2 mRNA vaccination. *J. Exp. Med.* **2022**, *220*, e20220258. [CrossRef]
141. Gao, Y.; Cai, C.; Wullimann, D.; Niessl, J.; Rivera-Ballesteros, O.; Chen, P.; Lange, J.; Cuapio, A.; Blennow, O.; Hansson, L.; et al. Immunodeficiency syndromes differentially impact the functional profile of SARS-CoV-2-specific T cells elicited by mRNA vaccination. *Immunity* **2022**, *55*, 1732–1746.e5. [CrossRef]
142. Gupta, S.; Agrawal, S.; Sandoval, A.; Su, H.; Tran, M.; Demirdag, Y. SARS-CoV-2-Specific and Functional Cytotoxic CD8 Cells in Primary Antibody Deficiency: Natural Infection and Response to Vaccine. *J. Clin. Immunol.* **2022**, *42*, 914–922. [CrossRef]
143. Barrios, Y.; Franco, A.; Alava-Cruz, C.; Cuesta-Martin, R.; Camara, C.; Matheu, V. Easy approach to detect cell immunity to COVID vaccines in common variable immunodeficiency patients. *Allergol. Immunopathol.* **2022**, *50*, 101–105. [CrossRef]
144. Sanchez, D.; Radigan, L.; Cunningham-Rundles, C. Assessing SARS-CoV-2 Antigen Specific T-cell Responses After mRNA Vaccination and/or Omicron Variant COVID-19 Infection in Patients with Primary Humoral Immunodeficiencies. *J. Allergy Clin. Immunol.* **2023**, *151*, AB195. [CrossRef]
145. Piano Mortari, E.; Pulvirenti, F.; Marcellini, V.; Terreri, S.; Salinas, A.F.; Ferrari, S.; Di Napoli, G.; Guadagnolo, D.; Sculco, E.; Albano, C.; et al. Functional CVIDs phenotype clusters identified by the integration of immune parameters after BNT162b2 boosters. *Front. Immunol.* **2023**, *14*, 1194225. [CrossRef]
146. Nourizadeh, M.; Feizabadi, E.; Mirmoghtadaei, M.; Mohammadi, A.; Fazlollahi, M.R.; Moradi, L.; Pourpak, Z. Antibody Production after COVID-19 Vaccination in Patients with Inborn Errors of Immunity. *Iran. J. Immunol.* **2023**, *20*, 400–409. [CrossRef]
147. Yam-Puc, J.C.; Hosseini, Z.; Horner, E.C.; Gerber, P.P.; Beristain-Covarrubias, N.; Hughes, R.; Lulla, A.; Rust, M.; Boston, R.; Ali, M.; et al. Age-associated B cells predict impaired humoral immunity after COVID-19 vaccination in patients receiving immune checkpoint blockade. *Nat. Commun.* **2023**, *14*, 3292. [CrossRef]
148. Van Leeuwen, L.P.M.; Grobben, M.; GeurtsvanKessel, C.H.; Ellerbroek, P.M.; De Bree, G.J.; Potjewijd, J.; Rutgers, A.; Jolink, H.; Van De Veerdonk, F.L.; Van Gils, M.J.; et al. Immune Responses 6 Months After mRNA-1273 COVID-19 Vaccination and the Effect of a Third Vaccination in Patients with Inborn Errors of Immunity. *J. Clin. Immunol.* **2023**, *43*, 1104–1117. [CrossRef]
149. Karabiber, E.; Atik, Ö.; Tepetam, F.M.; Ergan, B.; İlki, A.; Karakoç Aydıner, E.; Özen, A.; Özyer, F.; Barış, S. Clinical and immunological outcomes of SARS-CoV-2 infection in patients with inborn errors of immunity receiving different brands and doses of COVID-19 vaccines. *Tuberk. Toraks* **2023**, *71*, 236–249. [CrossRef]
150. Liu, J.; Chandrashekar, A.; Sellers, D.; Barrett, J.; Jacob-Dolan, C.; Lifton, M.; McMahan, K.; Sciacca, M.; VanWyk, H.; Wu, C.; et al. Vaccines elicit highly conserved cellular immunity to SARS-CoV-2 Omicron. *Nature* **2022**, *603*, 493–496. [CrossRef]
151. Steiner, S.; Schwarz, T.; Corman, V.M.; Gebert, L.; Kleinschmidt, M.C.; Wald, A.; Gläser, S.; Kruse, J.M.; Zickler, D.; Peric, A.; et al. SARS-CoV-2 T Cell Response in Severe and Fatal COVID-19 in Primary Antibody Deficiency Patients Without Specific Humoral Immunity. *Front. Immunol.* **2022**, *13*, 840126. [CrossRef]
152. Ameratunga, R.; Woon, S.-T.; Jordan, A.; Longhurst, H.; Leung, E.; Steele, R.; Lehnert, K.; Snell, R.; Brooks, A.E.S. Perspective: Diagnostic laboratories should urgently develop T cell assays for SARS-CoV-2 infection. *Expert Rev. Clin. Immunol.* **2021**, *17*, 421–430. [CrossRef]
153. Ameratunga, R.; Woon, S.-T.; Steele, R.; Lehnert, K.; Leung, E.; Edwards, E.S.J.; Brooks, A.E.S. Common Variable Immunodeficiency Disorders as a Model for Assessing COVID-19 Vaccine Responses in Immunocompromised Patients. *Front. Immunol.* **2021**, *12*, 798389. [CrossRef]
154. Labrador-Horrillo, M.; Franco-Jarava, C.; Garcia-Prat, M.; Parra-Martínez, A.; Antolín, M.; Salgado-Perandrés, S.; Aguiló-Cucurull, A.; Martinez-Gallo, M.; Colobran, R. Case Report: X-Linked SASH3 Deficiency Presenting as a Common Variable Immunodeficiency. *Front. Immunol.* **2022**, *13*, 881206. [CrossRef]
155. Kinoshita, H.; Durkee-Shock, J.; Jensen-Wachspress, M.; Kankate, V.; Lang, H.; Lazarski, C.A.; Keswani, A.; Webber, K.; Montgomery-Recht, K.; Walkiewicz, M.; et al. Robust Antibody and T Cell Responses to SARS-CoV-2 in Patients with Antibody Deficiency. *J. Clin. Immunol.* **2021**, *41*, 1146–1153. [CrossRef]

156. Reynolds, C.J.; Pade, C.; Gibbons, J.M.; Butler, D.K.; Otter, A.D.; Menacho, K.; Fontana, M.; Smit, A.; Sackville-West, J.E.; Cutino-Moguel, T.; et al. Prior SARS-CoV-2 infection rescues B and T cell responses to variants after first vaccine dose. *Science* **2021**, *372*, 1418–1423. [CrossRef]
157. Braun, J.; Loyal, L.; Frentsch, M.; Wendisch, D.; Georg, P.; Kurth, F.; Hippenstiel, S.; Dingeldey, M.; Kruse, B.; Fauchere, F.; et al. SARS-CoV-2-reactive T cells in healthy donors and patients with COVID-19. *Nature* **2020**, *587*, 270–274. [CrossRef]
158. Cuapio, A.; Boulouis, C.; Filipovic, I.; Wullimann, D.; Kammann, T.; Parrot, T.; Chen, P.; Akber, M.; Gao, Y.; Hammer, Q.; et al. NK cell frequencies, function and correlates to vaccine outcome in BNT162b2 mRNA anti-SARS-CoV-2 vaccinated healthy and immunocompromised individuals. *Mol. Med.* **2022**, *28*, 20. [CrossRef]
159. Evusheld (tixagevimab and cilgavimab) Dosing, Indications, Interactions, Adverse Effects, and More. Available online: https://reference.medscape.com/drug/evusheld-tixagevimab-cilgavimab-4000251 (accessed on 10 August 2023).
160. Zhang, J.; Zhang, H.; Sun, L. Therapeutic antibodies for COVID-19: Is a new age of IgM, IgA and bispecific antibodies coming? *mAbs* **2022**, *14*, 2031483. [CrossRef]
161. Zost, S.J.; Gilchuk, P.; Case, J.B.; Binshtein, E.; Chen, R.E.; Nkolola, J.P.; Schäfer, A.; Reidy, J.X.; Trivette, A.; Nargi, R.S.; et al. Potently neutralizing and protective human antibodies against SARS-CoV-2. *Nature* **2020**, *584*, 443–449. [CrossRef]
162. Pinto, D.; Park, Y.-J.; Beltramello, M.; Walls, A.C.; Tortorici, M.A.; Bianchi, S.; Jaconi, S.; Culap, K.; Zatta, F.; De Marco, A.; et al. Cross-neutralization of SARS-CoV-2 by a human monoclonal SARS-CoV antibody. *Nature* **2020**, *583*, 290–295. [CrossRef]
163. Tuccori, M.; Ferraro, S.; Convertino, I.; Cappello, E.; Valdiserra, G.; Blandizzi, C.; Maggi, F.; Focosi, D. Anti-SARS-CoV-2 neutralizing monoclonal antibodies: Clinical pipeline. *mAbs* **2020**, *12*, 1854149. [CrossRef]
164. Orange, J.; Hossny, E.; Weiler, C.; Ballow, M.; Berger, M.; Bonilla, F.; Buckley, R.; Chinen, J.; Elgamal, Y.; Mazer, B. Use of intravenous immunoglobulin in human disease: A review of evidence by members of the Primary Immunodeficiency Committee of the American Academy of Allergy, Asthma and Immunology. *J. Allergy Clin. Immunol.* **2006**, *117*, S525–S553. [CrossRef]
165. Therapeutic Goods Administration (TGA). Evusheld. Available online: https://www.tga.gov.au/resources/auspmd/evusheld (accessed on 10 August 2023).
166. Raphael, A.; Shamriz, O.; Lev, A.; Simon, A.J.; Tal, Y.; Somech, R.; Eisenberg, R.; Toker, O. SARS-CoV-2 spike antibody concentration in gamma globulin products from high-prevalence COVID-19 countries are transmitted to X-linked agammaglobulinemia patients. *Front. Immunol.* **2023**, *14*, 1156823. [CrossRef]
167. Park, H.; Gada, S. SARS-CoV-2 Antibody Profile of Immune Globulin Preparations. *J. Allergy Clin. Immunol.* **2022**, *149*, AB65. [CrossRef]
168. Cousins, K.; Sano, K.; Lam, B.; Röltgen, K.; Bhavsar, D.; Singh, G.; McRae, O.; Jeong, S.; Aboelregal, N.; Ho, H.; et al. Detection of SARS-CoV-2 Antibodies in Immunoglobulin Products. *J. Allergy Clin. Immunol. Pract.* **2023**, *11*, 2534–2541.e2. [CrossRef]
169. Schubert, M.; Bertoglio, F.; Steinke, S.; Heine, P.A.; Ynga-Durand, M.A.; Maass, H.; Sammartino, J.C.; Cassaniti, I.; Zuo, F.; Du, L.; et al. Human serum from SARS-CoV-2-vaccinated and COVID-19 patients shows reduced binding to the RBD of SARS-CoV-2 Omicron variant. *BMC Med.* **2022**, *20*, 102. [CrossRef]
170. Cox, M.; Peacock, T.P.; Harvey, W.T.; Hughes, J.; Wright, D.W.; COVID-19 Genomics UK (COG-UK) Consortium; Willett, B.J.; Thomson, E.; Gupta, R.K.; Peacock, S.J.; et al. SARS-CoV-2 variant evasion of monoclonal antibodies based on in vitro studies. *Nat. Rev. Microbiol.* **2023**, *21*, 112–124. [CrossRef]
171. Food and Drug Administration. Coronavirus (COVID-19) Update: FDA Authorizes Additional Monoclonal Antibody for Treatment of COVID-19. Available online: https://www.fda.gov/news-events/press-announcements/coronavirus-covid-19-update-fda-authorizes-additional-monoclonal-antibody-treatment-covid-19 (accessed on 25 April 2023).
172. Totschnig, D.; Augustin, M.; Niculescu, I.; Laferl, H.; Jansen-Skoupy, S.; Lehmann, C.; Wenisch, C.; Zoufaly, A. SARS-CoV-2 Pre-Exposure Prophylaxis with Sotrovimab and Tixagevimab/Cilgavimab in Immunocompromised Patients—A Single-Center Experience. *Viruses* **2022**, *14*, 2278. [CrossRef]
173. Martin-Blondel, G.; Marcelin, A.-G.; Soulié, C.; Kaisaridi, S.; Lusivika-Nzinga, C.; Dorival, C.; Nailler, L.; Boston, A.; Melenotte, C.; Gaube, G.; et al. Outcome of very high-risk patients treated by Sotrovimab for mild-to-moderate COVID-19 Omicron, a prospective cohort study (the ANRS 0003S COCOPREV study). *J. Infect.* **2022**, *84*, e101–e104. [CrossRef]
174. Gupta, A.; Gonzalez-Rojas, Y.; Juarez, E.; Crespo Casal, M.; Moya, J.; Rodrigues Falci, D.; Sarkis, E.; Solis, J.; Zheng, H.; Scott, N.; et al. Effect of Sotrovimab on Hospitalization or Death Among High-risk Patients With Mild to Moderate COVID-19: A Randomized Clinical Trial. *JAMA* **2022**, *327*, 1236–1246. [CrossRef]
175. Stadler, E.; Chai, K.L.; Schlub, T.E.; Cromer, D.; Polizzotto, M.N.; Kent, S.J.; Beecher, C.; White, H.; Turner, T.; Skoetz, N.; et al. Determinants of passive antibody efficacy in SARS-CoV-2 infection. *medRxiv* **2022**. [CrossRef]
176. Zheng, B.; Green, A.C.A.; Tazare, J.; Curtis, H.J.; Fisher, L.; Nab, L.; Schultze, A.; Mahalingasivam, V.; Parker, E.P.K.; Hulme, W.J.; et al. Comparative effectiveness of sotrovimab and molnupiravir for prevention of severe covid-19 outcomes in patients in the community: Observational cohort study with the OpenSAFELY platform. *BMJ* **2022**, *379*, e071932. [CrossRef]
177. Patel, V.; Yarwood, M.J.; Levick, B.; Gibbons, D.C.; Drysdale, M.; Kerr, W.; Watkins, J.D.; Young, S.; Pierce, B.F.; Lloyd, E.J.; et al. Characteristics and outcomes of patients with COVID-19 at high-risk of disease progression receiving sotrovimab, oral antivirals or no treatment in England. *medRxiv* **2022**. [CrossRef]

178. Zheng, B.; Tazare, J.; Nab, L.; Mehrkar, A.; MacKenna, B.; Goldacre, B.; Douglas, I.J.; Tomlinson, L.A. Comparative effectiveness of Paxlovid versus sotrovimab and molnupiravir for preventing severe COVID-19 outcomes in non-hospitalised patients: Observational cohort study using the OpenSAFELY platform. *medRxiv* **2023**. [CrossRef]
179. Harman, K.; Nash, S.G.; Webster, H.H.; Groves, N.; Hardstaff, J.; Bridgen, J.; Blomquist, P.B.; Hope, R.; Ashano, E.; Myers, R.; et al. Comparison of the risk of hospitalisation among BA.1 and BA.2 COVID-19 cases treated with sotrovimab in the community in England. *Influenza Other Respir. Viruses* **2023**, *17*, e13150. [CrossRef]
180. Cheng, M.M.; Reyes, C.; Satram, S.; Birch, H.; Gibbons, D.C.; Drysdale, M.; Bell, C.F.; Suyundikov, A.; Ding, X.; Maher, M.C.; et al. Real-World Effectiveness of Sotrovimab for the Early Treatment of COVID-19 During SARS-CoV-2 Delta and Omicron Waves in the USA. *Infect. Dis. Ther.* **2023**, *12*, 607–621. [CrossRef]
181. Martin-Blondel, G.; Marcelin, A.-G.; Soulié, C.; Kaisaridi, S.; Lusivika-Nzinga, C.; Dorival, C.; Nailler, L.; Boston, A.; Melenotte, C.; Cabié, A.; et al. Sotrovimab to prevent severe COVID-19 in high-risk patients infected with Omicron BA.2. *J. Infect.* **2022**, *85*, e104–e108. [CrossRef]
182. Zaqout, A.; Almaslamani, M.A.; Chemaitelly, H.; Hashim, S.A.; Ittaman, A.; Alimam, A.; Rustom, F.; Daghfal, J.; Abukhattab, M.; AlMukdad, S.; et al. Effectiveness of the neutralizing antibody sotrovimab among high-risk patients with mild-to-moderate SARS-CoV-2 in Qatar. *Int. J. Infect. Dis.* **2022**, *124*, 96–103. [CrossRef]
183. Case, J.B.; Mackin, S.; Errico, J.M.; Chong, Z.; Madden, E.A.; Whitener, B.; Guarino, B.; Schmid, M.A.; Rosenthal, K.; Ren, K.; et al. Resilience of S309 and AZD7442 monoclonal antibody treatments against infection by SARS-CoV-2 Omicron lineage strains. *Nat. Commun.* **2022**, *13*, 3824. [CrossRef]
184. Takashita, E.; Kinoshita, N.; Yamayoshi, S.; Sakai-Tagawa, Y.; Fujisaki, S.; Ito, M.; Iwatsuki-Horimoto, K.; Halfmann, P.; Watanabe, S.; Maeda, K.; et al. Efficacy of Antiviral Agents against the SARS-CoV-2 Omicron Subvariant BA.2. *N. Engl. J. Med.* **2022**, *386*, 1475–1477. [CrossRef]
185. Takashita, E.; Yamayoshi, S.; Halfmann, P.; Wilson, N.; Ries, H.; Richardson, A.; Bobholz, M.; Vuyk, W.; Maddox, R.; Baker, D.A.; et al. In Vitro Efficacy of Antiviral Agents against Omicron Subvariant BA.4.6. *N. Engl. J. Med.* **2022**, *387*, 2094–2097. [CrossRef] [PubMed]
186. Takashita, E.; Yamayoshi, S.; Simon, V.; van Bakel, H.; Sordillo, E.M.; Pekosz, A.; Fukushi, S.; Suzuki, T.; Maeda, K.; Halfmann, P.; et al. Efficacy of Antibodies and Antiviral Drugs against Omicron BA.2.12.1, BA.4, and BA.5 Subvariants. *N. Engl. J. Med.* **2022**, *387*, 468–470. [CrossRef]
187. Imai, M.; Ito, M.; Kiso, M.; Yamayoshi, S.; Uraki, R.; Fukushi, S.; Watanabe, S.; Suzuki, T.; Maeda, K.; Sakai-Tagawa, Y.; et al. Efficacy of Antiviral Agents against Omicron Subvariants BQ.1.1 and XBB. *N. Engl. J. Med.* **2023**, *388*, 89–91. [CrossRef]
188. Park, Y.-J.; Pinto, D.; Walls, A.C.; Liu, Z.; De Marco, A.; Benigni, F.; Zatta, F.; Silacci-Fregni, C.; Bassi, J.; Sprouse, K.R.; et al. Imprinted antibody responses against SARS-CoV-2 Omicron sublineages. *Science* **2022**, *378*, 619–627. [CrossRef]
189. Wu, M.Y.; Carr, E.J.; Harvey, R.; Mears, H.V.; Kjaer, S.; Townsley, H.; Hobbs, A.; Ragno, M.; Herman, L.S.; Adams, L.; et al. WHO's Therapeutics and COVID-19 Living Guideline on mAbs needs to be reassessed. *Lancet* **2022**, *400*, 2193–2196. [CrossRef] [PubMed]
190. Cao, Y.; Jian, F.; Wang, J.; Yu, Y.; Song, W.; Yisimayi, A.; Wang, J.; An, R.; Chen, X.; Zhang, N.; et al. Imprinted SARS-CoV-2 humoral immunity induces convergent Omicron RBD evolution. *Nature* **2022**, *641*, 521–529. [CrossRef] [PubMed]
191. Yue, C.; Song, W.; Wang, L.; Jian, F.; Chen, X.; Gao, F.; Shen, Z.; Wang, Y.; Wang, X.; Cao, Y. ACE2 binding and antibody evasion in enhanced transmissibility of XBB.1.5. *Lancet Infect. Dis.* **2023**, *23*, 278–280. [CrossRef] [PubMed]
192. Wang, Q.; Iketani, S.; Li, Z.; Liu, L.; Guo, Y.; Huang, Y.; Bowen, A.D.; Liu, M.; Wang, M.; Yu, J.; et al. Alarming antibody evasion properties of rising SARS-CoV-2 BQ and XBB subvariants. *Cell* **2023**, *186*, 279–286.e8. [CrossRef] [PubMed]
193. FDA. *FDA Updates Sotrovimab Emergency Use Authorization*; Food and Drug Administration: Silver Spring, MD, USA, 2022.
194. Loo, Y.-M.; McTamney, P.M.; Arends, R.H.; Abram, M.E.; Aksyuk, A.A.; Diallo, S.; Flores, D.J.; Kelly, E.J.; Ren, K.; Roque, R.; et al. The SARS-CoV-2 monoclonal antibody combination, AZD7442, is protective in nonhuman primates and has an extended half-life in humans. *Sci. Transl. Med.* **2022**, *14*, eabl8124. [CrossRef]
195. Stiasny, K.; Weseslindtner, L.; Heinzel, A.; Camp, J.V.; Oberbauer, R.; Reindl-Schwaighofer, R. SARS-CoV-2 Omicron BA.1/BA.2 Neutralization up to 8 Weeks After PrEP With Sotrovimab or Cilgavimab/Tixagevimab. *Transpl. Int.* **2022**, *35*, 10906. [CrossRef] [PubMed]
196. Bruel, T.; Hadjadj, J.; Maes, P.; Planas, D.; Seve, A.; Staropoli, I.; Guivel-Benhassine, F.; Porrot, F.; Bolland, W.-H.; Nguyen, Y.; et al. Serum neutralization of SARS-CoV-2 Omicron sublineages BA.1 and BA.2 in patients receiving monoclonal antibodies. *Nat. Med.* **2022**, *28*, 1297–1302. [CrossRef] [PubMed]
197. Benotmane, I.; Velay, A.; Gautier-Vargas, G.; Olagne, J.; Obrecht, A.; Cognard, N.; Heibel, F.; Braun-Parvez, L.; Keller, N.; Martzloff, J.; et al. Breakthrough COVID-19 cases despite prophylaxis with 150 mg of tixagevimab and 150 mg of cilgavimab in kidney transplant recipients. *Am. J. Transplant.* **2022**, *22*, 2675–2681. [CrossRef] [PubMed]
198. FDA. *FDA Announces Evusheld Is not Currently Authorized for Emergency Use in the U.S.*; Food and Drug Administration: Silver Spring, MD, USA, 2023.
199. AstraZeneca. *A Phase I/III Randomized, Double Blind Study to Evaluate the Safety and Neutralizing Activity of AZD5156/AZD3152 for Pre Exposure Prophylaxis of COVID 19 in Participants with Conditions Causing Immune Impairment*; Dana-Farber Cancer Institute: Boston, MA, USA, 2023.

200. First Participant Dosed in SUPERNOVA Phase I/III Trial Evaluating AZD5156, a Next-Generation Long-Acting Antibody Combination, for Prevention of COVID-19. Available online: https://www.astrazeneca-us.com/media/statements/2022/first-participant-dosed-in-supernova-phase-I-III-trial-evaluating-azd5156-a-next-generation-long-acting-antibody-combination-for-prevention-of-covid-19.html (accessed on 26 April 2023).
201. Davies, N.G.; Abbott, S.; Barnard, R.C.; Jarvis, C.I.; Kucharski, A.J.; Munday, J.D.; Pearson, C.A.B.; Russell, T.W.; Tully, D.C.; Washburne, A.D.; et al. Estimated Transmissibility and Impact of SARS-CoV-2 Lineage B.1.1.7 in England. *Science* **2021**, *372*, eabg3055. [CrossRef]
202. SARS-CoV-2 Variants of Concern as of 31 May 2024. Available online: https://www.ecdc.europa.eu/en/covid-19/variants-concern (accessed on 20 March 2023).
203. Davies, N.G.; Jarvis, C.I.; Edmunds, W.J.; Jewell, N.P.; Diaz-Ordaz, K.; Keogh, R.H. Increased Mortality in Community-Tested Cases of SARS-CoV-2 Lineage B.1.1.7. *Nature* **2021**, *593*, 270–274. [CrossRef]
204. Tegally, H.; Wilkinson, E.; Giovanetti, M.; Iranzadeh, A.; Fonseca, V.; Giandhari, J.; Doolabh, D.; Pillay, S.; San, E.J.; Msomi, N.; et al. Detection of a SARS-CoV-2 Variant of Concern in South Africa. *Nature* **2021**, *592*, 438–443. [CrossRef]
205. Cele, S.; Gazy, I.; Jackson, L.; Hwa, S.-H.; Tegally, H.; Lustig, G.; Giandhari, J.; Pillay, S.; Wilkinson, E.; Naidoo, Y.; et al. Escape of SARS-CoV-2 501Y.V2 from Neutralization by Convalescent Plasma. *Nature* **2021**, *593*, 142–146. [CrossRef]
206. Madhi, S.A.; Baillie, V.; Cutland, C.L.; Voysey, M.; Koen, A.L.; Fairlie, L.; Padayachee, S.D.; Dheda, K.; Barnabas, S.L.; Bhorat, Q.E.; et al. Efficacy of the ChAdOx1 nCoV-19 Covid-19 Vaccine against the B.1.351 Variant. *N. Engl. J. Med.* **2021**, *384*, 1885–1898. [CrossRef]
207. Planas, D.; Veyer, D.; Baidaliuk, A.; Staropoli, I.; Guivel-Benhassine, F.; Rajah, M.M.; Planchais, C.; Porrot, F.; Robillard, N.; Puech, J.; et al. Reduced Sensitivity of SARS-CoV-2 Variant Delta to Antibody Neutralization. *Nature* **2021**, *596*, 276–280. [CrossRef]
208. Faria, N.R.; Mellan, T.A.; Whittaker, C.; Claro, I.M.; Candido, D.D.S.; Mishra, S.; Crispim, M.A.E.; Sales, F.C.S.; Hawryluk, I.; McCrone, J.T.; et al. Genomics and Epidemiology of the P.1 SARS-CoV-2 Lineage in Manaus, Brazil. *Science* **2021**, *372*, 815–821. [CrossRef]
209. Dejnirattisai, W.; Zhou, D.; Supasa, P.; Liu, C.; Mentzer, A.J.; Ginn, H.M.; Zhao, Y.; Duyvesteyn, H.M.E.; Tuekprakhon, A.; Nutalai, R.; et al. Antibody Evasion by the P.1 Strain of SARS-CoV-2. *Cell* **2021**, *184*, 2939–2954.e9. [CrossRef]
210. Shiehzadegan, S.; Alaghemand, N.; Fox, M.; Venketaraman, V. Analysis of the Delta Variant B.1.617.2 COVID-19. *Clin. Pract.* **2021**, *11*, 778–784. [CrossRef]
211. Lopez Bernal, J.; Andrews, N.; Gower, C.; Gallagher, E.; Simmons, R.; Thelwall, S.; Stowe, J.; Tessier, E.; Groves, N.; Dabrera, G.; et al. Effectiveness of Covid-19 Vaccines against the B.1.617.2 (Delta) Variant. *N. Engl. J. Med.* **2021**, *385*, 585–594. [CrossRef]
212. Sheikh, A.; McMenamin, J.; Taylor, B.; Robertson, C. Public Health Scotland and the EAVE II Collaborators SARS-CoV-2 Delta VOC in Scotland: Demographics, Risk of Hospital Admission, and Vaccine Effectiveness. *Lancet* **2021**, *397*, 2461–2462. [CrossRef]
213. Stowe, J.; Andrews, N.; Kirsebom, F.; Ramsay, M.; Bernal, J.L. Effectiveness of COVID-19 Vaccines against Omicron and Delta Hospitalisation, a Test Negative Case-Control Study. *Nat. Commun.* **2022**, *13*, 5736. [CrossRef]
214. Nextstrain/Ncov/Open/Global/6m. Available online: https://nextstrain.org/ncov/open/global/6m (accessed on 20 March 2023).
215. Fan, Y.; Li, X.; Zhang, L.; Wan, S.; Zhang, L.; Zhou, F. SARS-CoV-2 Omicron Variant: Recent Progress and Future Perspectives. *Sig. Transduct. Target. Ther.* **2022**, *7*, 141. [CrossRef]
216. He, X.; Hong, W.; Pan, X.; Lu, G.; Wei, X. SARS-CoV-2 Omicron Variant: Characteristics and Prevention. *MedComm* **2021**, *2*, 838–845. [CrossRef]
217. Hui, K.P.Y.; Ho, J.C.W.; Cheung, M.-C.; Ng, K.-C.; Ching, R.H.H.; Lai, K.-L.; Kam, T.T.; Gu, H.; Sit, K.-Y.; Hsin, M.K.Y.; et al. SARS-CoV-2 Omicron Variant Replication in Human Bronchus and Lung Ex Vivo. *Nature* **2022**, *603*, 715–720. [CrossRef]
218. Rössler, A.; Knabl, L.; von Laer, D.; Kimpel, J. Neutralization Profile after Recovery from SARS-CoV-2 Omicron Infection. *N. Engl. J. Med.* **2022**, *386*, 1764–1766. [CrossRef]
219. Altarawneh, H.N.; Chemaitelly, H.; Hasan, M.R.; Ayoub, H.H.; Qassim, S.; AlMukdad, S.; Coyle, P.; Yassine, H.M.; Al-Khatib, H.A.; Benslimane, F.M.; et al. Protection against the Omicron Variant from Previous SARS-CoV-2 Infection. *N. Engl. J. Med.* **2022**, *386*, 1288–1290. [CrossRef]
220. Cao, Y.; Yisimayi, A.; Jian, F.; Song, W.; Xiao, T.; Wang, L.; Du, S.; Wang, J.; Li, Q.; Chen, X.; et al. BA.2.12.1, BA.4 and BA.5 Escape Antibodies Elicited by Omicron Infection. *Nature* **2022**, *608*, 593–602. [CrossRef]
221. Outbreak.Info SARS-CoV-2 Data Explorer. Available online: https://outbreak.info/ (accessed on 20 March 2023).
222. Zappa, M.; Verdecchia, P.; Angeli, F. Severe Acute Respiratory Syndrome Coronavirus 2 Evolution: How Mutations Affect XBB.1.5 Variant. *Eur. J. Intern. Med.* **2023**, *112*, 128–132. [CrossRef]
223. Uriu, K.; Ito, J.; Zahradnik, J.; Fujita, S.; Kosugi, Y.; Schreiber, G.; Sato, K. Enhanced Transmissibility, Infectivity, and Immune Resistance of the SARS-CoV-2 Omicron XBB.1.5 Variant. *Lancet Infect. Dis.* **2023**, *23*, 280–281. [CrossRef]
224. Qu, P.; Faraone, J.N.; Evans, J.P.; Zheng, Y.-M.; Carlin, C.; Anghelina, M.; Stevens, P.; Fernandez, S.; Jones, D.; Panchal, A.; et al. Extraordinary Evasion of Neutralizing Antibody Response by Omicron XBB.1.5, CH.1.1 and CA.3.1 Variants. *bioRxiv* **2023**. [CrossRef]
225. Luoma, E.; Rohrer, R.; Parton, H.; Hughes, S.; Omoregie, E.; Taki, F.; Wang, J.C.; Akther, S.; Amin, H.; Chang, C.; et al. *Notes from the Field:* Epidemiologic Characteristics of SARS-CoV-2 Recombinant Variant XBB.1.5—New York City, November 1, 2022–January 4, 2023. *MMWR Morb. Mortal. Wkly. Rep.* **2023**, *72*, 212–214. [CrossRef]

226. COVID XBB 1.16, Nicknamed as Arcturus, Is Spreading Faster than Its Ancestral Variants: Know More. *The Times of India*, 4 April 2023.
227. Tracking SARS-CoV-2 Variants. Available online: https://www.who.int/en/activities/tracking-SARS-CoV-2-variants/ (accessed on 17 March 2023).

vaccines

MDPI

Article

Seroprevalence of SARS-CoV-2 among Children Visiting a Tertiary Hospital during the Prevaccination Period, Southwest Region, Saudi Arabia

Ali Alsuheel Asseri [1,*] and Abdullah Alsabaani [2]

1 Department of Child Health, King Khalid University, Abha 62529, Saudi Arabia
2 Department of Family and Community Medicine, College of Medicine, King Khalid University, Abha 62529, Saudi Arabia
* Correspondence: alsoheel11@kku.edu.sa; Tel.: +966-500-186-013; Fax: +966-241-8139

Abstract: Background: In the early days of the COVID-19 pandemic, tests to ascertain whether individuals were infected with SARS-CoV-2 were often unavailable. One method to deal with this issue is to test for SARS-CoV-2 antibodies. This study sought to determine the seroprevalence of SARS-CoV-2 in children in Saudi Arabia before vaccines were available to them. Methods: This study was conducted among children who visited the tertiary Maternity and Children Hospital in Abha city, Saudi Arabia. Serum samples were screened for SARS-CoV-2-specific IgG, IgM, and IgA antibodies using ELISA. The crude and adjusted seroprevalence values among the studied children were calculated. Results: Among the 413 children studied, the ages of enrolled patients ranged from newborn to 12 years, with a median age of three years. We identified 127 (30.7%) seropositive children. IgG was exclusively positive in 43 (10.4%); IgM was exclusively positive in 8 (1.9%), and IgA was exclusively positive in 15 (3.6%) children. Conclusions: This study is the first to estimate the seroprevalence of SARS-CoV-2 among the pediatric population seeking medical care in southwestern Saudi Arabia. The findings shed light on the dynamics of virus transmission in the community and provide a good reference for future studies. Future research should examine factors related to SARS-CoV-2 infection and seroprevalence among pediatric populations.

Keywords: children; COVID-19; SARS-CoV-2; seroprevalence; COVID-19 serological testing

1. Introduction

COVID-19 is a highly contagious respiratory disease caused by SARS-CoV-2. The COVID-19 pandemic, which began in 2020, has had a devastating impact globally. As of July 2022, the World Health Organization (WHO) estimated that there were over 500 million cases of the virus and over 6 million deaths worldwide [1]. Additionally, during the pandemic through 2021, the WHO estimated that there were nearly 15 million additional deaths caused by both the virus itself and the impact of the pandemic on other health outcomes [2]. As of July 2022, the WHO also estimated that there had been nearly 800,000 cumulative cases of COVID-19 and over 9000 COVID-19 deaths in the Kingdom of Saudi Arabia [1]. Both the global and Saudi-specific estimates for deaths and cases are likely underestimated as cases of the disease go unreported. [3].

Cases of COVID-19 among children have received attention because they are often a very vulnerable population. Although children have a much lower case-fatality rate for COVID-19 compared to older populations [4], preventing infections among this population remains an important goal. In Saudi Arabia, one study estimates that children account for about 8% of cases [5], but the actual number may be higher due to underreporting. Additionally, these numbers may be underestimated because children are more likely to have asymptomatic infections and therefore not get tested [6].

Antibody testing for COVID-19 is a tool that can be used to determine the proportion of a population that has been infected with SARS-CoV-2. Antibody tests identify antibodies for SARS-CoV-2, which, in the prevaccine era, would most likely be caused by infection with the virus [7]. These antibodies are also present in asymptomatic individuals. There are limitations to the usage of antibody tests for COVID-19; they are not useful for identifying an active infection, and they can also result in false-positive and false-negative results. Additionally, some antibodies are cross-reactive with other viruses, which means a positive test result may not be due to a COVID-19 infection, but rather due to an infection with other viruses [7,8].

Previously, antibody studies were used to assess the proportion of asymptomatic COVID-19 infections. A systematic review of these studies estimated that around one-third of SARS-CoV-2 infections are asymptomatic [9]. A previous nationwide SARS-CoV-2 study in Saudi Arabia found that about 11% of the population had antibodies. In this study, the seroprevalence was much higher than the reported COVID-19 infection rate, and the seroprevalence was higher among healthcare workers [10]. In February of 2022, the United States Centers for Disease Control published the seroprevalence of SARS-CoV-2 among children between 0 and 11 years of age ranging between 40 and 75% [11].

There have been some studies that examined the presence of antibodies among children. These previous studies reported different seroprevalence values, ranging from a low value of 1.3% in Northern Cyprus [12] to 5.8% among school- and preschool-age children in Canada [13], 9.5% and 15.4% (for IgG) in Italy [14,15], and a high of 25.3% in Brazil [16]. Further seroprevalence studies among children in diverse geographic locations can provide additional details on SARS-CoV-2 infection among children. Therefore, this study sought to assess the seroprevalence for SARS-CoV-2 antibodies among a population of children who were admitted to hospital in Saudi Arabia. It also sought to determine whether the seroprevalence was associated with age group or gender.

2. Materials and Methods

2.1. Study Design, Setting, and Population

This is a cross-sectional study, the results of which are reported in accordance with the Guidelines for Strengthening the Reporting of Observational Studies in Epidemiology (STROBE) for Cross-sectional Studies [17]. The study was approved by the institutional review board of King Khalid University (approval number ECM#2021-5819), Abha, Saudi Arabia. The target population for this study is children attending Abha Maternity and Children Hospital (AMCH), a tertiary referral hospital in southwestern Saudi Arabia. The children who needed a blood test for any reason were included in this study. Written informed consent was obtained from all parents/guardians of the enrolled children. Inpatient, outpatient, and emergency department patients were included, based on two inclusion criteria: age less than 12 years of age and the need for a blood test for any reason. Patients were excluded for having risk factors for ongoing SARS-CoV-2 infection (typical symptoms, recent positive nasopharyngeal swab, contact with confirmed or suspected cases, and traveling abroad) and/or immunodeficiency, either primary or secondary. A total number of 413 children, who met the inclusion criteria, were sampled from the Serology Department at AMCH. Study data were obtained for patients seen between 1 October and 30 November 2021. An asymptomatic SARS-CoV-2 infection was defined as evident seropositivity in the absence of reported symptoms suggestive of COVID-19 (fever, chills, myalgia, ageusia, fatigue, anosmia, cough, and shortness of breath) [18].

2.2. Sampling Procedure and Processing

A sample of 454 children was planned to be included in the present study. The sample size was estimated based on an expected seroprevalence of 18% of COVID-19 antibodies in children [19], with an acceptable margin of error of 5% at a 95% confidence level and a design effect of 2. The sample size was determined using the Epi-Info 7 software (Centers for Disease Control and Prevention (CDC) in Atlanta, Georgia (US)), Serum samples were screened for SARS-CoV-2-specific IgG, IgM, and IgA antibodies using a commercially available indirect enzyme-linked immunosorbent assay (ELISA; Diapro, Milano, Italy). Two hundred microliters of the diluted (1:20 for IgM and 1:40 for IgG and IgA) test serum was added to microtiter plates containing 50 µL of neutralizing solution for IgM, 50 µL DILAS solution (the used assay diluent) for IgG and IgA along with a negative control in triplicate. A single positive control was added to the corresponding wells in the plates. One well was used as a blank in all plates for substrate addition only. The plates were sealed and incubated at 37 °C for 45 min. Plates were removed from the incubator and washed five times using an automatic ELISA plate washer 50 TS (BioTek® Instruments, Inc. Winooski, Vermont, USA). Then, 100 µL of anti-IgG, IgM, and IgA horseradish peroxidase conjugates was added to the corresponding plates. The plates were sealed and incubated again at 37 °C for 45 min. The plates were then rewashed as 100 µL of the substrate solution was added to all the wells and left for 15 min at room temperature, followed by 100 µL of stop solution. Wells were read at 450/620 nm using the ELISA reader (Humareader, Human company, Wiesbaden, Germany). The results were calculated as an antibody ratio in relation to standard cut-off values.

2.3. Statistical Analysis

The data were collected, managed, coded, and entered into the statistical software IBM SPSS version 22 (SPSS, Inc. Chicago, IL, USA). Frequency and percent distributions were calculated for all variables, including demographic data, clinical characteristics, and comorbidities. In addition, the mean with standard deviation was calculated for normally distributed quantitative variables, while the range and median with interquartile range (IQR) were calculated for skewed numerical variables. Adjusted seroprevalence among the studied children was calculated in addition to crude prevalence to account for screening test sensitivity and specificity as the test validity measures are not 100% with some probability for false-positive and false-negative results [20]. An analysis was conducted to test whether there was a relationship between serological findings and both age and gender. Finally, a logistic regression was used to test the odds of being seropositive according to age and gender.

3. Results

3.1. Characteristics of the Study Sample

Between 1 October and 30 November 2021, SARS-CoV-2-specific IgG, IgM, and IgA antibody levels were measured in 413 samples. The demographics and clinical characteristics of the enrolled children are shown in Table 1. Of the 413 children who were enrolled, 243 (58.8%) were male. The age range of enrolled patients was between newborn and 12 years of age, with a median age of three years (interquartile range, 1–7) years. School-age children (older than 5) were the most common age category (40%), and all age intervals were represented. Most of the children had Saudi citizenship (390, 94.4%). The inpatient department was the most common source for the analyzed samples. More than two thirds of the enrolled patients had comorbidities (342; 82.8%), with cardiopulmonary symptoms being the most frequently reported comorbidities.

Table 1. Demographics and clinical characteristics of the enrolled children.

Clinical Characteristic	Study Group n (%)
Age, median [IQR; min–max]	3 [1–7; 0–12]
Age categories in years	
<1	94 (22.8)
1–5	152 (36.8)
>5	167 (40.4)

Table 1. *Cont.*

Clinical Characteristic	Study Group n (%)
Gender	
Female	170 (41.2)
Male	243 (58.8)
Citizenship	
Saudi	390 (94.4)
Foreign	23 (5.6)
Department	
Outpatient	81 (39.5)
Emergency room/PICU	10 (4.9)
Inpatient	114 (55.6)
Comorbidities	
Yes	342 (82.8)
No	71 (17.2)

Data are shown as the median (interquartile range) or number (%) as appropriate. Pediatric Intensive Care Unit, PICU.

3.2. *SARS-CoV-2 IgG, IgM, and IgA Seroprevalence Results*

We identified 127 (30.7%) seropositive children out of the total of 413 children tested. As for seropositive children, IgG was exclusively positive in 43 (10.4%) children; IgM was exclusively positive in 8 (1.9%) children, and IgA was exclusively positive in 15 (3.6%) children. Sixteen (3.9%) were IgG- and IgA-positive; 28 (6.8%) were IgM- and IgG-positive; 1 (0.2%) was IgA- and IgM-positive, and 16 (3.9%) were IgM-, IgG- and IgA-positive (Figure 1).

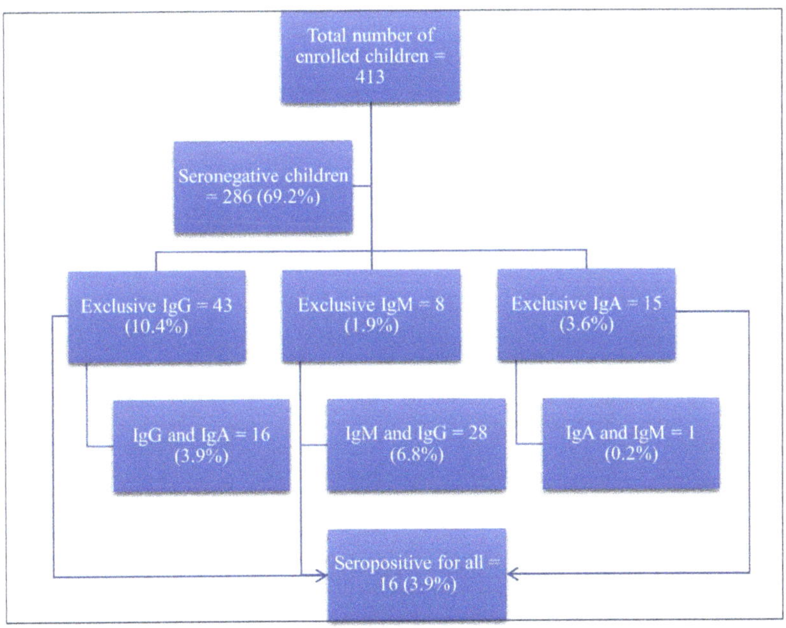

Figure 1. Flowchart of the seroprevalence among the study population.

Table 2 shows the crude seroprevalence and adjusted seroprevalence of COVID-19 antibodies among the children from whom the samples were tested. The adjusted prevalence for IgG antibodies was 26.6% (95% CI: 22.3–30.9%), that for IgM antibodies was 13.6% (95% CI:10.2–16.8%), and IgA antibody prevalence was 12.4% (95% CI: 9.2–15.6%). In total, seropositivity was found among 33.0% (95% CI: 28.5–37.4%) of the children from whom the samples were obtained.

Table 2. Crude and adjusted seroprevalence values of COVID-19 antibodies among children in Aseer region, Saudi Arabia.

Seroprevalence	No.	Crude Prevalence	Adjusted Prevalence	95% CI
IgG	103	24.9%	26.6%	22.3–30.9%
IgM	53	12.8%	13.6%	10.2–16.8%
IgA	48	11.6%	12.4%	9.2–15.6%
Seropositive	127	30.8%	33.0%	28.5–37.4%

CI: confidence interval.

3.3. *The Relation between Children's COVID-19 Seropositivity and Their Age and Gender*

Table 3 shows the crude and adjusted seroprevalence values of COVID-19 of children by their age and gender. The highest adjusted seroprevalence was found for children aged between 1 and 5 years 36.0% (95% CI: 28.4–43.6%), followed by school-age children (older than 5) 33.9% (95% CI: 26.7–41.1%) and children less than one year old 26.2% (95% CI: 17.3–35.1%). The adjusted seroprevalence was 35.9% (95% CI: 28.7–43.1%) among males and 30.8% (95% CI: 25.0–36.6%) among females.

Table 3. Crude and adjusted seroprevalences values of COVID-19 antibodies among children by their age and gender the in Aseer region, Saudi Arabia.

Variable	No.	Crude Prevalence (95% CI)	Adjusted Prevalence (95% CI)
Age in years			
- **<1**	23	24.5% (15.2–33.8%)	26.2% (17.3–35.1%)
- **1–5**	51	33.6% (25.4–40.3%)	36.0% (28.4–43.6%)
- **>5**	53	31.7% (24.6–38.7%)	33.9% (26.7–41.1%)
Gender			
- **Male**	70	55.1% (25.8–42.1%)	35.9% (28.7–43.1%)
- **Female**	57	44.9% (23.4–34.6%)	30.8% (25.0–36.6%)

CI: confidence interval.

Table 4 shows the crude and adjusted odds of the seropositivity of COVID-19 among children comparing males vs. females and different age groups. The odds of seropositivity adjusted for gender, age, and comorbidities was 1.54 (95% CI 0.86–2.74) for the 1–5-year-old age group compared to the children younger than 1 year old. Additionally, the rate of seropositivity for the age group >5 years was 1.41 (95% CI 0.79–2.5) compared with the children less than 1 year, while the rate of seropositivity among males was 1.25 (95% CI 0.8–1.87) compared to females. None of these comparisons was statistically significant. The crude odds ratios did not differ substantially from the adjusted odds ratios.

Table 4. Adjusted and crude relation between children's COVID-19 seropositivity and their age and gender.

Factors	COR	95% C.I for OR		AOR	95% C.I for OR	
		Lower	Upper		Lower	Upper
Age 1–5 Yrs. vs. <1 Yr.	1.56	0.874	2.779	1.54	0.86	2.74
Age > 5 Yrs. vs. <1 Yr.	1.44	0.810	2.543	1.41	0.79	2.5
Male vs. Female	1.25	0.82	1.89	1.20	0.80	1.87

COR: crude odds ratio; AOR: adjusted odds ratio, adjusting for age, gender, and the presence of commodities; CI: confidence interval.

4. Discussion

This study evaluated the seroprevalence of SARS-CoV-2 in 413 nonvaccinated children. To the best of the authors' knowledge, this is the first study on SARS-CoV-2 seroprevalence among children in southwest Saudi Arabia. Studies conducted among adult populations reported seroprevalence rates ranging from 1.4% to 50.2%. Other adult studies have also found different seroprevalence values [10,21–24]. This study was conducted before the Saudi MoH offered the COVID-19 vaccine for children between 5 and11 years of age, starting in February 2022. In southwest Saudi Arabia, we demonstrated a 33.0% adjusted seroprevalence rate of SARS-CoV-2 infection among hospital-based, nonvaccinated children aged 0–15 years. This result indicates that at least one in three unvaccinated children had acquired either symptomatic or asymptomatic COVID-19 infection within 18 months of the pandemic due to the presence of positive antibodies. The overall seroprevalence rate of SARS-CoV-2 among children in this study was higher than in other studies [13–16,19]. These previous studies showed a prevalence of 1.3% in Northern Cyprus [12], 5.8% among school- and preschool-age children in Canada [13], 9.5% to 15.4 (for IgG) in Italy [14,15], 27.1% in Saudi Arabia [19], and 25.3% in Brazil [16]. The higher prevalence in the current study could be explained by the fact that we conducted the study 18 months after the first reported case of COVID-19 in Saudi Arabia. The increase in seroprevalence in our study was consistent with the trend in confirmed cases in Saudi Arabia, with pediatric cases younger than 12 years of age increasing from 3% to 11% over a one-month period in May 2020 [5].

The SARS-CoV-2-specific IgG rate was 26.6%. In contrast, SARS-CoV-2-specific IgM and IgA were observed to be lower in the included children (13.6% and 12.4%, respectively). This indicates that a large number of children had previously been exposed to SARS-CoV-2. On the other hand, the presence of IgM and IgA suggests that many of the children may have had asymptomatic SARS-CoV, which is the most common manifestation of COVID-19 in children [24,25]. This is especially true as confirmed in previous studies, for the IgM and IgA classes of immunoglobulins specific to SARS-CoV-2 peak after two weeks following exposure to the virus, while the IgG peaks approximately at 28 days of infection [24–27].

The children who tested positive for SARS-CoV-2 IgM are suspected to have been infected by the virus in the period immediately prior to study since no vaccine is routinely used in this age group. No clinical disease was detected in these children on clinical observation, and consequently asymptomatic infection is suggested. An asymptomatic infection with SARS-CoV-2 is well-known and documented in various reports with an estimated prevalence of 30–50% of infections resulting in asymptomatic infection [24,25,28,29].

When comparing our study results with broad international studies that evaluated the seroprevalence of SARS-CoV-2 in children, the asymptomatic seropositivity rate found in our study is higher than the previously reported global seroprevalence, particularly within the first year of the pandemic, which was between 1 and 15% [5,12–16,20,21,30–32]. This variation may be explained by the fact that seropositivity is markedly influenced by various factors. These factors include variations in the study times and settings, sociodemographic criteria of the study participants, exposure risk, and implementation of school closures.

Although differences by age were not statistically significant, the current study revealed that children aged 1 to 5 years had the highest seroprevalence of SARS-CoV-2 (36.0% (28.4–43.6%)) compared to the other age groups of children tested. These children are considered to be in the preschool age group. This raises the issue that more attention should be paid to preventive care in this age group. In contrast, tested children younger than 1 year old had a seroprevalence of 26.2% (17.3–35.1%). Additionally, the study found a higher seroprevalence among males compared to females; however, this difference was not statistically significant. This finding is consistent with at least one other seroprevalence study from Saudi Arabia, which found a similar elevated seroprevalence among males compared to females [19]. While in this earlier study of adults, the higher seroprevalence may have been due to more exposure, such as work-related exposure among the male population, the reason for the increased seroprevalence among males in a pediatric population deserves more attention. A study from the United States estimated similar seroprevalence values for the population under 18 years of age for males and females [33].

Overall, the findings of the current study have public health implications, highlighting the importance of developing evidence-based guidelines for school closures and other social activities related to childhood during pandemics. This high seropositivity in children may provide a more accurate estimate of asymptomatic infections, which is needed to assess the spread of SARS-CoV-2 infection and gain a better understanding of local outbreaks of SARS-CoV-2 and how to control those outbreaks in the future. Pediatric hospitals may also need to implement more strict policies regarding infection control and the reduction in nosocomial infections since between 10 and 16% (IgM-positive) of visiting or admitted children had active asymptomatic infections with SARS-CoV-2.

Our study is limited by its hospital-based cross-sectional design. This design included patients with multiple comorbidities who needed frequent hospitalizations and were possibly exposed frequently to nosocomial infection. This may have led us to slightly overestimate the actual seroprevalence in the general child population. Data collection may also have suffered from a possible bias in the information collected from the medical records. Given the aforementioned limitations, we recommend community-based studies for the real estimation of the actual asymptomatic infection rate among the pediatric population in the country. In addition, the test used in this study does not have perfect sensitivity and specificity; although we adjusted for this issue in our analysis, it is still possible that some of those who tested positive for the presence of antibodies are false positives, and some of those who test negative for the presence of antibodies are false negatives. Furthermore, the presence of antibodies may decline over time; some children who were infected with SARS-CoV-2 early in the pandemic may not have tested positive because they no longer had detectable levels of antibodies. Moreover, SARS-CoV-2 antibodies have cross-reactivity with other viruses, such as MERS-CoV [8]. Some of the positive cases in this study may be due to infection with a virus other than SARS-CoV-2. Finally, the sample size of this study (413) was slightly below the required number based on our sample size calculation (454). This lower sample size may have impacted the precision of some of the estimates in this study and our ability to determine whether differences were statistically significant.

5. Conclusions

This is the first study identifying the seroprevalence of SARS-CoV-2 among a hospital-based pediatric population in the southwest region of Saudi Arabia. The observed rates likely reflect the patient population served by Abha Maternity and Children Hospital and do not necessarily apply to other centers. However, this study sheds light on the dynamics of viral transmission in the community of southwestern Saudi Arabia. It provides a good reference for future studies because of the large number of cases investigated, especially as future studies will be influenced by antibodies formed in response to vaccination. Future research should examine factors related to SARS-CoV-2 infection in pediatric populations and any protection afforded by the presence of SARS-CoV-2 antibodies from a previous infection.

Author Contributions: A.A.A. and A.A. designed the research, drafted the manuscript, interpreted the data, and performed the literature search and scientific overview of the manuscript. All authors have read and agreed to the published version of the manuscript.

Funding: This research was funded by the Institute of Research and Consulting Studies at King Khalid University through grant number # 16-2-S-2020.

Institutional Review Board Statement: This study was conducted according to the guidelines of the Declaration of Helsinki and approved by the Ethics Committee of King Khalid University with approval number (E.C.M. #2021-5819)-(HAPO-06-B-001) on 26 October 2021.

Informed Consent Statement: Informed consent was obtained from all the subjects involved in the study.

Data Availability Statement: The datasets used in this study are available from the corresponding authors upon request.

Acknowledgments: We thank the patients and their families for participation. In addition, the authors are thankful to the Deanship of Scientific Research and the Institute of Research and Consulting Studies at King Khalid University for supporting this research through grant number # 16-2-S-2020.

Conflicts of Interest: The authors declare no competing interest.

References

1. World Health Organization. Coronavirus (COVID-19) Dashboard. Available online: https://covid19.who.int/ (accessed on 12 July 2022).
2. World Health Organization. 14.9 Million Excess Deaths Associated with the COVID-19 Pandemic in 2020 and 2021. Available online: https://www.who.int/news/item/05-05-2022-14.9-million-excess-deaths-were-associated-with-the-covid-19-pandemic-in-2020-and-2021 (accessed on 14 July 2022).
3. Lau, H.; Khosrawipour, T.; Kocbach, P.; Ichii, H.; Bania, J.; Khosrawipour, V. Evaluating the massive underreporting and undertesting of COVID-19 cases in multiple global epicenters. *Pulmonology* **2021**, *27*, 110–115. [CrossRef] [PubMed]
4. Signorelli, C.; Odone, A. Age-specific COVID-19 case-fatality rate: No evidence of changes over time. *Int. J. Public Health* **2020**, *65*, 1435–1436. [CrossRef] [PubMed]
5. Alyami, M.H.; Naser, A.Y.; Orabi, M.A.A.; Alwafi, H.; Alyami, H.S. Epidemiology of COVID-19 in the Kingdom of Saudi Arabia: An Ecological Study. *Front. Public Health* **2020**, *8*, 506. [CrossRef] [PubMed]
6. Poletti, P.; Tirani, M.; Cereda, D.; Trentini, F.; Guzzetta, G.; Sabatino, G.; Marziano, V.; Castrofino, A.; Grosso, F.; Del Castillo, G.; et al. Association of Age With Likelihood of Developing Symptoms and Critical Disease Among Close Contacts Exposed to Patients With Confirmed SARS-CoV-2 Infection in Italy. *JAMA Netw. Open.* **2021**, *4*, e211085. [CrossRef]
7. Fei, Y.; Xu, H.; Zhang, X.; Musa, S.S.; Zhao, S.; He, D. Seroprevalence and infection attack rate of COVID-19 in Indian cities. *Infect. Dis. Model.* **2022**, *7*, 25–32. [CrossRef]
8. Jacofsky, D.; Jacofsky, E.M.; Jacofsky, M. Understanding Antibody Testing for COVID-19. *J. Arthroplast.* **2020**, *35*, S74–S81. [CrossRef]
9. Oran, D.P.; Topol, E.J. The Proportion of SARS-CoV-2 Infections That Are Asymptomatic: A Systematic Review. *Ann. Intern. Med.* **2021**, *174*, 655–662. [CrossRef]
10. Alharbi, N.K.; Alghnam, S.; Algaissi, A.; Albalawi, H.; Alenazi, M.W.; Albargawi, A.M.; Alharbi, A.G.; Alhazmi, A.; Al Qarni, A.; Alfarhan, A.; et al. Nationwide Seroprevalence of SARS-CoV-2 in Saudi Arabia. *J. Infect. Public Health* **2021**, *14*, 832–838. [CrossRef]
11. Kristie, E.N.; Clarke, J.M.J.; Deng, Y.; Nycz, E.; Lee, A.; Iachan, R.; Gundlapalli, A.V.; Hall, A.J.; MacNeil, A. Seroprevalence of Infection-Induced SARS-CoV-2 Antibodies—United States, September 2021–February 2022. *Morb. Mortal. Wkly. Rep. (MMWR)* **2022**, *71*, 606–608.
12. Gazi, U.; Sarioglu, A.A.; Ruh, E.; Sanlidag, B.; Dalkan, C.; Beyitler, I.; Suer, K.; Cakir, N.; Sayan, M.; Sanlidag, T. The pediatric asymptomatic SARS-CoV-2 IgG seropositivity in the Turkish Republic of Northern Cyprus. *Turk. J. Pediatr.* **2022**, *64*, 179–185. [CrossRef]
13. Zinszer, K.; McKinnon, B.; Bourque, N.; Pierce, L.; Saucier, A.; Otis, A.; Cheriet, I.; Papenburg, J.; Hamelin, M.E.; Charland, K.; et al. Seroprevalence of SARS-CoV-2 Antibodies Among Children in School and Day Care in Montreal, Canada. *JAMA Netw. Open* **2021**, *4*, e2135975. [CrossRef] [PubMed]
14. Comar, M.; Benvenuto, S.; Lazzerini, M.; Fedele, G.; Barbi, E.; Amaddeo, A.; Risso, F.M.; Strajn, T.; Di Rocco, P.; Stefanelli, P.; et al. Prevalence of SARS-CoV-2 infection in Italian pediatric population: A regional seroepidemiological study. *Ital. J. Pediatr.* **2021**, *47*, 131. [CrossRef] [PubMed]
15. Lazzerini, M.; Benvenuto, S.; Mariani, I.; Fedele, G.; Leone, P.; Stefanelli, P.; Vittori, G.; Schreiber, S.; Tommasini, A.; Rezza, G.; et al. Evolution of SARS-CoV-2 IgG Seroprevalence in Children and Factors Associated with Seroconversion: Results from a Multiple Time-Points Study in Friuli-Venezia Giulia Region, Italy. *Children* **2022**, *9*, 246. [CrossRef] [PubMed]

16. Cavalcante Pinto Junior, V.; Moura, L.; Cavalcante, R.C.; Lima, J.R.C.; Bezerra, A.S.; de Sousa Dantas, D.R.; Amaral, C.M.L.; Lima, D.F.; Junior, A.B.V.; Florindo Guedes, M.I. Prevalence of COVID-19 in children, adolescents and adults in remote education situations in the city of Fortaleza, Brazil. *Int. J. Infect. Dis.* **2021**, *108*, 20–26. [CrossRef]
17. von Elm, E.; Altman, D.G.; Egger, M.; Pocock, S.J.; Gotzsche, P.C.; Vandenbroucke, J.P.; Initiative, S. The Strengthening the Reporting of Observational Studies in Epidemiology (STROBE) Statement: Guidelines for reporting observational studies. *Int. J. Surg.* **2014**, *12*, 1495–1499. [CrossRef]
18. Marklund, E.; Leach, S.; Nystrom, K.; Lundgren, A.; Liljeqvist, J.A.; Nilsson, S.; Yilmaz, A.; Andersson, L.M.; Bemark, M.; Gisslen, M. Longitudinal Follow Up of Immune Responses to SARS-CoV-2 in Health Care Workers in Sweden With Several Different Commercial IgG-Assays, Measurement of Neutralizing Antibodies and CD4(+) T-Cell Responses. *Front. Immunol.* **2021**, *12*, 750448. [CrossRef]
19. Alhazmi, A.; Alamer, E.; Abdelwahab, S.; Khamjan, N.; Hamami, A.; Haddad, M.; Darraj, M.; Hashem, A.M.; Algaissi, A. Community-Based Seroprevalence of SARS-CoV-2 Antibodies following the First Wave of the COVID-19 Pandemic in Jazan Province, Saudi Arabia. *Int. J. Environ. Res. Public Health* **2021**, *18*, 2451. [CrossRef]
20. Sempos, C.T.; Tian, L. Adjusting Coronavirus Prevalence Estimates for Laboratory Test Kit Error. *Am. J. Epidemiol.* **2021**, *190*, 109–115. [CrossRef]
21. Banjar, A.; Al-Tawfiq, J.A.; Alruwaily, A.; Alserehi, H.; Al-Qunaibet, A.; Alaswad, R.; Almutlaq, H.; Almudaiheem, A.; Khojah, A.T.; Alsaif, F.; et al. Seroprevalence of antibodies to SARS-CoV-2 among blood donors in the early months of the pandemic in Saudi Arabia. *Int. J. Infect. Dis.* **2021**, *104*, 452–457. [CrossRef]
22. Almaghrabi, R.S.; Alsagheir, O.I.; Alquaiz, R.M.; Alhekail, O.Z.; Abaalkhail, A.M.; Alduaij, A.A.; Algwaiz, G.F.; Alkaff, M.A.; Althawadi, S.I. Seroprevalence of SARS-CoV-2 antibodies in healthcare workers at a tertiary care hospital in Riyadh, Saudi Arabia. *IJID Reg.* **2022**, *2*, 51–54. [CrossRef]
23. Almudarra, S.; Kamel, S.; Saleh, E.; Alaswad, R.; Alruwaily, A.; Almowald, S.; Alqunaibet, A.M.; Almudiaheem, A.; Almutlaq, H.; Alserehi, H.; et al. High seroprevalence of SARS-CoV-2 among high-density communities in Saudi Arabia. *Infection* **2022**, *50*, 643–649. [CrossRef] [PubMed]
24. Ali, A.S.; Al-Hakami, A.M.; Shati, A.A.; Asseri, A.A.; Al-Qahatani, S.M. Salient Conclusive Remarks on Epidemiology and Clinical Manifestations of Pediatric COVID-19: Narrative Review. *Front. Pediatr.* **2020**, *8*, 584694. [CrossRef] [PubMed]
25. Li, B.; Zhang, S.; Zhang, R.; Chen, X.; Wang, Y.; Zhu, C. Epidemiological and Clinical Characteristics of COVID-19 in Children: A Systematic Review and Meta-Analysis. *Front. Pediatr.* **2020**, *8*, 591132. [CrossRef] [PubMed]
26. Zervou, F.N.; Louie, P.; Stachel, A.; Zacharioudakis, I.M.; Ortiz-Mendez, Y.; Thomas, K.; Aguero-Rosenfeld, M.E. SARS-CoV-2 antibodies: IgA correlates with severity of disease in early COVID-19 infection. *J. Med. Virol.* **2021**, *93*, 5409–5415. [CrossRef] [PubMed]
27. Ma, H.; Zeng, W.; He, H.; Zhao, D.; Jiang, D.; Zhou, P.; Cheng, L.; Li, Y.; Ma, X.; Jin, T. Serum IgA, IgM, and IgG responses in COVID-19. *Cell Mol. Immunol.* **2020**, *17*, 773–775. [CrossRef]
28. Sah, P.; Fitzpatrick, M.C.; Zimmer, C.F.; Abdollahi, E.; Juden-Kelly, L.; Moghadas, S.M.; Singer, B.H.; Galvani, A.P. Asymptomatic SARS-CoV-2 infection: A systematic review and meta-analysis. *Proc. Natl. Acad. Sci. USA* **2021**, *118*, e2109229118. [CrossRef] [PubMed]
29. Hurst, J.H.; Heston, S.M.; Chambers, H.N.; Cunningham, H.M.; Price, M.J.; Suarez, L.; Crew, C.G.; Bose, S.; Aquino, J.N.; Carr, S.T.; et al. Severe Acute Respiratory Syndrome Coronavirus 2 Infections Among Children in the Biospecimens from Respiratory Virus-Exposed Kids (BRAVE Kids) Study. *Clin. Infect. Dis.* **2021**, *73*, e2875–e2882. [CrossRef]
30. Koirala, A.; Gidding, H.F.; Vette, K.; Macartney, K.; Group, P.S. The seroprevalence of SARS-CoV-2-specific antibodies in children, Australia, November 2020–March 2021. *Med. J. Aust.* **2022**, *217*, 43–45. [CrossRef]
31. Dethioux, L.; Dauby, N.; Montesinos, I.; Rebuffat, E.; Hainaut, M. SARS-CoV-2 seroprevalence in children and their family members, July-October 2020, Brussels. *Eur. J. Pediatr.* **2022**, *181*, 1009–1016. [CrossRef]
32. Smith, B.K.; Janowski, A.B.; Danis, J.E.; Harvey, I.B.; Zhao, H.; Dai, Y.N.; Farnsworth, C.W.; Gronowski, A.M.; Roper, S.; Fremont, D.H.; et al. Seroprevalence of SARS-CoV-2 Antibodies in Children and Adults in St. Louis, Missouri, USA. *mSphere* **2021**, *6*, e01207-20. [CrossRef]
33. Hobbs, C.V.; Drobeniuc, J.; Kittle, T.; Williams, J.; Byers, P.; Satheshkumar, P.S.; Inagaki, K.; Stephenson, M.; Kim, S.S.; Patel, M.M.; et al. Estimated SARS-CoV-2 Seroprevalence Among Persons Aged <18 Years-Mississippi, May-September 2020. *MMWR Morb. Mortal. Wkly. Rep.* **2021**, *70*, 312–315. [CrossRef] [PubMed]

vaccines

Article

Antibody Titers and Protection against Omicron (BA.1 and BA.2) SARS-CoV-2 Infection

Chloé Dimeglio [1,2,*], Marion Migueres [1,2], Naémie Bouzid [1], Sabine Chapuy-Regaud [1,2], Caroline Gernigon [3,4], Isabelle Da-Silva [1], Marion Porcheron [1], Guillaume Martin-Blondel [2,5], Fabrice Herin [3,4] and Jacques Izopet [1,2]

1 CHU Toulouse, Hôpital Purpan, Virology Laboratory, 31300 Toulouse, France
2 Toulouse Institute for Infectious and Inflammatory Diseases (INFINITy), 31300 Toulouse, France
3 Occupational Diseases Department, Toulouse University Hospital, 31000 Toulouse, France
4 UMR1295, Unité Mixte INSERM—Université Toulouse III Paul Sabatier, Centre for Epidemiology and Research in Population Health Unit (CERPOP), 31000 Toulouse, France
5 Infectious and Tropical Diseases Department, Toulouse University Hospital, 31300 Toulouse, France
* Correspondence: dimeglio.c@chu-toulouse.fr

Abstract: The emergence of the SARS-CoV-2 variants of concern has greatly influenced the immune correlates of protection, and there are little data about the antibody threshold concentrations to protect against infection with SARS-CoV-2 Omicron BA.1 or BA.2. We analyzed the antibody responses of 259 vaccinated healthcare workers, some of whom had been previously infected by SARS-CoV-2. The median follow-up was 179 days (IQR: 171–182) after blood collection. We detected 88 SARS-CoV-2 Omicron infections during the follow-up period, 55 (62.5%) with SARS-CoV-2 BA.1, and 33 (37.5%) with SARS-CoV-2 BA.2. A neutralizing antibody titer below 8 provided no protection against a BA.1 infection, a titer of 16 or 32 gave 73.2% protection, and a titer of 64 or 128 provided 78.4% protection. Conversely, the BA.2 infection rate did not vary as a function of anti-BA.2 neutralizing antibody titers. Binding antibody concentrations below 6000 BAU/mL provided no protection against Omicron BA.1 infection, 6000–20,000 BAU/mL provided 55.6% protection, and 20,000 or more provided 87.7% protection. There was no difference in BA.2 infection depending on the binding antibody concentration. Further studies are needed to investigate the relationship between antibody concentrations and infection with the Omicron BA.4/5 variants that are becoming predominant worldwide.

Keywords: SARS-CoV-2; Omicron; antibodies; protection; public health

1. Introduction

Since December 2020, the coronavirus disease 2019 (COVID-19) pandemic has been dominated by the emergence of severe acute respiratory syndrome coronavirus 2 (SARS-CoV-2) variants of concern (VOCs). The latest to date is the Omicron (B.1.1.529) variant, further divided into distinct sublineages: BA.1, BA.2, BA.3, BA.4, and BA.5. These new variants harboring numerous spike protein mutations, particularly in the receptor binding domain (RBD), have spread rapidly worldwide because they were more transmissible or more prone to immune escape.

The SARS-CoV-2 pandemic has resulted in substantial morbidity, mortality, and social disruption. However, vaccination and a previous infection provide a degree of protection against symptomatic, severe COVID-19 [1]. The vaccines presently available to protect against such infections all use the ancestral (Wuhan-like) virus or its spike protein as immunogen.

Serological diagnosis is becoming increasingly important in attempts to understand the extent to which COVID-19 is spreading in the community and to identify individuals who are immunized and potentially "protected" against re-infection. The most widely accepted marker of protection against a SARS-CoV-2 infection is the concentration of neutralizing antibody [2,3] that prevent viral infection mostly by blocking the early step of infection, viral entry, especially in interfering with virions binding to their receptor. There is also a correlation between the concentrations of neutralizing antibody and those of binding antibodies measured by immunoassays that use ancestral strain antigens [1–6]. The concentration of anti-spike IgG produced by vaccination or natural infection is associated with protection against infections of SARS-CoV-2 strains that were present before the Omicron variant emerged in November 2021 [7–9]. Goldblatt et al. used a random effects meta-analytic approach to calculate protective thresholds in WHO units for ancestral strain SARS-CoV-2 and Alpha (B.1.1.7) of 154 (95% CI 42, 559) and 171 (95% CI 57, 519) anti-S binding antibody units (BAU/mL), respectively [10]. It was consistent with the threshold of 141 BAU/mL conferring more than 89% protection, according to another study [7]. A slightly higher protective threshold of 264 BAU/mL was also proposed [8]. Gilbert et al. reported geometric mean neutralization titers ~247 IU/mL [9], compared to 1057 IU/mL in Khoury et al. [2], suggesting that different protection thresholds could be obtained depending on the neutralization assay used.

The emergence of these SARS-CoV-2 variants of concern (VOC) with increased transmissibility and the capacity to escape natural and vaccine immunity [11–14] has greatly influenced the immune correlates of protection. In late 2020, the Delta variant (B.1.617) was detected in India and spread rapidly worldwide, displacing other variants. Notable mutations in the B.1.617.2 variant included L452R, T478K, and E484Q in the S RBD. The combination of mutations in the Delta variant seems to impart the virus a selective advantage compared to the original virus and other variants, as evidenced by high transmissibility and infectivity, and immune evasion [11]. In late 2021, the B.1.1.529 variant emerged in Southern Africa and contains several mutations present in other variants, such as N501Y (Alpha), E484A~E484K (Beta and Gamma), and T478K (Delta), although in total it has more than 50 mutations with more than 30 identified in the S gene alone [15]. These mutations are associated with enhanced infectivity and transmissibility, and Omicron has also been demonstrated to escape neutralization by monoclonal antibodies, convalescent serum, and post-vaccine antibody [12]. Overall, with the exception of the Alpha VOC, the emerging VOCs have been associated with reductions in neutralizing activity of antibodies derived from previously infected or individuals who have undergone primary vaccination [16–19]. Evidence based on in vitro neutralization assays suggests that, for immune responses to Omicron in individuals who have already been exposed to ancestral SARS-CoV-2 antigens (whether through infection or vaccination), an Omicron correlate of protection may be higher than for ancestral SARS-CoV-2 or other VOCs, due to the reduced effectiveness of antibodies directed against the spike protein. To that point, Pfizer-BioNTech has reported a 25-fold reduction in neutralization titres against Omicron compared to ancestral SARS-CoV-2 in individuals vaccinated with two doses of BNT162b2 [20]. Studies from South Africa and Germany report a reduction in neutralization up to 41-fold [17], despite two or three doses of BNT162b2 or mRNA-1273 and previous infection. We therefore have determined the antibody threshold concentrations (binding and neutralizing antibodies) needed to protect against infection with SARS-CoV-2 Omicron BA.1 or BA.2.

2. Material and Methods

2.1. Patients

We analyzed the antibody responses of 259 vaccinated healthcare workers (HCWs), some of whom had been previously infected by SARS-CoV-2. Blood samples were taken 3–6 weeks (median: 4.2 weeks) after their last dose of vaccine (12 September 2021–13 October 2021) and before the Omicron variant arrived in France (December 2021–January 2022). The median follow-up was 179 days (IQR: 171–182) after blood collection. This study was approved by the French Research Ethics Committee Est-III (COVID BioToul, ID-RCB 2020-A01292-37, ClinicalTrials.gov Identifier: NCT04385108).

2.2. SARS-CoV-2 Detection, Variant Screening, and Genome Sequencing

Nucleic acids were extracted from nasopharyngeal swab samples on an MGI SP-960 instrument using the MGIEasy Nucleic Acid Extraction kit and amplified with the Thermofisher TaqPath RT-PCR assay (ThermoFisher, Waltham, MA, USA) on QuantStudio 5 Real-Time PCR systems. Positive results were then classified, according to the TaqPath S gene profile, as: S gene target failure (SGTF), S gene target late detection (SGTL), or non-SGTF/SGTL [21]. The SGTL profile was defined as a difference of at least 4 Ct between the N and S genes. The Omicron BA.1 variant was identified by its SGTF/SGTL TaqPath profiles (69–70 S gene deletion). Positive specimens with non-SGTF/SGTL profiles (only samples with N Ct $\leq$ 30) were then tested using the IDTM SARS-CoV-2/VOC Revolution Pentaplex assay (ID solutions, Montpellier, France). This multiplex RT-PCR assay targets the K417N, L452R, and E484K mutations. The Omicron BA.2 variant was identified by the presence of the K417N mutation. Our VOC screening strategy was validated by sequencing a large number of positive nasopharyngeal samples using the Pacific Biosciences (Pacbio) SMRT System [22].

2.3. Neutralizing and Binding Antibodies against SARS-CoV-2 Spike Protein

Neutralizing antibody (NAb) titers were measured by end-point dilution using Vero cells (ATCC, CCL-81™) [14] and clinical strains of SARS-CoV-2 Omicron BA.1 (EPI_ISL_10316329) and BA.2 (EPI_ISL_13540703). Anti-spike Immunoglobulin G (anti-S) concentrations were measured with an electrochemiluminescent assay, which is a binding antibody assay based on the RBD of the Spike protein (IgG II Quant, Alinity, Abbott, Sligo, Ireland) [4]. Raw data in AU/mL were converted in BAU/mL by using the conversion factor (0.142) recommended by the manufacturer.

2.4. Antibodies against SARS-CoV-2 Nucleocapsid Protein

Anti-nucleocapside (anti-N) antibodies were detected with an electrochemiluminescent assay (SARS-CoV-2 IgG, Alinity, Abbott, Sligo, Ireland). They can differentiate between natural and vaccine-derived sero reactivity.

2.5. Statistical Analysis

Correlations were identified using a Spearman test and groups were compared with the Chi^2 or Fisher's exact tests. Statistical significance was set at: p-value < 0.05.

The anonymized data were analyzed using Stata version 14 (StataCorp LP, College Station, TX, USA) and MATLAB 2018b.

3. Results

3.1. Population Characteristics and Vaccination Status

The 259 HCWs included 193 (74.5%) women (median age: 41.5, range: 21–61) and 66 (25.5%) men (median age: 41, range 22–61, $p > 0.05$ Wilcoxon rank test). 168 (64.9%) had been infected with SARS-CoV-2 before their vaccination (identified by positive PCR or the presence of anti-N antibodies at baseline). Most of them (152/168, 90.5%) had been given a BNT162b/BNT162b, 2-dose, vaccination schedule, while 16 (9.5%) others had a ChAdOx1-S/BNT162b schedule (Table 1). The majority (148/168, 88.1%) had only two doses of vaccine; 20/168 (11.9%) had a BNT162b booster (third dose) between 15 July and 30 August 2021. The 91 vaccinated HCWs with no previous infection included 8 (8.8%) given a ChAdOx1-S/ ChAdOx1-S schedule, 46 (50.5%) given ChAdOx1-S/BNT162b, and 37 (40.7%) given BNT162b/BNT162b (Table 1). Most of the 91 initially uninfected HCW (75, 82.4%) were given a BNT162b booster following 2-dose vaccination; the other 16 (11.6%) had only a primary vaccination (2 doses).

Table 1. HCW characteristics according to infectious status: infected then vaccinated or vaccinated without a past infection.

HCWs	Infected/Vaccinated	Vaccinated
N (%)	168 (64.9)	91 (35.1)
Age: Median (IQR)	39 (21–58)	42 (21–61)
Female: N (%)	130 (77.4)	63 (69.2)
Vaccines: *n* (%)		
BNT162b/BNT162b	152 (90.5)	37 (40.7)
ChadOx1-S/BNT162b	16 (9.5)	46 (50.5)
ChadOx1-S/ChadOx1-S	0	8 (8.8)
Vaccination status: *n* (%)		
-Primary vaccinated (2 doses)	148 (88.1)	16 (17.6)
-Primary vaccinated + booster dose	20 (11.9)	75 (82.4)

3.2. Occurrence of SARS-CoV-2 Infections

We detected 88 SARS-CoV-2 Omicron infections during the follow-up period, 55 (62.5%) with SARS-CoV-2 BA.1, and 33 (37.5%) with SARS-CoV-2 BA.2. No HCW required hospitalization for their SARS-CoV-2 Omicron infection.

The 36 (65.5%) BA.1 infections that occurred in vaccinated HCWs without prior infection included 29/75 (38.7%) detected within 44 days (median) after booster administration (range: 26–118 days), and 7/16 (43.8%) after complete vaccination without booster (Figure 1). The remaining 19 (34.5%) BA.1 infections occurred in HCWs infected with a strain of SARS-CoV-2 before their vaccination: 2/20 (10%) within 50 days (median, range 30–95) after booster administration, and 17/148 (10.6%) after 2-dose vaccination, no booster (Figure 1).

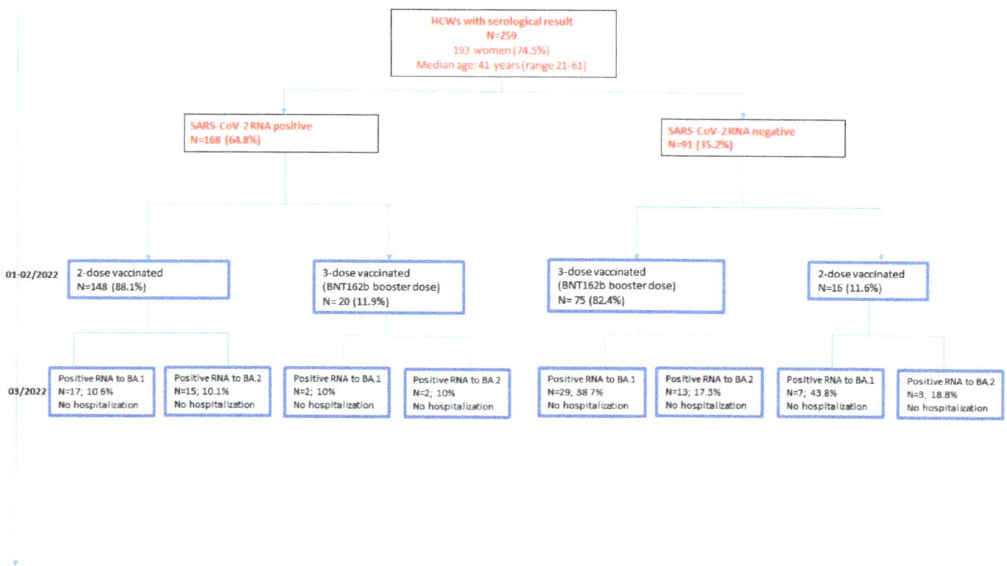

Figure 1. Study flowchart.

Similarly, 16 (48.5%) uninfected, vaccinated HCWs had BA.2 infections: 13/75 (17.3%) within 44 days (median, range: 17–74 days) after booster administration, and 3/16 (18.8%)

after complete vaccination without booster (Figure 1). The remaining 17 (51.5%) BA.2 infections occurred in HCWs infected with a strain of SARS-CoV-2 before their vaccination: 2/20 (10%) within 49 days (median, range 26–169 days) after a booster, and 15/148 (10.1%) after 2-dose vaccination (Figure 1).

3.3. Neutralizing Antibodies and Protection against SARS-CoV-2 BA.1 and BA.2

The median BA.1 neutralizing antibody (NAb) titer of the previously uninfected, vaccinated HCWs was 2 (IQR: 2–4) and their median anti-BA.2 NAb titer was 2 (IQR: 0–8) (Figure 2). The median anti-BA.1 titer in the infected-prior-to-vaccination HCWs was 8 (IQR: 4–16); it was 16 for BA.2 NAb (IQR: 16–32) (Figure 3). The correlation between the BA.1 and BA.2 neutralizing antibody titers was 0.78 ($p < 0.01$, Spearman test) among the previously uninfected, vaccinated HCWs and 0.86 ($p < 0.01$, Spearman test) among those infected before vaccination.

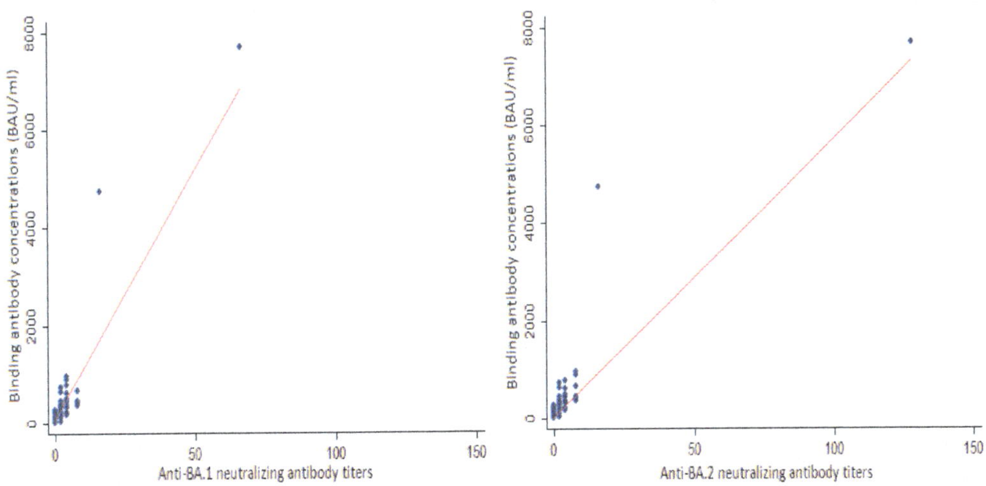

Figure 2. Binding antibody concentrations according to BA.1 and BA.2 neutralizing antibody titers among uninfected/vaccinated HCWs and trend curve (red line).

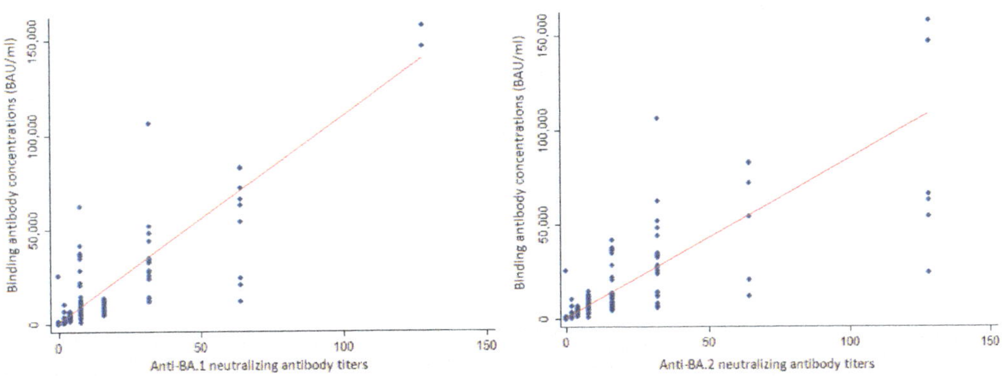

Figure 3. Binding antibody concentrations according to BA.1 and BA.2 neutralizing antibody titers among infected/vaccinated HCWs and trend curve (red line).

About one third of the HCWs whose anti-BA.1 NAb titer was below 8 (average: 28.4%, 95% CI: 19.9–38.2%) became infected with Omicron BA.1. In contrast, few (7%, [95% CI: 1.5–19.1%]) of those whose BA.1 NAb titer was 16–32, or those with NAb titers of 64 or 128 (6.2%, [95% CI: 1.6–30.2%]) became BA.1 infected ($p < 0.01$, Chi^2 test). An NAb titer below 8 provided no protection against a BA.1 infection, a titer of 16 or 32 gave 73.2% protection, and an NAb titer of 64 or 128 provided 78.4% protection (Figure 4).

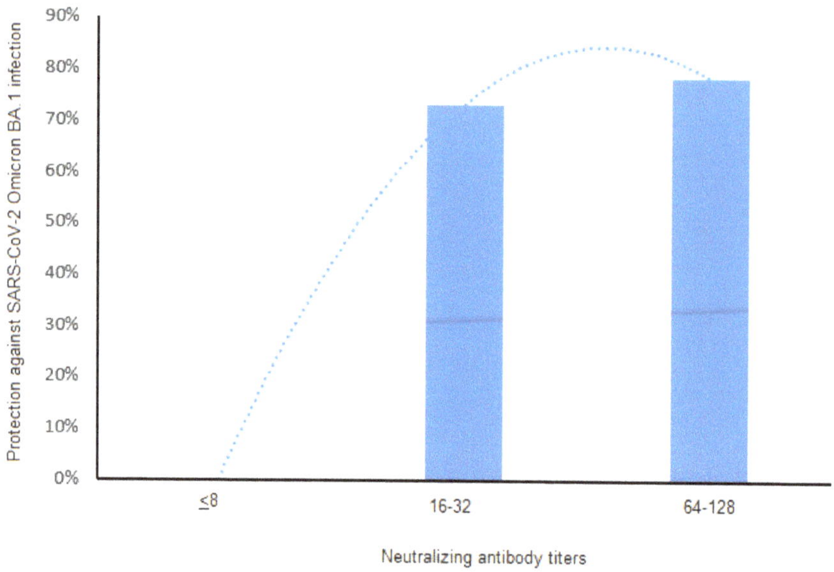

Figure 4. BA.1 neutralizing antibody titers and protection against SARS-CoV-2 Omicron BA.1 infection/re-infection with polynomial trend curve (dotted line).

Conversely, the BA.2 infection rate did not vary as a function of anti-BA.2 NAb titers. Only 6.9% (95% CI: 2.8–13.6%) of the HCWs with an anti-BA.2 NAb titer below 8 became infected with Omicron BA.2, as did 16.3% [95% CI: 6.8–30.7%] of those whose BA.2 NAb titer was 16–32, and 22.2% [95% CI: 2.8–60%] of those with an anti-BA.2 NAb titer of 64 or 128 ($p = 0.12$, Chi^2).

3.4. Binding Antibodies and Protection against SARS-CoV-2 BA.1 and BA.2

The correlations between the binding antibody (BAb) concentrations and the BA.1 and BA.2 NAb titers were 0.71 ($p < 0.01$, Spearman test) and 0.89 ($p < 0.01$, Spearman test), respectively. Of those HCWs who became infected with BA.1 between November 2021 and March 2022, 26.9% [95% CI: 19.8–35.1%] had a BAb concentration below 6000 BAU/mL, 12.1% [95% CI: 3.4–28.2%] had a BAb concentration of 6000–20,000 BAU/mL, and only 3.3% [95% CI: 0.4–11.3%] had a BAb concentrations of 20,000 BAU/mL or more ($p < 0.01$, Chi^2). BAb concentrations below 6000 BAU/mL provided no protection against Omicron BA.1 infection, 6000–20,000 BAU/mL provided 55.6% protection, and 20,000 or more provided 87.7% protection (Figure 5).

On the other hand, there was no difference in BA.2 infection depending on the BAb concentration: 9.2% [95% CI: 5–15.2%] of HCWs with a BAb concentration below 6000 BAU/mL became infected with BA.2 between November 2021 and March 2022, as did 12.1% [95% CI: 3.4–28.2%] of those HCWs with a BAb concentration of 6000–20,000 BAU/mL, and 6.6% [95% CI: 1.8–15.9%] of those whose BAb concentration was 20,000 BAU/mL and above ($p = 0.65$, Chi^2).

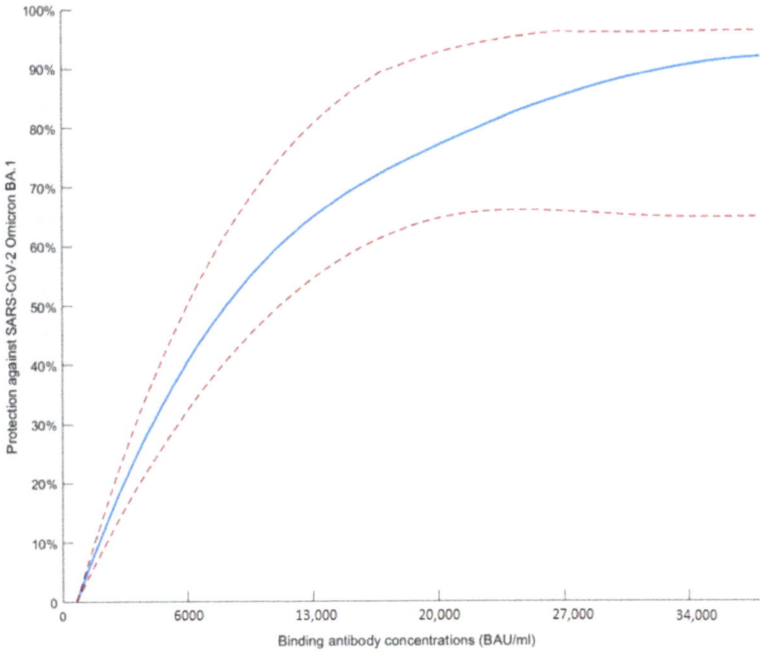

Figure 5. Binding antibody concentrations and protection against SARS-CoV-2 Omicron BA.1 infection/re-infection by spline interpolation (95% CI: dotted line).

3.5. Antibody Concentrations and Vaccination Status

Half the previously-infected HCWs (10/20, 50%) given a booster dose had an anti-BA.1 NAb titer above 64, as did only 5/148 (3.4%) of those given two doses ($p < 0.01$, Fisher's exact test). Those HCW given a booster dose (4/20, 20%) had BAb titers above 6000 BAU/mL, as did only 4/148 (2.7%) of those given two doses ($p < 0.01$, Fisher's exact test).

Only 1/75 (1.3%) of the HCWs who were not infected before vaccination and given a booster dose of vaccine had an anti-BA.1 NAb titer exceeding 64, or a BAb concentration above 6000 BAU/mL. None of the 16 vaccinated (2 doses, no booster) HCWs had a neutralizing antibody titer above 64 or a Bab concentration above 6000 BAU/mL.

4. Discussion

Several pre-oOmicron clinical [2,5,7–9] and animal [23] studies found that the neutralizing and binding antibody concentrations were good biomarkers of protection against a SARS-CoV-2 infection. We now find a similar relationship between the concentrations of anti-BA.1 binding and neutralizing antibodies and protection against a BA.1 SARS-CoV-2 infection.

We also find that there is no clear antibody concentration above which Omicron infection does not occur, in contrast to infections with the alpha variant or other earlier strains (D614G) [7]. Although we found an inverse link between the risk of a SARS-CoV-2 BA.1 infection and the anti-BA.1 NAb and Bab concentration, there seems to be no such link for BA.2. This could be due to differences in the time between antibody assay and SARS-CoV-2 BA.1 and BA.2 infections, or differences in the restrictions in place during the BA.1 wave (November 2021–February 2022) and BA.2 wave (March 2022–May 2022). Wearing masks and physical distancing were abolished in France on 14 March 2022, which could have resulted in greater exposure to BA.2 infections, even in HCWs with high anti-BA.2 NAb and BAb concentrations. The degree of protection conferred on this same HCW population by a NAb against the B.1.160 strain (D614G) varied slightly [7]. Titers of 64–128 anti-B.1.160 NAb conferred 94% protection against a D614G strain, and 64–128 anti-BA.1 NAb conferred 78.4% protection against BA.1. While an anti-B.1.160 NAb titer of 256 or more provided 100% protection, no HCW had anti-BA.1 or anti-BA.2 NAb titers greater than 256. A BAb concentration of 141 BAU/mL or more provided approximately 89.3% protection against infection with a D614G strain, and a BAb concentration of 1700 BAU/mL or more provided 100% protection. Our present results indicate that a concentration of 20,000 BAU/mL is needed for an equivalent degree of protection, approximately 142-times the 141 BAU/mL threshold concentration. This is probably due to differences in the antigenicity of the spike proteins in Omicron BA.1 and the ancestral SARS-CoV-2 strain used in current vaccines and immunoassays [24]. Similarly, 8.5 times more binding antibody is required to neutralize the Delta variant than to neutralize the Alpha variant [14]. Our results partially agree with those of a recent Danish study [25] that demonstated that the inverse relationship between the IgG level and the risk of contagion observed for the Delta variant demonstrated the protective effect of vaccines, but this association was not observed for the Omicron variant. This suggests that the quantitative level of anti-spike IgG has a limited impact on the risk of breakthrough infection with Omicron. Note, however, that the study did not distinguish between infections caused by the BA.1 strain or the BA.2 strain of Omicron. Another study on nursing home residents demonstrated correlates of protection between the level of (binding and neutralizing) antibodies and Omicron BA.2 infection [26]. A BA.2 NAb title below 8 provided 19.2% protection against Omicron BA.2, titles of 16 or 32 gave 85.3% protection and an NAb title of 64 or more provided 95.6% protection. A BAb concentration below 1000 BAU/mL provided only 25% protection against Omicron BA.2; 1000–6000 BAU/mL provided 77.9% protection; while >6000 provided 97.1% protection. It should be noted, however, that this population, which is particularly at risk, continued to benefit from restrictive sanitary measures, unlike the general population, and that in this study it was very little exposed to Omicron BA.1.

Although current vaccines reduce the risk of a symptomatic SARS-CoV-2 infection, hospitalization and death, their effectiveness against the Omicron variant [11,17,27,28] is altered due to lower neutralizing antibody titers. We found that a greater percentage of previously infected, vaccinated HCWs had high NAb and BAb titers than did uninfected vaccinated HCW. This is consistent with studies indicating that vaccination of previously infected individuals gives greater protection than the vaccination of naive individuals [29].

The limitations of this study concern both vaccination and antibody measurement. First, antibodies were not measured at the time of SARS-CoV-2 breakthrough. Waning antibody titers are associated with loss of protection [30] and the post-vaccination total antibody titer decreases faster in vaccinated people with no previous SARS-CoV-2 infection than in previously-infected, vaccinated individuals [30]. Second, all the HCWs were not given a booster vaccination at the time of analysis, particularly those HCWs who were infected before being vaccinated. The majority were given a complete (2-dose) schedule without booster. Third, we did not discriminate between infection and symptomatic disease. The antibody concentrations providing robust protection from severe infection require further investigation in other populations. Last, the contribution of the T-cell system to protection was not assessed.

5. Conclusions

This is, to our knowledge, the first study of protective antibody thresholds against infection with Omicron BA.1 and BA.2. We provide further evidence in a longitudinal cohort that robust antibody levels against the ancestral strain fail to establish sufficient protection against antigenically distant variants. Further, we demonstrate that a full booster vaccination schedule without infection may not adequately confer protection against breakthrough infection with the Omicron variant [25]. In order to achieve more robust immune protection and limit SARS-CoV-2 transmission, the next generation of SARS-CoV-2 vaccine preparations will include Omicron subvariant's spike determinants in addition to ancestral strain antigens [31].

While our results provide markers of protection against BA.1 infection, further studies are needed to investigate the relationship between antibody concentrations and infection with the Omicron BA.4/5 variants that are becoming predominant worldwide.

Author Contributions: Conceptualization, C.D., F.H., and J.I..; methodology, C.D.; software, C.D.; validation, C.D. and N.B.; formal analysis, C.D. and N.B.; investigation, G.M.-B.; resources, M.M., I.D.-S., M.P., F.H. and C.G.; data curation, M.M., I.D.-S., M.P. and S.C.-R.; writing—original draft preparation, C.D.; writing—review and editing, J.I.; visualization, M.M., N.B., S.C.-R., I.D.-S., M.P., C.G., G.M.-B., F.H. and J.I.; supervision, F.H. and J.I. All authors have read and agreed to the published version of the manuscript.

Funding: This research received no external funding.

Institutional Review Board Statement: The study was conducted in accordance with the Declaration of Helsinki, and approved by the Institutional Review Board (or Ethics Committee) of CHU de Toulouse (COVID BioToul, ID-RCB 2020-A01292-37, ClinicalTrials.gov Identifier: NCT04385108).

Informed Consent Statement: Informed consent was obtained from all subjects involved in.

Data Availability Statement: The data that support the findings of this study are available from the corresponding author upon reasonable request.

Acknowledgments: The English text was edited by Owen Parkes.

Conflicts of Interest: The authors declare no conflict of interest.

References

1. Bok, K.; Sitar, S.; Graham, B.S.; Mascola, J.R. Accelerated COVID-19 vaccine development: Milestones, lessons, and prospects. *Immunity* **2021**, *54*, 1636–1651. [CrossRef] [PubMed]
2. Khoury, D.S.; Cromer, D.; Reynaldi, A.; Schlub, T.E.; Wheatley, A.K.; Juno, J.A.; Subbarao, K.; Kent, S.J.; Triccas, J.A.; Davenport, M.P. Neutralizing antibody levels are highly predictive of immune protection from symptomatic SARS-CoV-2 infection. *Nat. Med.* **2021**, *27*, 1205–1211. [CrossRef] [PubMed]
3. Cromer, D.; Steain, M.; Reynaldi, A.; Schlub, T.E.; Wheatley, A.K.; Juno, J.A.; Kent, S.J.; Triccas, J.A.; Khoury, D.S.; Davenport, M.P. Neutralising antibody titres as predictors of protection against SARS-CoV-2 variants and the impact of boosting: A meta-analysis. *Lancet Microbe* **2022**, *3*, e52–e61. [CrossRef]
4. Chapuy-Regaud, S.; Miédougé, M.; Abravanel, F.; Da Silva, I.; Porcheron, M.; Fillaux, J.; Diméglio, C.; Izopet, J. Evaluation of Three Quantitative Anti-SARS-CoV-2 Antibody Immunoassays. *Microbiol. Spectr.* **2021**, *9*, e0137621. [CrossRef]
5. Bergwerk, M.; Gonen, T.; Lustig, Y.; Amit, S.; Lipsitch, M.; Cohen, C.; Mandelboim, M.; Levin, E.G.; Rubin, C.; Indenbaum, V.; et al. Covid-19 breakthrough infections in vaccinated health care workers. *N. Engl. J. Med.* **2021**, *385*, 1474–1484. [CrossRef] [PubMed]
6. Resman Rus, K.; Korva, M.; Knap, N.; Avšič Županc, T.; Poljak, M. Performance of the rapid high-throughput automated electrochemiluminescence immunoassay targeting total antibodies to the SARS-CoV-2 spike protein receptor binding domain in comparison to the neutralization assay. *J. Clin. Virol.* **2021**, *139*, 104820. [CrossRef]
7. Dimeglio, C.; Herin, F.; Martin-Blondel, G.; Miedougé, M.; Izopet, J. Antibody titers and protection against a SARS-CoV-2 infection. *J. Infect.* **2022**, *84*, 248–288. [CrossRef] [PubMed]
8. Feng, S.; Phillips, D.J.; White, T.; Sayal, H.; Aley, P.K.; Bibi, S.; Dold, C.; Fuskova, M.; Gilbert, S.C.; Hirsch, I.; et al. Correlates of protection against symptomatic and asymptomatic SARS-CoV-2 infection. *Nat. Med.* **2021**, *27*, 2032–2040. [CrossRef]
9. Gilbert, P.B.; Montefiori, D.C.; McDermott, A.B.; Fong, Y.; Benkeser, D.; Deng, W.; Zhou, H.; Houchens, C.R.; Martins, K.; Jayashankar, L.; et al. Immune correlates analysis of the mRNA-1273 COVID-19 vaccine efficacy clinical trial. *Science* **2022**, *375*, 43–50. [CrossRef]
10. Goldblatt, D.; Alter, G.; Crotty, S.; Plotkin, S.A. Correlates of protection against SARS-CoV-2 infection and COVID-19 disease. *Immunol. Rev.* **2022**, *310*, 6–26. [CrossRef]
11. Planas, D.; Veyer, D.; Baidaliuk, A.; Staropoli, I.; Guivel-Benhassine, F.; Rajah, M.M.; Planchais, C.; Porrot, F.; Robillard, N.; Puech, J.; et al. Reduced sensitivity of SARS-CoV-2 variant Delta to antibody neutralization. *Nature* **2021**, *596*, 276–280. [CrossRef] [PubMed]
12. Planas, D.; Saunders, N.; Maes, P.; Guivel-Benhassine, F.; Planchais, C.; Buchrieser, J.; Bolland, W.H.; Porrot, F.; Staropoli, I.; Lemoine, F.; et al. Considerable escape of SARS-CoV-2 Omicron to antibody neutralization. *Nature* **2022**, *602*, 671–675. [CrossRef] [PubMed]

13. Kuhlmann, C.; Mayer, C.K.; Claassen, M.; Maponga, T.; Burgers, W.A.; Keeton, R.; Riou, C.; Sutherland, A.D.; Suliman, T.; Shaw, M.L.; et al. Breakthrough infections with SARS-CoV-2 omicron despite mRNA vaccine booster dose. *Lancet* **2022**, *399*, 625–626. [CrossRef]
14. Dimeglio, C.; Herin, F.; Da-Silva, I.; Gernigon, C.; Porcheron, M.; Chapuy-Regaud, S.; Izopet, J. Decreased Efficiency of Neutralizing Antibodies from Previously Infected or Vaccinated Individuals against the B.1.617.2 (Delta) SARS-CoV-2 Variant. *Microbiol. Spectr.* **2022**, *10*, e0270621. [CrossRef] [PubMed]
15. Callaway, E. Heavily mutated Omicron variant puts scientists on alert. *Nature.* **2021**, *600*, 21. [CrossRef]
16. Chen, X.; Chen, Z.; Azman, A.S.; Sun, R. Neutralizing antibodies against SARS-CoV-2 variants induced by natural infection or vaccination: A systematic review and pooled meta-analysis. *Clin. Infect. Dis* **2021**, *73*, 1722–1732. [CrossRef]
17. Cele, S.; Jackson, L.; Khoury, D.S.; Khan, K.; Moyo-Gwete, T.; Tegally, H.; San, J.E.; Cromer, D.; Scheepers, C.; Amoako, D.G.; et al. Omicron extensively but incompletely escapes Pfizer BNT162b2 neutralization. *Nature* **2021**, *602*, 654–656. [CrossRef]
18. Schmidt, F.; Muecksch, F.; Weisblum, Y.; da Silva, J.; Bednarski, E.; Cho, A.; Wang, Z.; Gaebler, C.; Caskey, M.; Nussenzweig, M.C.; et al. Plasma neutralization of the SARS-CoV-2 Omicron variant. *N. Engl. J. Med.* **2022**, *386*, 599–601. [CrossRef]
19. Gallais, F.; Gantner, P.; Bruel, T.; Velay, A.; Planas, D.; Wendling, M.-J.; Bayer, S.; Solis, M.; Laugel, E.; Reix, N.; et al. Evolution of antibody responses up to 13 months after SARS-CoV-2 infection and risk of reinfection. *EBioMedicine* **2021**, *71*, 103561. [CrossRef]
20. Pfizer. Pfizer and BioNTech Provide Update on Omicron Variant 2021 [Updated Wednesday December 08, 2021]. Available online: https://www.pfizer.com/news/press-release/press-release-detail/pfizer-and-biontech-provide-update-omicron-variant (accessed on 14 September 2022).
21. Migueres, M.; Lhomme, S.; Trémeaux, P.; Dimeglio, C.; Ranger, N.; Latour, J.; Dubois, M.; Nicot, F.; Miedouge, M.; Mansuy, J.M.; et al. Evaluation of two RT-PCR screening assays for identifying SARS-CoV-2 variants. *J. Clin. Virol.* **2021**, *143*, 104969. [CrossRef]
22. Migueres, M.; Dimeglio, C.; Mansuy, J.M.; Abravanel, F.; Raymond, S.; Latour, J.; Jeanne, N.; Ranger, N.; Lhomme, S.; Saune, K.; et al. The influence of the nasopharyngeal viral load on the spread of the Omicron BA.2 variant. *Clin. Infect. Dis.* **2022**, ciac563. [CrossRef] [PubMed]
23. McMahan, K.; Yu, J.; Mercado, N.B.; Loos, C.; Tostanoski, L.H.; Chandrashekar, A.; Liu, J.; Peter, L.; Atyeo, C.; Zhu, A.; et al. Correlates of protection against SARS-CoV-2 in rhesus macaques. *Nature* **2021**, *590*, 630–634. [CrossRef] [PubMed]
24. McCallum, M.; Czudnochowski, N.; Rosen, L.E.; Zepeda, S.K.; Bowen, J.E.; Walls, A.C.; Hauser, K.; Joshi, A.; Stewart, C.; Dillen, J.R.; et al. Structural basis of SARS-CoV-2 Omicron immune evasion and receptor engagement. *Science* **2022**, *375*, 864–868. [CrossRef] [PubMed]
25. Stærke, N.B.; Reekie, J.; Nielsen, H.; Benfield, T.; Wiese, L.; Knudsen, L.S.; Iversen, M.B.; Iversen, K.; Fogh, K.; Bodilsen, J.; et al. Levels of SARS-CoV-2 antibodies among fully vaccinated individuals with Delta or Omicron variant breakthrough infections. *Nat. Commun.* **2022**, *13*, 4466. [CrossRef] [PubMed]
26. Dimeglio, C.; Trémeaux, P.; Herin, F.; Da-Silva, I.; Porcheron, M.; Martin-Blondel, G.; Gernigon, C.; Chapuy-Regaud, S.; Villars, H.; Izopet, J. Post-vaccination SARS-CoV-2 antibody kinetics and protection duration against Omicron in elderly population. *J. Infect.* **2022**, S0163-4453(22)00522-9. [CrossRef]
27. Cao, Y.; Wang, J.; Jian, F.; Xiao, T.; Song, W.; Yisimayi, A.; Huang, W.; Li, Q.; Wang, P.; An, R.; et al. Omicron escapes the majority of existing SARS-CoV-2 neutralizing antibodies. *Nature* **2022**, *602*, 657–663. [CrossRef]
28. Dejnirattisai, W.; Huo, J.; Zhou, D.; Zahradník, J.; Supasa, P.; Liu, C.; Duyvesteyn, H.M.E.; Ginn, H.M.; Mentzer, A.J.; Tuekprakhon, A.; et al. SARS-CoV-2 Omicron-B.1.1.529 leads to widespread escape from neutralizing antibody responses. *Cell* **2022**, *185*, 467–484.e15. [CrossRef]
29. Hall, V.; Foulkes, S.; Insalata, F.; Kirwan, P.; Saei, A.; Atti, A.; Wellington, E.; Khawam, J.; Munro, K.; Cole, M.; et al. Protection against SARS-CoV-2 after Covid-19 Vaccination and Previous Infection. *N. Engl. J. Med.* **2022**, *386*, 1207–1220. [CrossRef]
30. Dimeglio, C.; Herin, F.; Da-Silva, I.; Porcheron, M.; Martin-Blondel, G.; Chapuy-Regaud, S.; Izopet, J. Post-vaccination SARS-CoV-2 antibody kinetics and protection duration. *Clin. Infect. Dis* **2021**, ciab984. [CrossRef]
31. Li, X. Omicron: Call for updated vaccines. *J. Med. Virol.* **2022**, *94*, 1261–1263. [CrossRef]

vaccines

MDPI

Communication

No Significant Association between 25-OH Vitamin D Status and SARS-CoV-2 Antibody Response after COVID-19 Vaccination in Nursing Home Residents and Staff

Eline Meyers [1], Evelien De Smet [2], Hanne Vercruysse [3], Steven Callens [4], Elizaveta Padalko [1,5], Stefan Heytens [6], Linos Vandekerckhove [2], Piet Cools [1,*,†] and Wojciech Witkowski [2,*,†]

1 Department of Diagnostic Sciences, Faculty of Medicine and Health Sciences, Ghent University, 9000 Ghent, Belgium; eline.meyers@ugent.be (E.M.)
2 HIV Cure Research Center, Department of Internal Medicine and Pediatrics, Ghent University Hospital, Ghent University, 9000 Ghent, Belgium
3 Research and Analytics, Liantis, 8000 Bruges, Belgium
4 Department of Internal Medicine and Pediatrics, Ghent University Hospital, Ghent University, 9000 Ghent, Belgium
5 Department of Medical Microbiology, Ghent University Hospital, 9000 Ghent, Belgium
6 Department of Public Health and Primary Care, Faculty of Medicine and Health Sciences, Ghent University, 9000 Ghent, Belgium
* Correspondence: piet.cools@ugent.be (P.C.); wojciech.witkowski@ugent.be (W.W.)
† These authors contributed equally to this work.

Abstract: Vitamin D is an essential nutrient for various physiological functions, including immunity. While it has been suggested that higher vitamin D levels/supplementation are associated with a better immune response to COVID-19 vaccination, conflicting data exist. Therefore, we aimed to investigate the association between vitamin D (25-hydroxyvitamin D) deficiency/supplementation, and SARS-CoV-2 antibody responses post-vaccination in nursing home residents (NHRs) and staff (NHS). Blood samples were collected from 115 NHRs and 254 NHS at baseline and 14 days after primary course BNT162b2 vaccination. Baseline samples were assessed for serum 25-hydroxyvitamin D levels, while follow-up samples were analyzed for spike protein S1 receptor-binding domain (S1RBD) IgG antibody concentrations and 50% pseudoneutralization titers. Vitamin D supplementation status was obtained from NHRs medical records. We compared immune responses between (severe) vitamin D-deficient and -sufficient NHRs/NHS and between supplemented and non-supplemented NHRs, stratified for history of SARS-CoV-2 infection and participant type. No significant differences in either binding or neutralizing COVID-19 vaccine antibody response were found between groups. The prevalence of vitamin D deficiency (<20 ng/mL) was 45% (95% CI: 36–54%) among NHRs and 60% (95% CI: 54–66%) among NHS. Although we showed that vitamin D status may not be related to a better COVID-19 vaccine antibody response, addressing the high prevalence of vitamin D deficiency in the nursing home population remains important.

Keywords: vitamin D; 25-hydroxyvitamin D; older adults; nursing home residents; nursing homes; SARS-CoV-2; COVID-19 vaccination

1. Background

Vitamin D is a crucial nutrient involved in multiple physiological processes, including immunity [1–8]. By interacting with both adaptive (T-/B-cells) and innate immune cells (monocytes/dendritic cells), vitamin D can co-regulate immune cell differentiation and cytokine production, which is essential for effective immunogenicity against microbial infections [9,10]. When an individual's 25-hydroxyvitamin D (25(OH)D) serum levels decrease below 20 ng/mL, we commonly speak of a pathological condition, referred to as vitamin D deficiency [11]. Previous studies have shown that vitamin D deficiency is associated with increased susceptibility to viral infections such as influenza, Respiratory Syncytial Virus (RSV), and Human Immunodeficiency Virus (HIV) [12–14]. Recently, different studies have shown that vitamin D may also play a role in protecting against coronavirus disease 19 (COVID-19), with higher levels of vitamin D and/or vitamin D supplementation being linked to better survival rates, less severe disease outcomes, and protection against infection [15–23]. In addition, a limited number of studies have investigated the association between vitamin D levels and COVID-19 vaccine-induced immune responses. Here, contrasting findings exist. Most studies report that vitamin D levels and/or supplementation are not associated with COVID-19 vaccine immunogenicity [24–27]. However, some report a positive association between vitamin D levels/supplementation and COVID-19 vaccine antibody responses [28,29].

While the relationship between vitamin D levels and COVID-19 vaccine immunogenicity has been investigated by a limited number of studies in healthy adults, little is known about this association in older adults, such as nursing home residents (NHRs). This population is particularly vulnerable to vitamin D deficiency, which is a major public health problem in the NHR population [30–33]. Moreover, older adults living in nursing homes (NHs) are known to exhibit impaired antibody responses to COVID-19 vaccination, compared to younger healthy individuals [34,35]. In light of this evidence, we conducted a study to investigate vitamin D status in nursing home residents and nursing home staff, 14 days after receiving two doses of the Pfizer/BioNTech BNT162b2 COVID-19 vaccine. Our aim was to determine whether (severe) vitamin D deficiency or treatment with vitamin D supplementation is associated with severe acute respiratory syndrome coronavirus 2 (SARS-CoV-2) antibody responses following vaccination.

2. Materials and Methods

2.1. Study Design and Population

The current study is a secondary analysis of data from a study that aimed to assess BNT162b2 vaccine immune response in nursing home residents, and has been described in detail elsewhere [35]. In brief, a total of 138 NHRs and 312 nursing home staff (NHS) from six Flemish NHs were recruited between 18 January and 4 March 2021. Venous blood was collected on the day of administration of the first BNT162b2 vaccine dose (baseline) and 14 days after administration of the second dose (follow-up). Baseline samples were used to assess history of SARS-CoV-2 infection and 25(OH)D levels, while follow-up samples were used to assess vaccine antibody response.

2.2. Ethics

This study was approved by the Ethical Committee of Ghent University Hospital (reference number BC-07665) and conducted according to the principles of the Declaration of Helsinki. Participants were informed about the study goals and procedures before written consent was obtained. A confidential counselor, such as a nurse, signed for participants who were incapable of signing the consent form, such as residents with dementia, whose consent was given by their legal representative.

2.3. Sample Collection

Approximately 5 mL of venous blood was obtained from each participant. Serum tubes were transported to the Laboratory of Clinical Microbiology of the Ghent University Hospital (Ghent, Belgium) within six hours after blood collection. There, serum tubes were centrifuged at 2000× g for 8 min and stored at 4 °C. The next day, serum was aliquoted and frozen at −20 °C until further analysis.

2.4. Antibody Detection

In the baseline samples, SARS-CoV-2 nucleocapsid protein (NCP)-specific immunoglobulin G (IgG)-binding antibodies were detected using a semi-quantitative enzyme-linked immune sorbent assay (ELISA) (EUROIMMUN, Lübeck, Germany) according to the manufacturer's instructions. Results were expressed in optical density (OD) ratio. Samples that exceeded an OD ratio of 0.8 were considered seropositive, and therefore considered as previously SARS-CoV-2 infected. In the follow-up samples, SARS-CoV-2 spike protein S1 receptor-binding domain (S1RBD)-specific IgG-binding antibody concentrations were detected using a quantitative ELISA assay (ImmunoDiagnostics, Hong Kong), which we have previously validated [36]. Results were expressed in International Units/mL (IU/mL).

2.5. Pseudovirus Neutralization Assay

The neutralizing capacities of SARS-CoV-2 vaccine-induced antibodies were assessed using a pseudovirus (recombinant immunodeficiency virus 1 SG3ΔEnv) neutralization assay, as described before [35]. The highest antibody serum dilution resulting in 50% pseudovirus neutralization was reported as the 50% pseudovirus neutralization titer.

2.6. 25-Hydroxyvitamin D Detection and Supplementation

A metabolite of vitamin D, serum 25(OH)D, was measured using a quantitative ELISA assay with 6-point calibration (EUROIMMUN, Lübeck, Germany) according to the manufacturer's instructions at baseline. The EUROIMMUN assay kit reliably detects 25(OH)D3 and 25(OH)D2. Vitamin D deficiency and severe vitamin D deficiency were defined as a 25(OH)D serum concentration below 20 ng/mL and 12 ng/mL, respectively [11,37]. Data on the use of vitamin D supplementation was obtained from the medical records for NHRs only.

2.7. Statistical Analysis

Differences in S1RBD IgG response and 50% pseudoneutralization titer (both post-vaccination) between vitamin-D-deficient and -sufficient participants were assessed using 20 ng/mL (deficiency) and 12ng/mL (severe deficiency) of serum 25(OH)D levels as cut-off. The analysis was stratified for participant type (NHRs/NHS) and infection status, as these factors were previously shown to affect vaccine antibody response [35]. Mann–Whitney U tests were performed to assess statistically significant differences (p-value ≤ 0.05) between groups (vitamin D sufficiency vs. deficiency and supplemented vs. non-supplemented). No multiplicity adjustments were carried out. Samples with a 50% pseudoneutralization titer of 0.00 were adjusted to a value of 0.01 in order to plot them on a logarithmic scale. The proportions of vitamin-D-deficient NHRs and NHS are reported with 95% confidence intervals (95% CI). All statistical analyses were performed in Graphpad Prism Version 9.3 (GraphPad Software, San Diego, CA, USA).

3. Results

3.1. Participant Characteristics

From all recruited participants (138 NHRs and 312 NHS), data from 115 NHRs and 254 NHS from five different NHs were included in the current analysis (participants with missing data regarding their age and/or information on vitamin D supplementation were excluded). Sociodemographic and participant characteristics of the study population are summarized in Table 1. The median age for NHRs was 89 years old, and 81% were female. The median age for NHS was 51 years old and 82% were female. A high prevalence of vitamin D deficiency was observed in our study population, with 45% (95% CI: 36–54%) of NHRs and 60% (95% CI: 54–66%) of NHS having serum 25(OH)D levels below 20 ng/mL. A total of 24% and 11% of NHRs and NHS, respectively, had severe vitamin D deficiency (<12 ng/mL). Median 25(OH)D levels and interquartile range was 20.80 ng/mL (16.85–24.75) and 18.19 ng/mL (14.94–23.02) for NHRs and NHS, respectively. Among NHRs, 37% ($n = 42$) received vitamin D supplementation. 25(OH)D levels were significantly higher in supplemented NHRs (27.97 ng/mL; 24.82–33.49), compared to non-supplemented NHRs (13.39 ng/mL; 10.82–22.42) ($p < 0.0001$).

Table 1. Participant characteristics of nursing home residents and staff.

	Nursing Home Residents (n = 115)	Nursing Home Staff (n = 254)
Sociodemographic characteristics		
Female, n (%)	93 (81%)	208 (82%)
Age, median (interquartile range)	89 (86–93)	51 (36–63)
25(OH)D		
25(OH)D serum concentration (ng/mL), median (interquartile range)	20.80 (16.85–24.75)	18.19 (14.94–23.02)
25(OH)D serum concentration non-supplemented (ng/mL), median (interquartile range)	13.39 (10.82–22.42)	NA
25(OH)D serum concentration supplemented (ng/mL), median (interquartile range)	27.97 (24.82–33.49)	NA
25(OH)D serum concentration previous SARS-CoV-2 infection (ng/mL), median (interquartile range)	19.71 (11.52–28.29)	18.52 (16.90–20.82)
25(OH)D serum concentration no history of SARS-CoV-2 infection (ng/mL), median (interquartile range)	22.56 (13.13–26.69)	18.22 (14.94–23.26)
25-OH Vitamin D deficiency (<20 ng/mL), n (%; 95% CI)	52 (45%; 36–54%)	153 (60%; 54–66%)
25-OH Vitamin D severe deficiency (<12 ng/mL), n (%; 95% CI)	28 (24%; 17–33%)	27 (11%; 7–15%)
Vitamin D supplementation, n (%)	42 (37%)	NA
SARS-CoV-2		
Previous SARS-CoV-2 infection, n (%) [a]	26 (23%)	29 (11%)
SARS-CoV-2 IgG concentration post-vaccination, geometric mean (interquartile range)	388.24 (82.15–2237.43)	2286.64 (1630.52–4521.25)
SARS-CoV-2 50% pseudoneutralization titer, median (interquartile range)	20.96 (2.35–153.3)	124.00 (61.71–271.48)
Prevalence seroconversion after vaccination, n (%)	102 (89%)	250 (98%)

[a] Assessed by detection of anti-nucleocapsid protein IgG in baseline samples.

3.2. COVID-19 Vaccine Binding and Neutralizing Antibody Responses in Vitamin-D-Deficient versus Sufficient NHRs and NHS

SARS-CoV-2 S1RBD IgG levels and 50% pseudoneutralization titers measured 14 days after the second dose of the BNT162b2 vaccine were compared between vitamin-D-deficient (<20 ng/mL) and vitamin D sufficient (≥20 ng/mL) participants, stratified per participant type and infection status. No significant differences in either binding or neutralizing antibody response were found between vitamin-D-deficient participants compared to participants with vitamin D sufficiency, not for residents nor for staff (Figure 1). In addition, when applying a cutoff of 12 ng/mL 25(OH)D serum concentration for severe vitamin D deficiency, no significant differences in binding/neutralizing antibody response between groups were observed ($p > 0.05$, Supplementary Figure S1).

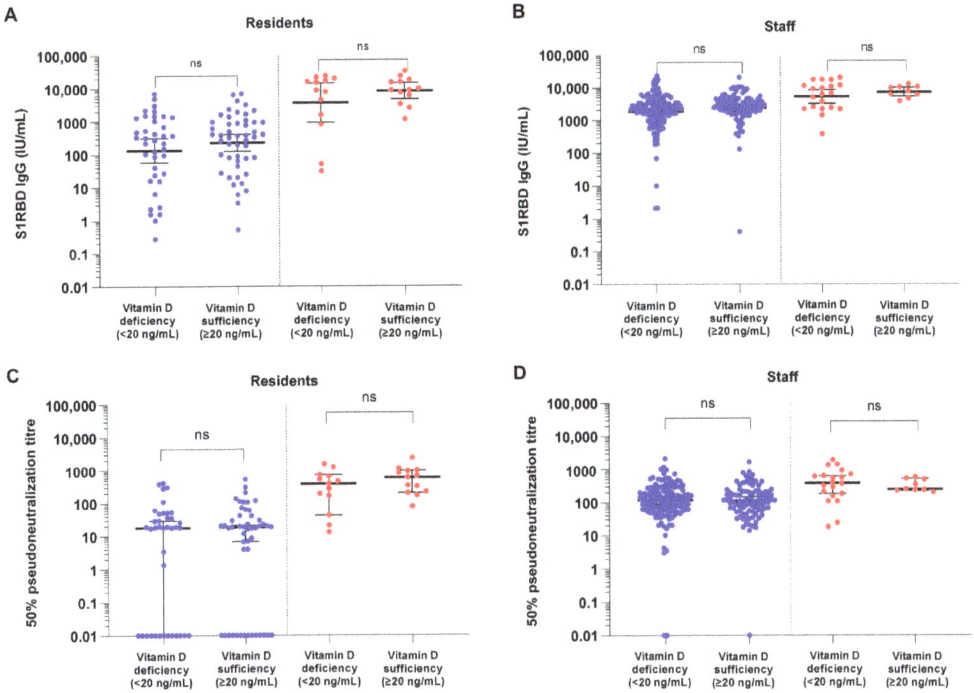

Figure 1. S1RBD IgG antibody concentration (International Unit/mL) (**A**,**B**) and 50% pseudoneutralization titer (**C**,**D**) 14 days after BNT162b2 vaccination among 25-OH vitamin-D-deficient (<20 ng/mL) and 25-OH vitamin D sufficient (≥20 ng/mL) nursing home residents (**A**,**C**) and nursing home staff (**B**,**D**). Data is presented stratified for infection naïve participants (blue) and previously infected participants (red). Bold horizontal lines with error bars represent the geometric mean S1RBD IgG antibody concentration and median 50% pseudoneutralization titer per group with 95% confidence intervals. ns: not significant at the 0.05 level. Samples with a 50% pseudoneutralization titer of 0.00 were adjusted to a value of 0.01 in order to plot them on a logarithmic scale.

3.3. COVID-19 Vaccine Binding and Neutralizing Antibody Responses in Vitamin D Supplemented NHRs versus Non-Supplemented NHR

We compared post-vaccination S1RBD IgG antibody concentrations and 50% pseudoneutralization titers between vitamin D supplemented and non-supplemented NHRs. No significant differences in post-vaccination S1RBD IgG levels nor 50% pseudoneutralization titers were found between NHRs treated with vitamin D supplements compared to non-supplemented NHRs (Figure 2).

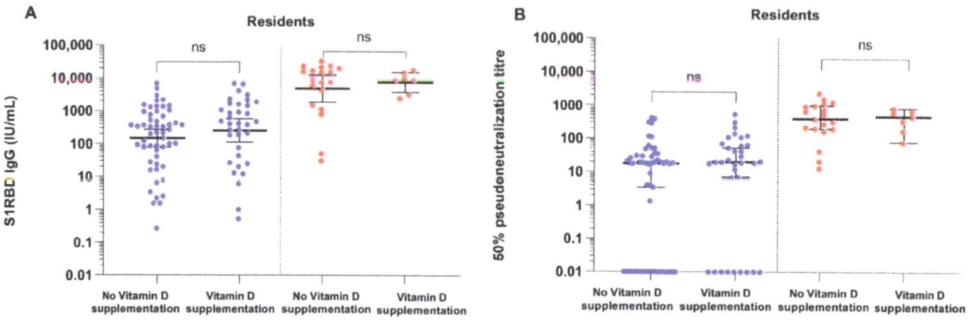

Figure 2. S1RBD IgG antibody concentrations (International Unit/mL) (**A**) and 50% pseudoneutralization titers (**B**) 14 days after BNT162b2 vaccination among vitamin D supplemented and non-supplemented nursing home residents. Data is presented stratified for infection naïve residents (blue) and previously infected residents (red). Bold horizontal lines with error bars represent the geometric mean S1RBD IgG antibody concentration and median 50% pseudoneutralization titer per group with 95% confidence intervals. ns: not significant at the 0.05 level. Samples with a 50% pseudoneutralization titer of 0.00 were adjusted to a value of 0.01 in order to plot them on a logarithmic scale.

4. Discussion

In the current study, we aimed to investigate the potential association between vitamin D deficiency/vitamin D supplementation and SARS-CoV-2 antibody responses in NHRs and NHS following two doses of the BNT162b2 COVID-19 vaccine. Our findings show that neither (severe) vitamin D deficiency nor treatment with vitamin D supplementation were associated with antibody responses, either binding (S1RBD IgG) or neutralizing (50% pseudovirus neutralization titer), after COVID-19 vaccination in NHRs and NHS.

Our results are in line with what most other report concerning the association between vitamin D status, deficiency and/or supplementation and SARS-CoV-2 immune responses following vaccination in healthy adults. The majority of previous studies have similarly found no association between vitamin D and different immune endpoints following COVID-19 vaccination, such as binding antibodies, neutralizing antibodies, antibody decline and cellular responses [24–27]. Yet, a limited pair of studies report conflicting findings. One study found that vitamin D levels were positively associated with antibody response two weeks following a single BNT162b2 dose [28]. However, this study was limited by a small sample size and did not measure the antibody response after the two doses of the BNT162b2 vaccine, which is the recommended vaccine schedule. Moreover, their data show that 8 weeks following a single vaccine dose, differences in antibody response are no longer observed between the deficient/insufficient/replete groups. Another study identified regular intake of vitamin D supplementation as a predictor for SARS-CoV-2 seropositivity at a median of 8.6 weeks after COVID-19 vaccination in a population-based study [29]. Nevertheless, the association between use of vitamin D supplements and antibody levels as a continuous variable was not found there.

Supporting our data, other evidence can be found in studies investigating the association between vitamin D and antibody responses following vaccination against other viral infections, such as influenza. These studies have similarly demonstrated that neither vitamin D supplementation, vitamin D levels nor vitamin D deficiency, were associated with post-influenza vaccination antibody levels in both younger as older adults [38–41]. One study in particular, investigating the effect of vitamin D supplementation in nursing home residents, found that vitamin D supplementation did not affect antibody responses upon influenza vaccination, however, it did increase certain inflammatory cytokine levels post-vaccination [38].

A secondary interesting finding of the current study is the prevalence of vitamin D deficiency measured in our randomly recruited study population in Flanders, Belgium. We found that 45% (95% CI: 36–54%) of NHRs and 60% (95% CI: 54–66%) of NHS were vitamin D deficient (<20 ng/mL), and 24% (95% CI: 17–33%) of NHRs and 11% (95% CI: 7–15%) of NHS severe vitamin D deficient (<12 ng/mL). Other observational studies in a general European population have similarly reported a prevalence of vitamin D deficiency (<20 ng/mL) of ~40% and severe vitamin D deficiency (<12 ng/mL) of 13% [37,42]. In NHR populations, the prevalence of vitamin D deficiency is generally known to be even higher, with prevalence measured up to 94% in non-supplemented individuals [30]. One other study, dated from 2012, assessed the prevalence of vitamin D deficiency among NHRs from 53 NHs in Belgium, and reported a prevalence of 75.6% [43]. Multiple factors are known to affect vitamin D status in older adults, for example, poor daylight exposure, inadequate dietary intake, poor renal function, or reduced gut absorption due to ageing [30]. In our study population, however, 37% of NHRs were being treated with vitamin D supplements, which could explain the relatively low prevalence of vitamin D deficiency, compared to what others reported. Although we did not collect data on vitamin D supplementation in NHS, it could be speculated that a lower percentage of NHS were under vitamin D supplementation, which could explain the higher prevalence of vitamin D deficiency in NHS compared to NHRs. Regardless, Belgian guidelines recommend a daily intake of 800–2000 international units of vitamin D supplementation for all institutionalized elderly people [44]. Additionally, it is important to note that >80% of our study population were female, and the prevalence of vitamin D deficiency is known to be higher in women, with the highest difference observed between men and women in young adolescence and middle age [45]. Moreover, it should be noted that, although the observed prevalence of vitamin D deficiency was higher in NHS than NHRs, more NHRs had severe vitamin D deficiency.

Although vitamin D deficiency is highly prevalent among NHRs, and generally, older adults are known to have decreased immune responses following COVID-19 vaccination [30,34,35,46], our study suggests that vitamin D deficiency may not be the primary factor contributing to the observed impaired immune responses in nursing home residents following COVID-19 vaccination. In the literature, several studies have demonstrated that there is a negative association between vitamin D levels and COVID-19 severity in a pre-vaccination context [15–20], yet, our findings show that vitamin D is not associated with antibody levels two weeks after vaccination with the BNT162b2 COVID-19 vaccine. Most likely, other mechanisms exist through which vitamin D induces better COVID-19 outcomes. One study has suggested that vitamin D acts as a protecting agent by suppression of pro-inflammatory cytokines, which were shown to be negatively correlated with vitamin D levels [47]. Additionally, other mechanisms have been suggested by which vitamin D acts protectively against severe COVID-19, like induction of the transcription of the antimicrobial peptides cathelicidin and defensin [48]. Nevertheless, more fundamental research will be needed to fully understand how vitamin D status is associated with COVID-19 severity. Additionally, it is important to emphasize that, although vitamin D status may not be related to a better COVID-19 vaccine antibody response, it remains important to address the high prevalence of vitamin D deficiency among the nursing home population, as vitamin-D-deficient older adults are at high risk for multiple pathological conditions, e.g., cognitive decline, depression, osteoporosis, and increased risk of falling [49–53].

Limitations

The current study assessed the association between vitamin D levels/supplementation and COVID-19 vaccine-induced antibody responses in a large sample of NHRs and NHS, however this study has limitations. Firstly, the results in this study were obtained by an observational study design, and not an experimental study design with controlled treatment groups. Moreover, we considered vitamin D blood levels as sufficient when 25(OH)D serum concentrations were 20 ng/mL or more. However, different classifications exist, as levels between 20 and 29 ng/mL are often categorized as insufficient, and those of 30 ng/mL or more as sufficient [8]. In our observations, not many participants had 25(OH)D levels that exceeded 30 ng/mL. Therefore, the effects 25(OH)D levels in the higher range of healthy blood levels, could not be investigated. Nevertheless, circulating serum 25(OH)D levels are known as a robust and reliable marker of vitamin D status [54]. Additionally, data on the use of vitamin D supplementation at baseline was obtained for NHRs from their medical record, however, no data were collected concerning the dosing and duration of supplementation.

5. Conclusions

Several studies have demonstrated a negative association between vitamin D status and COVID-19 severity in a pre-vaccination context. In the present study, we aimed to investigate whether (severe) vitamin D deficiency/treatment with vitamin D supplementation is associated with the SARS-CoV-2 antibody response measured 14 days after two doses of the BNT162b2 vaccine, in 115 NHRs and 254 NHS from 5 Belgian NHs. We found that neither (severe) vitamin D deficiency, nor vitamin D supplementation was associated with binding or neutralizing COVID-19 vaccine antibody response. Secondly, we found a high prevalence of vitamin D deficiency (<20 ng/mL) of 45% (95% CI: 36–54%) among NHRs and 60% (95% CI: 54–66%) among NHS, and severe vitamin D deficiency (<12 ng/mL) of 24% (95% CI: 17–33%) among NHRs and 11% (95% CI: 7–15%) among NHS. Although vitamin D status may not be related to a better COVID-19 vaccine antibody response, it remains important to address the high prevalence of vitamin D deficiency among the nursing home population, as vitamin-D-deficient older adults are at high risk for multiple other pathological conditions. More fundamental research will be needed to fully understand how vitamin D is associated with COVID-19 severity.

Supplementary Materials: The following supporting information can be downloaded at: https://www.mdpi.com/article/10.3390/vaccines11081343/s1, Figure S1: S1RBD IgG antibody concentration (International Unit/mL).

Author Contributions: Conceptualization, W.W., P.C. and L.V.; methodology, W.W., P.C. and L.V.; validation, E.M., W.W. and P.C.; formal analysis, E.M. and W.W.; investigation, H.V., S.H., E.D.S., W.W., E.M., E.P. and S.C.; resources, P.C. and W.W.; data curation, P.C., W.W. and E.M.; writing—original draft preparation, E.M.; writing—review and editing, W.W., L.V., E.P. and S.C.; visualization, E.M.; supervision, W.W., P.C. and L.V.; project administration, P.C. and W.W.; funding acquisition, L.V. and P.C. All authors have read and agreed to the published version of the manuscript.

Funding: P.C. and L.V. received funding from the Special Research Fund of Ghent University. (BOF.COV.2020.0010.01 and BOF.COV.2020.0009.01, respectively). L.V. is supported by the Research Foundation Flanders (Linos Vandekerckhove, grant 1.8.020.09.N.00) and the Collen-Francqui Research Professor Mandate. E.M. is supported by the Research Foundation Flanders (PhD fellowship Strategic Basic Research, 1SD2524N). The sample analysis was supported by the Research Foundation Flanders (FWO-OPR.2020.0113.01).

Institutional Review Board Statement: The study was conducted in accordance with the Declaration of Helsinki, and approved by the Ethics Committee of the Ghent University Hospital (reference number BC-07665).

Informed Consent Statement: Written informed consent has been obtained from the study participants to publish this paper. Each participant signed an informed consent form after being informed about the goal of the study and the sampling procedures by the management of the NH. A confidential counsellor, such as a nurse, signed for participants who were incapable of signing the consent form, such as residents with dementia whose consent was given by their legal representative.

Data Availability Statement: The data presented in this study are available on request from the corresponding authors.

Acknowledgments: The authors wish to thank all residents and their families, staff and management from the nursing homes that participated in the study.

Conflicts of Interest: The authors declare no conflict of interest.

References

1. Bikle, D.D. Vitamin D and Bone. *Curr. Osteoporos. Rep.* **2012**, *10*, 151–159. [CrossRef] [PubMed]
2. Ceglia, L. Vitamin D and its role in skeletal muscle. *Curr. Opin. Clin. Nutr. Metab. Care* **2009**, *12*, 628–633. [CrossRef] [PubMed]
3. Wrzosek, M.; Łukaszkiewicz, J.; Wrzosek, M.; Jakubczyk, A.; Matsumoto, H.; Piątkiewicz, P.; Radziwoń-Zaleska, M.; Wojnar, M.; Nowicka, G. Vitamin D and the central nervous system. *Pharmacol. Rep.* **2013**, *65*, 271–278. [CrossRef]
4. Miliku, K.; Vinkhuyzen, A.; Blanken, L.M.; McGrath, J.J.; Eyles, D.W.; Burne, T.H.; Hofman, A.; Tiemeier, H.; AP Steegers, E.; Gaillard, R.; et al. Maternal vitamin D concentrations during pregnancy, fetal growth patterns, and risks of adverse birth outcomes. *Am. J. Clin. Nutr.* **2016**, *103*, 1514–1522. [CrossRef] [PubMed]
5. DeLuca, G.C.; Kimball, S.M.; Kolasinski, J.; Ramagopalan, S.V.; Ebers, G.C. Review: The role of vitamin D in nervous system health and disease. *Neuropathol. Appl. Neurobiol.* **2013**, *39*, 458–484. [CrossRef] [PubMed]
6. Sîrbe, C.; Rednic, S.; Grama, A.; Pop, T.L. An Update on the Effects of Vitamin D on the Immune System and Autoimmune Diseases. *Int. J. Mol. Sci.* **2022**, *23*, 9784. [CrossRef]
7. Muresan, G.C.; Hedesiu, M.; Lucaciu, O.; Boca, S.; Petrescu, N. Effect of Vitamin D on Bone Regeneration: A Review. *Medicina* **2022**, *58*, 1337. [CrossRef]
8. Charoenngam, N.; Shirvani, A.; Holick, M.F. Vitamin D for skeletal and non-skeletal health: What we should know. *J. Clin. Orthop. Trauma* **2019**, *10*, 1082–1093. [CrossRef]
9. Gunville, C.F.; Mourani, P.M.; Ginde, A.A. The Role of Vitamin D in Prevention and Treatment of Infection. *Inflamm. Allergy-Drug Targets* **2013**, *12*, 239–245. [CrossRef]
10. Aranow, C. Vitamin D and the Immune System. *J. Investig. Med.* **2011**, *59*, 881–886. [CrossRef]
11. Holick, M.F. Vitamin D Deficiency. *N. Engl. J. Med.* **2007**, *357*, 266–281. [CrossRef] [PubMed]
12. Moan, J.E.; Dahlback, A.; Ma, L.; Juzeniene, A. Influenza, solar radiation and vitamin D. *Dermato-Endocrinology* **2009**, *1*, 308–310. [CrossRef] [PubMed]
13. Sudfeld, C.R.; Wang, M.; Aboud, S.; Giovannucci, E.L.; Mugusi, F.M.; Fawzi, W.W. Vitamin D and HIV Progression among Tanzanian Adults Initiating Antiretroviral Therapy. *PLoS ONE* **2012**, *7*, e40036. [CrossRef] [PubMed]
14. McNally, J.D.; Sampson, M.; Matheson, L.A.; Hutton, B.; Little, J. Vitamin D receptor (VDR) polymorphisms and severe RSV bronchiolitis: A systematic review and meta-analysis. *Pediatr. Pulmonol.* **2013**, *49*, 790–799. [CrossRef]
15. Annweiler, G.; Corvaisier, M.; Gautier, J.; Dubée, V.; Legrand, E.; Sacco, G.; Annweiler, C. Vitamin D Supplementation Associated to Better Survival in Hospitalized Frail Elderly COVID-19 Patients: The GERIA-COVID Quasi-Experimental Study. *Nutrients* **2020**, *12*, 3377. [CrossRef]
16. Campi, I.; Gennari, L.; Merlotti, D.; Mingiano, C.; Frosali, A.; Giovanelli, L.; Torlasco, C.; Pengo, M.F.; Heilbron, F.; Soranna, D.; et al. Vitamin D and COVID-19 severity and related mortality: A prospective study in Italy. *BMC Infect. Dis.* **2021**, *21*, 566. [CrossRef]
17. Baktash, V.; Hosack, T.; Zahari, N.; Shah, S.; Kandiah, P.; Van den Abbeele, K.; Mandal, A.K.J.; Missouris, C.G. Vitamin D status and outcomes for hospitalised older patients with COVID-19. *Postgrad. Med. J.* **2020**, *97*, 1149. [CrossRef]
18. Radujkovic, A.; Hippchen, T.; Tiwari-Heckler, S.; Dreher, S.; Boxberger, M.; Merle, U. Vitamin D Deficiency and Outcome of COVID-19 Patients. *Nutrients* **2020**, *12*, 2757. [CrossRef]
19. Pereira, M.; Dantas Damascena, A.D.; Galvão Azevedo, L.M.G.; de Almeida Oliveira, T.D.A.; da Mota Santana, J.D.M. Vitamin D deficiency aggravates COVID-19: Systematic review and meta-analysis. *Crit. Rev. Food Sci. Nutr.* **2022**, *62*, 1308–1316. [CrossRef]
20. Wang, Z.; Joshi, A.; Leopold, K.; Jackson, S.; Christensen, S.; Nayfeh, T.; Mohammed, K.; Creo, A.; Tebben, P.; Kumar, S. Association of vitamin D deficiency with COVID-19 infection severity: Systematic review and meta-analysis. *Clin. Endocrinol.* **2021**, *96*, 281–287. [CrossRef]
21. Merzon, E.; Tworowski, D.; Gorohovski, A.; Vinker, S.; Cohen, A.G.; Green, I.; Frenkel-Morgenstern, M. Low plasma 25(OH) vitamin D level is associated with increased risk of COVID-19 infection: An Israeli population-based study. *FEBS J.* **2020**, *287*, 3693–3702. [CrossRef]
22. Kaufman, H.W.; Niles, J.K.; Kroll, M.H.; Bi, C.; Holick, M.F. SARS-CoV-2 positivity rates associated with circulating 25-hydroxyvitamin D levels. *PLoS ONE* **2020**, *15*, e0239252. [CrossRef]
23. Gibbons, J.B.; Norton, E.C.; McCullough, J.S.; Meltzer, D.O.; Lavigne, J.; Fiedler, V.C.; Gibbons, R.D. Association between vitamin D supplementation and COVID-19 infection and mortality. *Sci. Rep.* **2022**, *12*, 19397. [CrossRef] [PubMed]
24. Jolliffe, D.A.; Vivaldi, G.; Chambers, E.S.; Cai, W.; Li, W.; Faustini, S.E.; Gibbons, J.M.; Pade, G.; Coussens, A.K.; Richter, A.K.; et al. Vitamin D Supplementation Does Not Influence SARS-CoV-2 Vaccine Efficacy or Immunogenicity: Sub-Studies Nested within the CORONAVIT Randomised Controlled Trial. *Nutrients* **2022**, *14*, 3821. [CrossRef]
25. Chillon, T.S.; Demircan, K.; Heller, R.A.; Hirschbil-Bremer, I.M.; Diegmann, J.; Bachmann, M.; Moghaddam, A.; Schomburg, L. Relationship between Vitamin D Status and Antibody Response to COVID-19 mRNA Vaccination in Healthy Adults. *Biomedicines* **2021**, *9*, 1714. [CrossRef]
26. Öztürk, R.; Yılmaz, N.S.; Ulukanlıgil, M. The relationship between serum vitamin D and antibody response following two doses of inactivated COVID-19 vaccine. *Turk. J. Biochem.* **2022**, *47*, 665–671. [CrossRef]
27. Parthymou, A.; Habeos, E.E.; Habeos, G.I.; Deligakis, A.; Livieratos, E.; Marangos, M.; Chartoumpekis, D.V. Factors associated with anti-SARS-CoV-2 antibody titres 3 months post-vaccination with the second dose of BNT162b2 vaccine: A longitudinal observational cohort study in western Greece. *BMJ Open* **2022**, *12*, e057084. [CrossRef] [PubMed]

28. Piec, I.; Cook, L.; Dervisevic, S.; Fraser, W.D.; Ruetten, S.; Berman, M.; English, E.; John, W.G. Age and vitamin D affect the magnitude of the antibody response to the first dose of the SARS-CoV-2 BNT162b2 vaccine. *Curr. Res. Transl. Med.* **2022**, *70*, 103344. [CrossRef]
29. Jolliffe, D.A.; Faustini, S.E.; Holt, H.; Perdek, N.; Maltby, S.; Talaei, M.; Greenig, M.; Vivaldi, G.; Tydeman, F.; Symons, J.; et al. Determinants of Antibody Responses to SARS-CoV-2 Vaccines: Population-Based Longitudinal Study (COVIDENCE UK). *Vaccines* **2022**, *10*, 1601. [CrossRef]
30. Feehan, O.; Magee, P.J.; Pourshahidi, L.K.; Armstrong, D.J.; McSorley, E.M. Vitamin D deficiency in nursing home residents: A systematic review. *Nutr. Rev.* **2022**, *81*, 804–822. [CrossRef]
31. Arnljots, R.; Thorn, J.; Elm, M.; Moore, M.; Sundvall, P.-D. Vitamin D deficiency was common among nursing home residents and associated with dementia: A cross sectional study of 545 Swedish nursing home residents. *BMC Geriatr.* **2017**, *17*, 229. [CrossRef]
32. Goldberg, T.H.; Hassan, T.; Grant, R. High Prevalence of Vitamin D Deficiency in Elderly Nursing Home Patients Despite Vitamin Supplements. *J. Am. Med. Dir. Assoc.* **2008**, *9*, B15. [CrossRef]
33. Bruyere, O.; Decock, C.; Delhez, M.; Collette, J.; Reginster, J.-Y. Highest Prevalence of Vitamin D Inadequacy in Institutionalized Women Compared with Noninstitutionalized Women: A Case–Control Study. *Women Health* **2009**, *5*, 49–54. [CrossRef]
34. Meyers, E.; Deschepper, E.; Duysburgh, E.; De Rop, L.; De Burghgraeve, T.; Van Ngoc, P.; Digregorio, M.; Delogne, S.; Coen, A.; De Clercq, N.; et al. Declining Prevalence of SARS-CoV-2 Antibodies among Vaccinated Nursing Home Residents and Staff Six Months after the Primary BNT162b2 Vaccination Campaign in Belgium: A Prospective Cohort Study. *Viruses* **2022**, *14*, 2361. [CrossRef] [PubMed]
35. Witkowski, W.; Gerlo, S.; De Smet, E.; Wejda, M.; Acar, D.; Callens, S.; Heytens, S.; Padalko, E.; Vercruysse, H.; Cools, P.; et al. Humoral and Cellular Responses to COVID-19 Vaccination Indicate the Need for Post-Vaccination Testing in Frail Population. *Vaccines* **2022**, *10*, 260. [CrossRef] [PubMed]
36. Meyers, E.; Coen, A.; De Sutter, A.; Padalko, E.; Callens, S.; Vandekerckhove, L.; Witkowski, W.; Heytens, S.; Cools, P. Diagnostic performance of the SARS-CoV-2 S1RBD IgG ELISA (Immuno Diagnostics) for the quantitative detection of SARS-CoV-2 antibodies on dried blood spots. *J. Clin. Virol.* **2022**, *155*, 105270. [CrossRef]
37. Amrein, K.; Scherkl, M.; Hoffmann, M.; Neuwersch-Sommeregger, S.; Köstenberger, M.; Berisha, A.T.; Martucci, G.; Pilz, S.; Malle, O. Vitamin D deficiency 2.0: An update on the current status worldwide. *Eur. J. Clin. Nutr.* **2020**, *74*, 1498–1513. [CrossRef]
38. Goncalves-Mendes, N.; Talvas, J.; Dualé, C.; Guttmann, A.; Corbin, V.; Marceau, G.; Sapin, V.; Brachet, P.; Evrard, B.; Laurichesse, H.; et al. Impact of Vitamin D Supplementation on Influenza Vaccine Response and Immune Functions in Deficient Elderly Persons: A Randomized Placebo-Controlled Trial. *Front. Immunol.* **2019**, *10*, 65. [CrossRef]
39. Lee, R.U.; Won, S.H.; Hansen, C.; Crum-Cianflone, N.F. 25-hydroxyvitamin D, influenza vaccine response and healthcare encounters among a young adult population. *PLoS ONE* **2018**, *13*, e0192479. [CrossRef]
40. Sundaram, M.E.; Talbot, H.K.; Zhu, Y.; Griffin, M.R.; Spencer, S.; Shay, D.K.; Coleman, L.A. Vitamin D is not associated with serologic response to influenza vaccine in adults over 50 years old. *Vaccine* **2013**, *31*, 2057–2061. [CrossRef]
41. Sadarangani, S.P.; Young, B.E.; Lian, W.; Phua, H.P.; Chen, M.I.-C.; Barr, I.; Yeo, T.W.; Dalan, R.; Chow, A. DYNAMIC cohort study evaluating metabolic predictors of influenza vaccine immune response in older adults. *NPJ Vaccines* **2022**, *7*, 135. [CrossRef]
42. Cashman, K.D.; Dowling, K.G.; Škrabáková, Z.; Gonzalez-Gross, M.; Valtueña, J.; De Henauw, S.; Moreno, L.; Damsgaard, C.T.; Michaelsen, K.F.; Mølgaard, C.; et al. Vitamin D deficiency in Europe: Pandemic? *Am. J. Clin. Nutr.* **2016**, *103*, 1033–1044. [CrossRef] [PubMed]
43. Verhoeven, V.; Vanpuyenbroeck, K.; Lopez-Hartmann, M.; Wens, J.; Remmen, R. Walk on the sunny side of life—Epidemiology of hypovitaminosis D and mental health in elderly nursing home residents. *J. Nutr. Health Aging* **2011**, *16*, 417–420. [CrossRef]
44. BCFI. Formularium Ouderenzorg: Vitamine D. Available online: https://farmaka.bcfi.be/nl/formularium/282 (accessed on 14 June 2023).
45. Arshad, S.; Zaidi, S.J.A. Vitamin D levels among children, adolescents, adults, and elders in Pakistani population: A cross-sectional study. *BMC Public Health* **2022**, *22*, 2040. [CrossRef]
46. Kweder, H.; Eidi, H. Vitamin D deficiency in elderly: Risk factors and drugs impact on vitamin D status. *Avicenna J. Med.* **2018**, *8*, 139–146. [CrossRef] [PubMed]
47. Bayraktar, N.; Turan, H.; Bayraktar, M.; Ozturk, A.; Erdoğdu, H. Analysis of serum cytokine and protective vitamin D levels in severe cases of COVID-19. *J. Med. Virol.* **2021**, *94*, 154–160. [CrossRef]
48. Tomaszewska, A.; Rustecka, A.; Lipińska-Opałka, A.; Piprek, R.P.; Kloc, M.; Kalicki, B.; Kubiak, J.Z. The Role of Vitamin D in COVID-19 and the Impact of Pandemic Restrictions on Vitamin D Blood Content. *Front. Pharmacol.* **2022**, *13*, 836738. [CrossRef]
49. Meehan, M.; Penckofer, S. The Role of Vitamin D in the Aging Adult. *J. Aging Gerontol.* **2014**, *2*, 60–71. [CrossRef]
50. Ling, Y.; Xu, F.; Xia, X.; Dai, D.; Xiong, A.; Sun, R.; Qiu, L.; Xie, Z. Vitamin D supplementation reduces the risk of fall in the vitamin D deficient elderly: An updated meta-analysis. *Clin. Nutr.* **2021**, *40*, 5531–5537. [CrossRef]
51. Llewellyn, D.J.; Lang, I.A.; Langa, K.M.; Muniz-Terrera, G.; Phillips, C.L.; Cherubini, A.; Ferrucci, L.; Melzer, D. Vitamin D and Risk of Cognitive Decline in Elderly Persons. *Arch. Intern. Med.* **2010**, *170*, 1135–1141. [CrossRef]
52. Miller, J.W.; Harvey, D.J.; Beckett, L.A.; Green, R.; Farias, S.T.; Reed, B.R.; Olichney, J.M.; Mungas, D.M.; DeCarli, C. Vitamin D Status and Rates of Cognitive Decline in a Multiethnic Cohort of Older Adults. *JAMA Neurol.* **2015**, *72*, 1295–1303. [CrossRef] [PubMed]

53. Lapid, M.; Takahashi, P.Y.; Cha, S.S. Vitamin D and depression in geriatric primary care patients. *Clin. Interv. Aging* **2013**, *8*, 509–514. [CrossRef] [PubMed]
54. Cashman, K.D.; van den Heuvel, E.G.; Schoemaker, R.J.W.; Prévéraud, D.P.; Macdonald, H.M.; Arcot, J. 25-Hydroxyvitamin D as a Biomarker of Vitamin D Status and Its Modeling to Inform Strategies for Prevention of Vitamin D Deficiency within the Population. *Adv. Nutr.* **2017**, *8*, 947–957. [CrossRef] [PubMed]

vaccines

MDPI

Article

Effects of Severe Acute Respiratory Syndrome Coronavirus Vaccination on Reinfection: A Community-Based Retrospective Cohort Study

Hyerin Gim [1,2], Seul Lee [1], Haesook Seo [1], Yumi Park [3] and Byung Chul Chun [2,4,*]

1 Infectious Disease Research Center, Citizens' Health Bureau, Seoul Metropolitan Government, Seoul 04524, Republic of Korea; linflower@seoul.go.kr (H.G.); seul0710@gmail.com (S.L.); 27723@seoul.go.kr (H.S.)
2 Department of Epidemiology & Health Informatics, Graduate School of Public Health, Korea University, Seoul 02841, Republic of Korea
3 Citizens' Health Bureau, Seoul Metropolitan Government, Seoul 04524, Republic of Korea; soandho1@hanmail.net
4 Department of Preventive Medicine, Korea University College of Medicine, Seoul 02841, Republic of Korea
* Correspondence: chun@korea.ac.kr; Tel.: +82-02-2286-1169

Abstract: Background: Coronavirus disease 2019 (COVID-19) is a disease that is characterized by frequent reinfection. However, the factors influencing reinfection remain poorly elucidated, particularly regarding the effect of COVID-19 vaccination on preventing reinfection and its effects on symptomatology and the interval until reinfection. Methods: This retrospective cohort study examined patients with severe acute respiratory syndrome coronavirus reinfection between January 2020 and February 2022. This study included patients aged >17 years who were reinfected at least 90 days between two infections with severe acute respiratory syndrome coronavirus. The main outcome measure was a reduction in symptoms during reinfection, and reinfection interval. Results: Overall, 712 patients (average age: 40.52 ± 16.41 years; 312 males) were included. The reduction rate of symptoms at reinfection than that at first infection was significantly higher in the vaccinated group than in the unvaccinated group ($p < 0.001$). The average reinfection interval was 265.81 days. The interval between the first and second infection was 63.47 days longer in the vaccinated group than in the unvaccinated group. The interval was also 57.23 days, significantly longer in the asymptomatic group than in the symptomatic group ($p < 0.001$). Conclusions: Besides its role in preventing severe acute respiratory syndrome coronavirus infection, vaccination reduces the rate of symptomatic reinfection and increases the reinfection interval; thus, it is necessary to be vaccinated even after a previous infection. The findings may inform the decision to avail COVID-19 vaccination.

Keywords: COVID-19; epidemiology; reinfection; vaccination; symptoms

1. Introduction

Patients vaccinated against coronavirus disease 2019 (COVID-19) generally have a significantly lower risk of recurrent infection, symptomatic disease, and severity [1–4]. However, studies comparing clinical symptoms and severity in the same person are scarce. Further, for reinfection case confirmation, real-time polymerase chain reaction (RT-PCR) testing was only performed for the symptomatic cases in previous studies [3,5], and among COVID-19 cases, 40.5% were asymptomatic [6]. A bias in the studies of asymptomatic cases is likely. With the Omicron variant's emergence, which is known to have a high percentage of asymptomatic infections compared with the other variants [7–9], the proportion of completely asymptomatic cases may be much larger. Therefore, it is necessary to study populations of asymptomatic and symptomatic cases in a community-based retrospective cohort.

Severe acute respiratory syndrome coronavirus (SARS-CoV-2) infection or vaccination suppresses reinfection by increasing neutralizing antibodies [10,11]. In previous studies, natural immunity was shown to lower the risk of reinfection [12,13] and 20-month hospitalization [14]. Natural Killer cells (NK cells) play a major role in preventing viral infections and eliminating tumors, as well as for the work of the immune system [15]. Natural immunity such as NK cell and vaccination immunity reduce reinfection [14] and lower the risk of additional 9-month hospitalization [12]. The COVID-19 reinfection interval, which is the interval between consecutive infections, is the period from the first infection date to reinfection and represents the body's immune protection period against reinfection [10,16]. The reinfection interval after the first SARS-CoV-2 infection was found to be 6–8 months [17]. A protection period of more than 1 year is achieved when vaccination is performed despite SARS-CoV-2 infection [18]. During the Omicron variant spread, protective immunity against COVID-19 was reduced to 28.6–35.6% 10 weeks after vaccination [19]. As the COVID-19 pandemic continues and reinfection is likely to become more common [20], studying the reinfection interval is important.

To reduce infection numbers, SARS-CoV-2 vaccination in Korea began on 26 February 2021, focusing first on the elderly, immunocompromised population and healthcare workers, and then expanding to the rest of the population. Overall, 87.9% of the Korean population [21] and 87.7% of the population in Seoul have received basic vaccination (two doses of messenger ribonucleic acid (mRNA) and ChAdOx1 vaccine, one dose of Ad26.COV2.S) [22].

This study aimed to analyze the effect of SARS-CoV-2 vaccination on symptoms and severity during reinfection and identify the effects of vaccination on the reinfection interval.

2. Materials and Methods

2.1. Study Design and Cohort Construction

This was a retrospective cohort study conducted on first-infected Seoul citizens. The observation period was from 1 January 2020 to 24 February 2022. SARS-CoV-2 infection data were compiled and refined according to the Seoul Metropolitan Government's data, and vaccine information was provided by the Korea Centers for Disease Control and Prevention (KCDC). The sampling frame was the total population aged 18 years or older residing in Seoul. The study defined pandemic periods per national genomic surveillance as follows: Pre-Delta, 1 January 2020 to 30 June 2021; Delta, 1 July to 31 December 2021; and Omicron, 1 January to 30 April 2022 [23].

2.2. Study Cases

Infection cases only included those confirmed positive by RT-PCR testing during the study period. Reinfection cases were defined as $\geq$2 positive confirmations in the same person and an interval of at least 90 days between the first infection and reinfection dates, following the National Institutes of Health and the literature [11,24–26]. There were some cases of third infection among the study subjects; however, only reinfection was considered in this study. The reinfection interval was defined as the interval between consecutive infections confirmed by RT-PCR testing, and not the date of symptom onset, to prevent the omission of asymptomatic cases.

All SARS-CoV-2 vaccination records are uploaded and managed in real-time through the Disease Control and Prevention Integrated Management System in South Korea. Using this system, vaccinated patients were identified as those who had completed basic vaccination [27,28] (e.g., two doses of the mRNA and ChAdOx1 vaccine, one dose for Ad26.COV2.S) against COVID-19 between 26 February 2021 and 24 February 2022. Only licensed vaccines in Korea, with proven effectiveness in preventing infection [29–34] (ChAdOx1—Oxford University/AstraZeneca vaccine, Ad26.COV2.S—Johnson & Johnson (Janssen) vaccine, BNT162b2—BioNTech (Pfizer) vaccine, and mRNA-1273—Moderna vaccine), were included. The number of people vaccinated with the mRNA type of vaccine was 957, and with the vector type of vaccine was 231, and this included vaccinations from the 1st to the

4th round (Table S1). Those who had not completed basic vaccination were considered unvaccinated ($n = 202$). The vaccine data in the KCDC were documented along with the vaccination date, vaccine type, sex, and age. The collected infection and vaccination data were integrated to confirm the precedent relationship between the two datasets (Table S2). Patients infected within 14 days after vaccination were considered unvaccinated [35,36].

2.3. Data Selection

This retrospective cohort study was a public health investigation and research on infectious diseases targeting Korea, legally mandatory following the Infectious Disease Prevention Act (Nos. 14,316 [37] and 30,743 [38]). The Seoul Metropolitan Government conducted COVID-19 tests free of charge for anyone who had been in contact with a COVID-19 patient or wanted to be tested for suspected COVID-19 from November 2020 to 1 October 2022 [39]. With this, the COVID-19 test rate showed an increasing trend over time, and by 24 February 2022, the number of tests exceeded 32 million (the number that most Seoul citizens had received a COVID-19 RT-PCR test) [39]. The study outcome index was reinfection, and the secondary outcome index was the reinfection interval. The endpoint for the vaccine effectiveness was defined as the occurrence of COVID-19 reinfection, and for individuals who did not experience reinfection, the endpoint was set as the end of the study period, which was 24 February 2022. Potential confounding factors included sex, age, period of variant predominance, symptoms, underlying comorbidities, vaccination, and the effect of each variable combination.

The presence or absence of symptoms and severity during infection and reinfection were investigated using the same tool [40]. This study included information on sex, age, infection date, and symptoms and severity during infection. Fifteen symptoms were recorded, and the symptoms were further analyzed in three categories: systemic, including fever (>38 °C), muscle pain, chills, headache, malaise and fatigue, allergic reaction, and dizziness; local, including cough, sputum, sore throat, rhinorrhea, gastrointestinal disorder, and chest pain; and neurological, including the loss of smell and taste. Following the KCDC guidelines [41], severity was classified by Seoul city patient management teams of doctors during occurrence into three stages: asymptomatic and mild, if the situation immediately after the first infection did not interfere with daily life and oxygen therapy was unnecessary, even if it interfered with daily life; moderate, in cases of nasal tube or mask oxygen treatment; and severe, depending on the use of non-invasive ventilation, high-flow oxygen therapy, invasive ventilation, multi-organ damage, use of extracorporeal membrane oxygenation, or continuous renal replacement therapy. The clinical symptoms and their severity were assessed following the same guidelines [41].

2.4. Statistical Analysis

This study used the chi-square test or Fisher's exact test to compare differences between the vaccinated and unvaccinated groups to determine the vaccination's effect on reducing the number of clinical symptoms at first infection and reinfection. Cochran–Mantel–Haenszel analysis was performed to confirm differences in proportions of symptoms and severity according to vaccination status. Given that severity information was unavailable in some patients, the chi-square analysis was performed by classifying these patients into two groups: asymptomatic or mild group, and moderate or severe group. To determine the effect of time of the reinfection interval by sex, age, presence of symptoms, vaccination, and underlying morbidities, Kaplan–Meier analyses were performed, and multivariate regression analysis was performed with variables showing significant results in the Kaplan–Meier analysis. Age groups were divided into 10-year intervals (18–19, 20–29, 30–39, 40–49, 50–59, 60–69, 70–79, ≤80), where the 10s group included those aged 18–19 years. All results were estimated with 95% confidence intervals (CIs), and p values < 0.05 indicated statistical significance. All statistical analyses were performed using the Statistical Package for the Social Sciences software (version 24.0, IBM Corp., Armonk, NY, USA).

As this is an ongoing study with analysis triggered by novel circumstances, such as the emergence of the Omicron variant and increased reinfection, the sample sizes were not calculated before its initiation. Instead, the final sample size was calculated considering the inclusion and exclusion criteria.

2.5. Ethical Consideration

This study used secondary data approved by the Public Institutional Review Board designated by the Ministry of Health and Welfare of the Republic of Korea (IRB Approval Number: P01-202107-21-075). Patient consent was not required in this study. The results were reported following the STROBE guidelines [42] (Table S3). All authors confirmed the accuracy and completeness of the data and the study's originality.

3. Results

3.1. General Characteristics

Among the patients aged >17 years, 488,455 patients with SARS-CoV-2 infection con-firmed with RT-PCR testing were identified. Among these, 447,223 cases of infection were initially eligible, and 712 cases satisfying the definition of reinfection were included in the final analyses (Figure S1). Among the included patients, 43.8% were male, and the average age was 40.52 ± 16.41 years. A total of 510 individuals (71.6%) belonged to the vaccinated group, and no significant differences in gender distribution and most underlying comorbidities were observed between the vaccinated and unvaccinated groups. However, significant differences were found between the groups in terms of two underlying morbidities: hypertension and respiratory diseases. The majority (31.3%) of the patients with reinfection were in their 20s, while a minority (1.4%) were in their 80s (Table 1). The distribution of primary infection was 44.7% Pre-Delta and 55.3% Delta variants, and the distribution of reinfection was 7.3% Delta and 92.7% Omicron variants (Figure S2 and Tables S5 and S6).

Table 1. General characteristics of the study population based on vaccination status.

Characteristics	Total		Unvaccinated		Vaccinated		*p*-Value [a]
	No.	%	No.	%	No.	%	
Total	712	100.0	202	28.4	510	71.6	
Age							
Age (years), mean (SD)	40.52	16.4	36.91	14.84	41.95	16.80	<0.001
18–19	22	3.1	13	6.4	9	1.8	0.002
20–29	223	31.3	67	33.2	156	30.6	
30–39	135	19.0	48	23.8	87	17.1	
40–49	131	18.4	30	14.9	101	19.8	
50–59	80	11.2	22	10.9	58	11.4	
60–69	82	11.5	16	7.9	66	12.9	
70–79	29	4.1	4	2.0	25	4.9	
≥80	10	1.4	2	1.0	8	1.6	
Sex							
Female	400	56.2	110	54.5	290	56.9	0.31
Male	312	43.8	92	45.5	220	43.1	
Underlying morbidity							
Total	162	22.8	43	21.3	119	23.3	
Having an underlying morbidity, mean (SD)	1.46	0.79	1.26	0.64	1.53	0.83	0.10
Allergic disease	2	1.2	0	0.0	2	1.7	0.51
Cancer	6	3.7	1	2.3	5	4.2	0.46
Cardiovascular system disease	11	6.8	1	2.3	10	8.4	0.13
Cerebrovascular disease	6	3.7	2	4.7	4	3.4	0.55
Diabetes mellitus	39	24.1	8	18.6	31	26.1	0.18
Endocrine disease	7	4.3	3	7.0	4	3.4	0.32
Hypertension	62	38.3	11	25.6	51	42.9	0.03
Immunocompromised disease	3	1.9	2	4.7	1	0.8	0.16

Table 1. *Cont.*

Characteristics	Total		Unvaccinated		Vaccinated		*p*-Value [a]
	No.	%	No.	%	No.	%	
Kidney disease	6	3.7	3	7.0	3	2.5	0.23
Liver disease	2	1.2	0	0.0	2	1.7	0.51
Mental disorder	14	8.6	2	4.7	12	10.1	0.19
Respiratory system disease	28	17.3	13	30.2	15	12.6	0.03

[a] *p*-value from chi-square test or Fisher's exact test.

This study includes patients with SARS-CoV-2 reinfection aged >17 years and who had an interval of at least 90 days between two infections between January 2020 and February 2022.

3.2. Descriptive Data

3.2.1. Changes in Symptoms and Severity upon Reinfection According to Vaccination

In the unvaccinated group, during the reinfection compared to the first infection, the proportion of systemic symptoms decreased significantly by 23.08% ($p < 0.001$). In the vaccinated group, during the reinfection compared to the first infection, the proportion of systemic symptoms decreased significantly by 35.16%; local symptoms also significantly decreased by 11.39% during the reinfection compared to the first infection and neurological symptoms decreased by 11.03% ($p < 0.001$) (Table 2). An analysis according to vaccination status showed that the symptom reduction rate during reinfection compared to that during the first infection was significantly higher in the vaccinated than in the unvaccinated group ($p < 0.001$). The systemic symptom reduction rate, local symptom reduction rate, and neurological symptom reduction rate were significantly higher by 12.1%, 4.1%, and 5.2%, respectively ($p < 0.05$). The symptom reduction rates during reinfection for loss of smell and chills were significantly higher by 5.7% and 5.5%, respectively ($p < 0.001$) in the vaccinated group, and the symptom reduction rate for cough was significantly higher by 6.2% in the unvaccinated group ($p = 0.022$) (Table 2, Figure S3 and Table S7).

Table 2. Changes in apparent symptom frequencies between the first infection and reinfection of COVID-19 according to vaccination status.

	Unvaccinated (n = 202)				*p* Value	Vaccinated (n = 510)				*p* Value	Difference in Proportions of Symptoms According to Vaccination Status [a]		
	1st Infection		2nd Infection			1st Infection		2nd Infection					
	No.	%	No.	%		No.	%	No.	%		Diff %	Diff *p* Value	OR (95% CI [b])
Symptom													
No	36	17.82	79	39.11	<0.001	107	20.98	220	43.14	<0.001	−0.87	<0.001	0.35 (0.27–0.44)
Yes	166	82.18	123	60.89		403	79.02	290	56.86				
Symptom type													
Systemic symptom	95	57.23	42	34.15	<0.001	232	57.57	65	22.41	<0.001	−12.08	<0.001	0.26 (0.20–0.34)
Fever	66	39.76	24	19.51	<0.001	139	34.49	32	11.03	0.001	−3.21	<0.001	0.28 (0.20–0.38)
Myalgia	51	30.72	20	16.26	0.003	110	27.30	34	11.72	<0.001	−1.12	<0.001	0.38 (0.27–0.53)
Chills	38	22.89	17	13.82	0.04	92	22.83	24	8.28	<0.001	−5.48	<0.001	0.37 (0.25–0.54)
Headache	46	27.71	24	19.51	0.07	95	23.57	38	13.10	<0.001	−2.27	<0.001	0.53 (0.38–0.74)
Malaise and fatigue	5	3.01	4	3.25	0.58	28	6.95	6	2.07	0.002	−5.12	0.02	0.40 (0.20–0.83)
Allergic	0	0.00	2	1.63	0.18	1	0.25	2	0.69	0.38	−1.19	0.21	5.56 (0.62–50.0)
Dizziness	1	0.60	1	0.81	0.67	5	1.24	1	0.34	0.21	−1.11	0.54	0.46 (0.09–2.28)
Local symptom	112	67.47	74	60.16	0.12	278	68.98	167	57.59	<0.001	−4.08	0.001	0.64 (0.49–0.84)

Table 2. *Cont.*

	Unvaccinated (n = 202)				p Value	Vaccinated (n = 510)				p Value	Difference in Proportions of Symptoms According to Vaccination Status [a]		
	1st Infection No.	1st Infection %	2nd Infection No.	2nd Infection %		1st Infection No.	1st Infection %	2nd Infection No.	2nd Infection %		Diff %	Diff p Value	OR (95% CI [b])
Cough	83	50.00	47	38.21	0.03	163	40.45	101	34.83	0.08	6.17	0.02	0.73 (0.56–0.95)
Sputum	41	24.70	27	21.95	0.34	86	21.34	69	23.79	0.25	5.20	0.79	1.05 (0.78–1.42)
Sore throat	68	40.96	53	43.09	0.40	150	37.22	117	40.34	0.23	0.99	0.41	1.13 (0.87–1.46)
Rhinorrhea	11	6.63	16	13.01	0.05	32	7.94	20	6.90	0.36	−7.42	0.59	1.17 (0.73–1.85)
Gastro symptom	2	1.20	1	0.81	0.61	6	1.49	4	1.38	0.59	0.28	0.98	0.86 (0.28–2.65)
Chest pain	1	0.60	1	0.81	0.67	4	0.99	3	1.03	0.62	−0.17	0.85	1.11 (0.30–4.14)
Neurological symptom	15	9.04	4	3.25	0.08	50	12.41	4	1.38	<0.001	−5.24	<0.001	0.15 (0.07–0.32)
Loss of smell	6	3.61	3	2.44	0.42	32	7.94	3	1.03	<0.001	−5.74	<0.001	0.21 (0.09–0.49)
Loss of taste	11	6.63	2	1.63	0.04	29	7.20	2	0.69	<0.001	−1.51	<0.001	0.13 (0.05–0.36)
Severity [c]	(n = 193)		(n = 78)			(n = 495)		(n = 153)					
Mild or Lower	188	97.41	74	94.87	0.24	483	97.58	150	98.04	0.51	−3.00	0.86	1.21 (0.49–2.98)
Moderate or Severe	5	2.59	4	5.13		12	2.42	3	1.96				

Data are presented as n or %. [a] "Difference in proportions of symptoms according to vaccination status" means differences in proportions of a decrease in symptoms when confirming the comparison of first and second infection symptoms and the type of symptoms in the same person in comparison with the vaccinated group and the unvaccinated group, respectively. Cochran–Mantel–Haenszel analysis was performed to confirm the difference in proportions of symptoms and severity according to vaccination status. [b] CI, confidence interval. [c] Severity classified into two groups: asymptomatic or mild, and moderate or severe. Patients had been residents of Seoul since 1 January 2020. All patients were reinfected with SARS-CoV-2.

3.2.2. Influencing Factors of Reinfection Interval

The average reinfection interval was 265.78 (95% CI: 253.81–277.76) days. The reinfection interval by age group increased gradually from 234.59 days for those in their 10s to 322.22 days for those in their 60s ($p < 0.001$). The reinfection interval was significantly longer in the vaccinated group than in the unvaccinated group (283.79 days vs. 220.32 days, $p < 0.001$) and was significantly shorter in the symptomatic group than in the asymptomatic group (254.29 days vs. 311.52 days, $p < 0.001$). The reinfection intervals of different sexes and underlying comorbidities were similar (Table 3). The evaluation of vaccine effectiveness by vaccine type is presented in Table S8. Nevertheless, it is essential to approach the interpretation of these results with caution due to substantial differences in vaccination timing, target populations, and the number of vaccinated individuals among various vaccines (Table S4). Multivariate regression analysis included sex, age, presence of symptoms at the first infection, and vaccination; variables with significant results in the Kaplan–Meier analysis were used. During the Pre-Delta period, the reinfection interval increased significantly by 0.838 days for every 10-year increase in age and was significantly higher by 30.964 days in the vaccinated group than in the unvaccinated group (all $p < 0.05$). However, during the Delta period, reinfection intervals did not change significantly, with or without vaccination (Table 4).

Table 3. Distribution of the intervals for reinfection by age, underlying comorbidities, symptoms at the first infection, period of variant predominance, and vaccination status.

Reinfection Interval	No.	Median	IQR [a]	Mean (95% CI [b])	*p*-Value [c]
Total	712	164.50	129.00–419.00	265.78 (253.81–277.76)	
Age group, years					
18–19	22	147.00	134.00–358.25	234.59 (176.54–292.65)	0.003
20–29	223	157.00	129.00–387.00	237.83 (218.03–257.63)	
30–39	135	154.00	121.00–397.00	242.21 (217.21–267.22)	
40–49	131	170.00	128.00–425.00	279.54 (250.60–308.49)	
50–59	80	308.00	132.50–430.00	301.14 (262.24–340.04)	
60–69	82	361.00	148.00–438.50	322.22 (285.46–358.97)	
70–79	29	152.00	120.50–452.00	284.48 (219.27–349.69)	
≥80	10	186.00	110.25–466.75	295.90 (179.57–412.23)	
Vaccination					
Unvaccinated	202	141.00	119.00–323.25	220.32 (199.25–241.38)	<0.001
Vaccinated	510	218.00	133.75–424.00	283.79 (269.63–297.96)	
Presence of symptoms (1st infection)					
No	143	356.00	144.00–432.00	311.52 (284.57–338.46)	0.005
Yes	569	158.00	127.60–413.00	254.29 (241.11–267.47)	
Period of variant predominance					
Pre-Delta period	319	425.00	376.00–463.00	428.44 (417.34–439.53)	<0.001
Delta period	393	133.00	113.00–151.00	133.76 (131.05–136.47)	
Sex					
Female	400	165.00	129.50–421.75	268.48 (252.18–284.78)	0.22
Male	312	161.00	128.00–416.00	262.33 (244.77–279.89)	
Presence of underlying morbidity					
No	550	161.00	131.00–414.00	260.31 (246.98–273.63)	0.16
Yes	162	221.00	122.75–431.00	284.38 (257.78–310.99)	

Data are presented as *n* or %. [a] IQR, interquartile range. [b] CI, confidence interval. [c] Kaplan–Meier analyses were performed to determine the effect of time of the reinfection interval by sex, age, presence of symptoms, vaccination, and underlying morbidities. Patients had been residents of Seoul since 1 January 2020. All patients were reinfected with SARS-CoV-2.

Table 4. Multivariate regression analysis of the reinfection interval using sex, age, presence of symptoms at the first infection, and vaccination as variables.

	Coefficient	95% CI [a]		Standard Error	*p*-Value [b]
Pre-Delta period					
Sex	−12.446	−34.685	9.794	11.303	0.23
Age	0.838	0.172	1.504	0.339	0.01
Presence of symptoms at the first infection	7.274	−17.792	32.34	12.739	0.57
Vaccination	30.964	3.594	58.335	13.911	0.03
Delta period					
Sex	−0.269	−5.742	5.205	2.783	0.92
Age	−0.223	−0.397	−0.051	0.088	0.01
Presence of symptoms at the first infection	−3.839	−11.698	4.019	3.997	0.34
Vaccination	5.141	−0.67	10.953	2.956	0.08

[a] CI, confidence interval. [b] Multivariate regression analysis was performed with significant variables in the Kaplan–Meier analysis. Patients had been residents of Seoul since 1 January 2020. All patients were reinfected with SARS-CoV-2.

4. Discussion

This paired comparison study was conducted to confirm the effect of vaccination on the symptoms, severity, and reinfection interval of SARS-CoV-2 in the same person. In this study, patients who received vaccination showed a higher proportion of asymptomatic cases and milder symptoms during reinfection compared to those who were unvaccinated. Additionally, the reinfection interval was observed to be prolonged.

The reduction rate of symptoms upon reinfection compared to the first infection was significantly higher by 0.9% in the vaccinated group, consistent with previous findings that vaccination is significantly associated with symptomatic SARS-CoV-2 infection reduction [43]. Further, the reduction in systemic, local, and neurological symptoms was significantly higher in the vaccinated group than in the unvaccinated group. In the vaccinated group, the reduction rates of fever, myalgia, chills, headache, malaise and fatigue, and loss of smell and taste at reinfection were significantly higher than those in the unvaccinated group. The difference in proportions of moderate or severe cases according to vaccination status was insignificant.

However, to the best of our knowledge, previous studies have not compared the symptoms and severity between the first and second infections in the same patients in community-based cohort, and changes in detailed clinical symptoms of reinfection according to vaccination status have also not been studied to date. Nevertheless, the results of this study, conducted on the same patients, support the previous studies indicating that vaccination reduces the severity of reinfection [44,45]. However, a cohort study conducted in Denmark revealed that two vaccine doses offered merely a restricted and brief shield against SARS-CoV-2 infection with Omicron. Consequently, further ongoing research is warranted [46].

Vaccination status, presence of symptoms during the first infection, date of the first infection, and age difference significantly affected the reinfection interval. The reinfection interval gradually increased with age until the 60s. It was 63.47 days longer for the vaccinated group than that for the unvaccinated group, and 57.23 days longer for the asymptomatic group than for the symptomatic group. In multivariate regression analysis, during the Pre-Delta period, the reinfection interval increased significantly by 0.838 days for each 10-year increase in age and was significantly longer by 30.964 days for the vaccinated group. During the Delta period, the reinfection interval decreased significantly by 0.223 days for each 10-year increase in age. Vaccination during the Pre-Delta period significantly affected the reinfection interval, but vaccination during the Delta period did not. The reason for the impact of the reinfection interval during the pre-delta stage is believed to be twofold. Firstly, the SARS-CoV-2 infectivity became stronger during the

Delta stage [47–49], and secondly, the vaccine effectiveness was reduced in preventing SARS-CoV-2 infections during the Delta stage [50,51]. We were able to identify almost all of the secondary infections, regardless of the vaccination status, as we observed all subjects under the same conditions. Therefore, even if there were more cases of infections, there might have been differences in the effectiveness of the vaccine during the Pre-Delta and Delta stages. Furthermore, the effectiveness of the vaccine has continuously varied according to viral mutations [51,52]. In addition, this is identical to previous studies that showed that regardless of whether infection occurred before or after vaccination, the gradual decline in antibody titers according to hybrid immunity resulted in a decline in immunity, eventually losing protection against SARS-CoV-2 variant strains [4,11,14,53]. While many studies, including this research, support the effectiveness of the vaccine [1–4,10,11], there are also studies that suggest the vaccine afforded less protection, and effectiveness was not demonstrated [54].

To the best of our knowledge, no previous study has analyzed the influence of various factors on the reinfection interval through multivariate regression analysis. Also, in a previous study on a single variable, no relationship between age at first infection and reinfection was found [55]. By adding various variables to the results of previous studies, the current study confirmed that age can affect the reinfection interval. A previous study found that vaccination increased neutralizing antibodies that suppressed infection and increased immunity [10], supporting the hypothesis that vaccinations led to longer intervals for reinfection in the Pre-Delta period. Nevertheless, the efficacy of these vaccines has not been firmly established through long-term studies, and it cannot fully account for the impact of unmeasured factors. Consequently, akin to the situation observed with the previous BCG vaccine [56], the vaccine's effectiveness is beneficial rather than fully sufficient. However, there are few studies on how sex, symptoms at the first infection, underlying comorbidity, and vaccination affect the reinfection interval, and further research is needed.

This study had some limitations. First, as a study targeting Seoul citizens, it did not represent all reinfection cases. Nevertheless, a cohort was established for all patients infected with SARS-CoV-2, and reinfection cases were observed. Furthermore, since the same person was examined for symptoms and severity was measured with the same tool, as many confounding factors as possible were eliminated. Therefore, reinfected individuals can be considered representative by establishing an all-inclusive cohort within the community. Second, when analyzing the reinfection interval, Kaplan–Meier and Cox proportional hazards models were considered, but the vaccination effect decreased over time and did not satisfy the assumption of Cox proportional hazards analysis. Therefore, we used multivariate regression analysis, divided by two peaks according to the duration of the outbreak of the variant virus during the first infection, instead of Cox proportional hazards analysis. Third, since the SARS-CoV-2 infection date was based on the date of confirmation in the RT-PCR test, it may be unclear when exactly the infection occurred. However, since the SARS-CoV-2 infection date was determined by applying the same criteria to all infected patients, there would be no difference between vaccinated and unvaccinated patients. Additionally, this study is an observational epidemiological study without the use of placebo vaccines, which limited our ability to exclude the influence of nonidentical infection pressure. However, the factors influencing the vaccine's efficacy were symmetrically distributed between the vaccine and non-vaccine groups, and there was no evidence of reverse surveillance bias in disease monitoring. Lastly, although the non-specific effects of COVID-19 vaccination have been discussed and acknowledged [57,58], the assessment of the vaccine's non-specific effects was not within the primary scope of this study, as our primary objective was not to confirm their impact. Moreover, the potential for false positives and the challenge of differentiating between various respiratory infections also could potentially affect the interpretation of the results.

5. Conclusions

As COVID-19 spreads, it is important to understand the patterns and characteristics of reinfection cases, confirm vaccine protection, and encourage unvaccinated infected persons to become vaccinated. It was confirmed that vaccination relieved the clinical symptoms during reinfection. In particular, systemic and neurological symptoms were significantly reduced during reinfection in the vaccinated group. The factors influencing the reinfection interval were age, the presence of symptoms during the first infection, and vaccination. In the Pre-Delta period, age and vaccination had a significant effect on the reinfection interval, and in the Delta period, age had a significant effect.

Supplementary Materials: The following supporting information can be downloaded at: https://www.mdpi.com/article/10.3390/vaccines11091408/s1, Figure S1: Flow chart for the identification of COVID-19 reinfection; Figure S2: Distribution of the date of first infection and reinfection including vaccination information by the variant virus epidemic period; Figure S3: Reduced proportion of apparent symptoms between the first infection and reinfection of SARS-CoV-2 according to vaccination status; Table S1: Number of persons vaccinated with a particular type of vaccine; Table S2: Classification of vaccinated and non-vaccinated groups according to the order of COVID-19 vaccination and infection; Table S3: STROBE Statement—Checklist of items that should be included in reports of cohort studies; Table S4: General characteristics of the vaccinated population based on the vaccination type; Table S5: Comparison of characteristics of primary and secondary vaccination by the variant virus epidemic period on a weekly basis; Table S6: Comparison of characteristics of primary and secondary vaccination during the variant virus epidemic period on a monthly basis; Table S7: Comparison of differences in symptoms after first confirmation and reconfirmation according to vaccination status (present/absent); Table S8: Distribution of the intervals for reinfection by type of vaccine.

Author Contributions: Conceptualization, H.G. and B.C.C.; methodology, H.G. and B.C.C.; software, H.G. and B.C.C.; validation, B.C.C.; formal analysis, H.G.; investigation, H.G., S.L. and B.C.C.; resources, H.G. and S.L.; data curation, H.G. and S.L.; writing—original draft preparation, H.G.; writing—review and editing, H.G. and B.C.C.; visualization, H.G.; supervision, H.S., Y.P. and B.C.C.; project administration, H.G.; funding acquisition, H.S., Y.P. and B.C.C. All authors have read and agreed to the published version of the manuscript.

Funding: This research received no external funding.

Institutional Review Board Statement: The study was approved by the Public Institutional Review Board designated by the Ministry of Health and Welfare of the Republic of Korea (IRB Approval Number: P01-202107-21-075).

Informed Consent Statement: Patient consent was waived because only secondary deidentified data were used.

Data Availability Statement: The data used in this study are unavailable due to privacy restrictions.

Acknowledgments: We extend our gratitude to the Big Data Team of the Korea Disease Control and Prevention Agency for their valuable contributions.

Conflicts of Interest: The authors declare no conflict of interest.

References

1. Flacco, M.E.; Acuti Martellucci, C.; Baccolini, V.; De Vito, C.; Renzi, E.; Villari, P.; Manzoli, L. COVID-19 vaccines reduce the risk of SARS-CoV-2 reinfection and hospitalization: Meta-analysis. *Front. Med.* **2022**, *9*, 1023507. [CrossRef] [PubMed]
2. Gazit, S.; Shlezinger, R.; Perez, G.; Lotan, R.; Peretz, A.; Ben-Tov, A.; Herzel, E.; Alapi, H.; Cohen, D.; Muhsen, K.; et al. The incidence of SARS-CoV-2 reinfection in persons with naturally acquired immunity with and without subsequent receipt of a single dose of BNT162b2 vaccine: A retrospective cohort study. *Ann. Intern. Med.* **2022**, *175*, 674–681. [CrossRef] [PubMed]
3. Kirsebom, F.C.; Andrews, N.; Stowe, J.; Toffa, S.; Sachdeva, R.; Gallagher, E.; Groves, N.; O'Connell, A.M.; Chand, M.; Ramsay, M.; et al. COVID-19 vaccine effectiveness against the omicron (BA. 2) variant in England. *Lancet Infect. Dis.* **2022**, *22*, 931–933. [CrossRef] [PubMed]

4. Altarawneh, H.N.; Chemaitelly, H.; Hasan, M.R.; Ayoub, H.H.; Qassim, S.; AlMukdad, S.; Coyle, P.; Yassine, H.M.; Al-Khatib, H.A.; Bensilmane, F.M.; et al. Protection against the Omicron variant from previous SARS-CoV-2 infection. *N. Engl. J. Med.* **2022**, *386*, 1288–1290. [CrossRef]
5. Murugesan, M.; Mathews, P.; Paul, H.; Karthik, R.; Mammen, J.J.; Rupali, P. Protective effect conferred by prior infection and vaccination on COVID-19 in a healthcare worker cohort in South India. *PLoS ONE* **2022**, *17*, e0268797. [CrossRef] [PubMed]
6. Ma, Q.; Liu, J.; Liu, Q.; Kang, L.; Liu, R.; Jing, W.; Wu, Y.; Liu, M. Global percentage of asymptomatic SARS-CoV-2 infections among the tested population and individuals with confirmed COVID-19 diagnosis: A systematic review and meta-analysis. *JAMA Netw. Open* **2021**, *4*, e2137257. [CrossRef] [PubMed]
7. Meo, S.; Meo, A.; Al-Jassir, F.; Klonoff, D. Omicron SARS-CoV-2 new variant: Global prevalence and biological and clinical characteristics. *Eur. Rev. Med. Pharmacol. Sci.* **2021**, *25*, 8012–8018. [CrossRef] [PubMed]
8. Yu, W.; Guo, Y.; Zhang, S.; Kong, Y.; Shen, Z.; Zhang, J. Proportion of asymptomatic infection and nonsevere disease caused by SARS-CoV-2 Omicron variant: A systematic review and analysis. *J. Med. Virol.* **2022**, *94*, 5790–5801. [CrossRef]
9. Shang, W.; Kang, L.; Cao, G.; Wang, Y.; Gao, P.; Liu, J.; Liu, M. Percentage of asymptomatic infections among SARS-CoV-2 omicron variant-positive individuals: A systematic review and meta-analysis. *Vaccines* **2022**, *10*, 1049. [CrossRef]
10. Khoury, D.S.; Cromer, D.; Reynaldi, A.; Schlub, T.E.; Wheatley, A.K.; Juno, J.A.; Subbarao, K.; Kent, S.J.; Triccas, J.A.; Davenport, M.P. Neutralizing antibody levels are highly predictive of immune protection from symptomatic SARS-CoV-2 infection. *Nat. Med.* **2021**, *27*, 1205–1211. [CrossRef]
11. Bellusci, L.; Grubbs, G.; Zahra, F.T.; Forgacs, D.; Golding, H.; Ross, T.M.; Khurana, S. Antibody affinity and cross-variant neutralization of SARS-CoV-2 Omicron BA. 1, BA. 2 and BA. 3 following third mRNA vaccination. *Nat. Commun.* **2022**, *13*, 4617. [CrossRef] [PubMed]
12. Nordström, P.; Ballin, M.; Nordström, A. Risk of SARS-CoV-2 reinfection and COVID-19 hospitalisation in individuals with natural and hybrid immunity: A retrospective, total population cohort study in Sweden. *Lancet Infect. Dis.* **2022**, *22*, 781–790. [CrossRef] [PubMed]
13. Hammerman, A.; Sergienko, R.; Friger, M.; Beckenstein, T.; Peretz, A.; Netzer, D.; Yaron, S.; Arbel, R. Effectiveness of the BNT162b2 vaccine after recovery from COVID-19. *N. Engl. J. Med.* **2022**, *386*, 1221–1229. [CrossRef] [PubMed]
14. Goldberg, Y.; Mandel, M.; Bar-On, Y.M.; Bodenheimer, O.; Freedman, L.S.; Ash, N.; Alroy-Preis, S.; Huppert, A.; Milo, R. Protection and waning of natural and hybrid immunity to SARS-CoV-2. *N. Engl. J. Med.* **2022**, *386*, 2201–2212. [CrossRef] [PubMed]
15. Zimmer, J.; Jurišić, V. Special Issue "New Developments in Natural Killer Cells for Immunotherapy". *Cells* **2023**, *12*, 1496. [CrossRef] [PubMed]
16. Bates, T.A.; Leier, H.C.; McBride, S.K.; Schoen, D.; Lyski, Z.L.; Lee, D.X.; Messer, W.B.; Curlin, M.E.; Tafesse, F.G. An extended interval between vaccination and infection enhances hybrid immunity against SARS-CoV-2 variants. *JCI Insight* **2023**, *8*, e165265. [CrossRef] [PubMed]
17. Chivese, T.; Matizanadzo, J.T.; Musa, O.A.; Hindy, G.; Furuya-Kanamori, L.; Islam, N.; Al-Shebly, R.; Shalaby, R.; Habibullah, M.; Al-Marwani, T.A.; et al. The prevalence of adaptive immunity to COVID-19 and reinfection after recovery—A comprehensive systematic review and meta-analysis. *Pathog. Glob. Health* **2022**, *116*, 269–281. [CrossRef] [PubMed]
18. Hall, V.; Foulkes, S.; Insalata, F.; Kirwan, P.; Saei, A.; Atti, A.; Wellington, E.; Khawam, J.; Munro, K.; Cole, M.; et al. Protection against SARS-CoV-2 after COVID-19 vaccination and previous infection. *N. Engl. J. Med.* **2022**, *386*, 1207–1220. [CrossRef]
19. Andrews, N.; Stowe, J.; Kirsebom, F.; Toffa, S.; Rickeard, T.; Gallagher, E.; Gower, C.; Kall, M.; Groves, N.; O'Connell, A.M.; et al. COVID-19 vaccine effectiveness against the Omicron (B. 1.1. 529) variant. *N. Engl. J. Med.* **2022**, *386*, 1532–1546. [CrossRef]
20. Townsend, J.P.; Hassler, H.B.; Wang, Z.; Miura, S.; Singh, J.; Kumar, S.; Ruddle, N.H.; Galvani, A.P.; Dornburg, A. The durability of immunity against reinfection by SARS-CoV-2: A comparative evolutionary study. *Lancet Microbe* **2021**, *2*, e666–e675. [CrossRef]
21. Korea Disease Control and Prevention Agency. COVID-19 Vaccination Dashboard. Available online: https://ncv.kdca.go.kr/eng/ (accessed on 31 May 2023).
22. Seoul Metropolitan Government. COVID-19 Vaccination Status. Available online: https://www.seoul.go.kr/coronaV/coronaStatus.do?menu_code=47 (accessed on 31 May 2023).
23. Jang, E.J.; Choe, Y.J.; Yun, G.W.; Wang, S.; Cho, U.J.; Yi, S.; Lee, S.; Park, Y.J. Reinfection with SARS-CoV-2 in general population, South Korea; nationwide retrospective cohort study. *J. Med. Virol.* **2022**, *94*, 5589–5592. [CrossRef]
24. Arteaga-Livias, K.; Panduro-Correa, V.; Pinzas-Acosta, K.; Perez-Abad, L.; Pecho-Silva, S.; Espinoza-Sánchez, F.; Dámaso-Mata, B.; Rodriguez-Morales, A.J. COVID-19 reinfection? A suspected case in a Peruvian patient. *Travel Med. Infect. Dis.* **2021**, *39*, 101947. [CrossRef] [PubMed]
25. Yahav, D.; Yelin, D.; Eckerle, I.; Eberhardt, C.S.; Wang, J.; Cao, B.; Kaiser, L. Definitions for coronavirus disease 2019 reinfection, relapse and PCR re-positivity. *Clin. Microbiol. Infect.* **2021**, *27*, 315–318. [CrossRef] [PubMed]
26. Abu-Raddad, L.J.; Chemaitelly, H.; Bertollini, R. Severity of SARS-CoV-2 reinfections as compared with primary infections. *N. Engl. J. Med.* **2021**, *385*, 2487–2489. [CrossRef] [PubMed]
27. Korea Disease Control and Prevention Agency. Revision of COVID-19 Vaccination Standards and Related FAQ Information (27 October 2022). Available online: https://ncv.kdca.go.kr/board.es?mid=a12101000000&bid=0031#content (accessed on 31 May 2023).
28. Creech, C.B.; Walker, S.C.; Samuels, R.J. SARS-CoV-2 vaccines. *JAMA* **2021**, *325*, 1318–1320. [CrossRef] [PubMed]

29. Falsey, A.R.; Sobieszczyk, M.E.; Hirsch, I.; Sproule, S.; Robb, M.L.; Corey, L.; Neuzil, K.M.; Hahn, W.; Hunt, J.; Mulligan, M.J.; et al. Phase 3 safety and efficacy of AZD1222 (ChAdOx1 nCoV-19) COVID-19 vaccine. *N. Engl. J. Med.* **2021**, *385*, 2348–2360. [CrossRef] [PubMed]
30. Baden, L.R.; El Sahly, H.M.; Essink, B.; Kotloff, K.; Frey, S.; Novak, R.; Diemert, D.; Spector, S.A.; Rouphael, N.; Creech, C.B.; et al. Efficacy and safety of the mRNA-1273 SARS-CoV-2 vaccine. *N. Engl. J. Med.* **2021**, *384*, 403–416. [CrossRef] [PubMed]
31. Thomas, S.J.; Moreira, E.D., Jr.; Kitchin, N.; Absalon, J.; Gurtman, A.; Lockhart, S.; Perez, J.L.; Marc, G.P.; Polack, F.P.; Zerbini, C.; et al. Safety and efficacy of the BNT162b2 mRNA COVID-19 vaccine through 6 months. *N. Engl. J. Med.* **2021**, *385*, 1761–1773. [CrossRef]
32. Patel, R.; Kaki, M.; Potluri, V.S.; Kahar, P.; Khanna, D. A comprehensive review of SARS-CoV-2 vaccines: Pfizer, moderna & Johnson & Johnson. *Hum. Vaccines Immunother.* **2022**, *18*, 2002083. [CrossRef]
33. Sadoff, J.; Gray, G.; Vandebosch, A.; Cárdenas, V.; Shukarev, G.; Grinsztejn, B.; Goepfert, P.A.; Truyers, C.; Fennema, H.; Spiessens, B.; et al. Safety and efficacy of single-dose Ad26. COV2. S vaccine against COVID-19. *N. Engl. J. Med.* **2021**, *384*, 2187–2201. [CrossRef]
34. Voysey, M.; Clemens, S.A.C.; Madhi, S.A.; Weckx, L.Y.; Folegatti, P.M.; Aley, P.K.; Angus, B.; Baillie, V.L.; Barnabas, S.L.; Bhorat, Q.E.; et al. Safety and efficacy of the ChAdOx1 nCoV-19 vaccine (AZD1222) against SARS-CoV-2: An interim analysis of four randomised controlled trials in Brazil, South Africa, and the UK. *Lancet* **2021**, *397*, 99–111. [CrossRef] [PubMed]
35. Chemaitelly, H.; Yassine, H.M.; Benslimane, F.M.; Al Khatib, H.A.; Tang, P.; Hasan, M.R.; Malek, J.A.; Coyle, P.; Ayoub, H.H.; Kanaani, Z.A.; et al. mRNA-1273 COVID-19 vaccine effectiveness against the B. 1.1. 7 and B. 1.351 variants and severe COVID-19 disease in Qatar. *Nat. Med.* **2021**, *27*, 1614–1621. [CrossRef] [PubMed]
36. Thompson, M.G.; Burgess, J.L.; Naleway, A.L.; Tyner, H.L.; Yoon, S.K.; Meece, J.; Olsho, L.E.; Caban-Martinez, A.J.; Fowlkes, A.; Lutrick, K.; et al. Interim estimates of vaccine effectiveness of BNT162b2 and mRNA-1273 COVID-19 vaccines in preventing SARS-CoV-2 infection among health care personnel, first responders, and other essential and frontline workers—Eight US locations, December 2020–March 2021. *Morb. Mortal. Wkly. Rep.* **2021**, *70*, 495–500. [CrossRef]
37. Ministry of Government Legislation of Republic of Korea. Infectious Disease Control and Prevention Act. Available online: https://www.law.go.kr/LSW/lsInfoP.do?lsiSeq=188080&viewCls=engLsInfoR&urlMode=engLsInfoR&chrClsCd=010203#0000 (accessed on 31 May 2023).
38. Ministry of Government Legislation of Republic of Korea. Enforcement Decree of the Infectious Disease Control and Prevention Act. Available online: https://elaw.klri.re.kr/kor_service/lawView.do?hseq=54657&lang=ENG (accessed on 31 May 2023).
39. Seoul Metropolitan Government. The Daily News Review about Seoul Response to COVID-19. Available online: https://www.seoul.go.kr/coronaV/coronaStatus.do?menu_code=07 (accessed on 31 May 2023).
40. Korea Disease Control and Prevention Agency. Basic and In-Depth Investigation of COVID-19 (Translated into 16 Languages). Available online: https://www.kcda.go.kr/board/board.es?mid=a20507030000&bid=0020 (accessed on 31 May 2023).
41. Korea Disease Control and Prevention Agency. Coronavirus Infectious Disease-19 Response Guidelines 13-1. Available online: https://ncov.kdca.go.kr/duBoardList.do?brdld=2&brdGubun=28 (accessed on 31 May 2023).
42. Von Elm, E.; Altman, D.G.; Egger, M.; Pocock, S.J.; Gøtzsche, P.C.; Vandenbroucke, J.P. The Strengthening the Reporting of Observational Studies in Epidemiology (STROBE) statement: Guidelines for reporting observational studies. *Lancet* **2007**, *370*, 1453–1457. [CrossRef] [PubMed]
43. Rotshild, V.; Hirsh-Raccah, B.; Miskin, I.; Muszkat, M.; Matok, I. Comparing the clinical efficacy of COVID-19 vaccines: A systematic review and network meta-analysis. *Sci. Rep.* **2021**, *11*, 22777. [CrossRef] [PubMed]
44. Goldberg, Y.; Mandel, M.; Bar-On, Y.M.; Bodenheimer, O.; Freedman, L.; Haas, E.J.; Milo, R.; Alroy-Preis, S.; Ash, N.; Huppert, A. Waning immunity after the BNT162b2 vaccine in Israel. *N. Engl. J. Med.* **2021**, *385*, e85. [CrossRef] [PubMed]
45. Chatterjee, P.; Anand, T.; Singh, K.J.; Rasaily, R.; Singh, R.; Das, S.; Singh, H.; Praharaj, I.; Gangakhedkar, R.R.; Bhargava, B.; et al. Healthcare workers & SARS-CoV-2 infection in India: A case-control investigation in the time of COVID-19. *Indian J. Med. Res.* **2020**, *151*, 459–467. [CrossRef]
46. Gram, M.A.; Emborg, H.-D.; Schelde, A.B.; Friis, N.U.; Nielsen, K.F.; Moustsen-Helms, I.R.; Legarth, R.; Hoa Lam, J.U.; Chaine, M.; Malik, A.Z.; et al. Vaccine effectiveness against SARS-CoV-2 infection or COVID-19 hospitalization with the Alpha, Delta, or Omicron SARS-CoV-2 variant: A nationwide Danish cohort study. *PLoS Med.* **2022**, *19*, e1003992. [CrossRef]
47. Public Health England. SARS-CoV-2 Variants of Concern and Variants under Investigation in England. Technical Briefing 2021; p. 23, Report No. 15. 11 June 2021. Available online: https://assets.publishing.service.gov.uk/government/uploads/system/uploads/attachment_data/file/993879/Variants_of_Concern_VOC_Technical_Briefing_15.pdf (accessed on 31 May 2023).
48. Fisman, D.N.; Tuite, A.R. Evaluation of the relative virulence of novel SARS-CoV-2 variants: A retrospective cohort study in Ontario, Canada. *Can. Med. Assoc. J.* **2021**, *193*, e1619–e1625. [CrossRef]
49. Sheikh, A.; McMenamin, J.; Taylor, B.; Robertson, C. SARS-CoV-2 Delta VOC in Scotland: Demographics, risk of hospital admission, and vaccine effectiveness. *Lancet* **2021**, *397*, 2461–2462. [CrossRef]
50. Lopez Bernal, J.; Andrews, N.; Gower, C.; Gallagher, E.; Simmons, R.; Thelwall, S.; Stowe, J.; Tessier, E.; Groves, N.; Dabrera, G.; et al. Effectiveness of COVID-19 vaccines against the B. 1.617. 2 (Delta) variant. *N. Engl. J. Med.* **2021**, *385*, 585–594. [CrossRef]
51. Pouwels, K.B.; Pritchard, E.; Matthews, P.C.; Stoesser, N.; Eyre, D.W.; Vihta, K.D.; House, T.; Hay, J.; Bell, J.I.; Newton, J.N.; et al. Effect of Delta variant on viral burden and vaccine effectiveness against new SARS-CoV-2 infections in the UK. *Nat. Med.* **2021**, *27*, 2127–2135. [CrossRef] [PubMed]

52. Nielsen, K.F.; Moustsen-Helms, I.R.; Schelde, A.B.; Gram, M.A.; Emborg, H.D.; Nielsen, J.; Hansen, C.H.; Andersen, M.A.; Meaidi, M.; Wohlfahrt, J.; et al. Vaccine effectiveness against SARS-CoV-2 reinfection during periods of Alpha, Delta, or Omicron dominance: A Danish nationwide study. *PLoS Med.* **2022**, *19*, e1004037. [CrossRef]
53. Bates, T.A.; McBride, S.K.; Leier, H.C.; Guzman, G.; Lyski, Z.L.; Schoen, D.; Winders, B.; Lee, J.Y.; Lee, D.X.; Messer, W.B.; et al. Vaccination before or after SARS-CoV-2 infection leads to robust humoral response and antibodies that effectively neutralize variants. *Sci. Immunol.* **2022**, *7*, eabn8014. [CrossRef] [PubMed]
54. Shrestha, N.K.; Burke, P.C.; Nowacki, A.S.; Simon, J.F.; Hagen, A.; Gordon, S.M. Effectiveness of the Coronavirus Disease 2019 Bivalent Vaccine. *Open Forum Infect. Dis.* **2023**, *10*, ofad209. [CrossRef] [PubMed]
55. Qureshi, A.I.; Baskett, W.I.; Huang, W.; Lobanova, I.; Hasan Naqvi, S.; Shyu, C.-R. Reinfection with severe acute respiratory syndrome coronavirus 2 (SARS-CoV-2) in patients undergoing serial laboratory testing. *Clin. Infect. Dis.* **2022**, *74*, 294–300. [CrossRef] [PubMed]
56. Hatherill, M.; Cobelens, F. Infant BCG vaccination is beneficial, but not sufficient. *Lancet Glob. Health* **2022**, *10*, e1220–e1221. [CrossRef] [PubMed]
57. Aaby, P.; Netea, M.G.; Benn, C.S. Beneficial non-specific effects of live vaccines against COVID-19 and other unrelated infections. *Lancet Infect. Dis.* **2023**, *23*, e34–e42. [CrossRef]
58. Benn, C.S.; Schaltz-Buchholzer, F.; Nielsen, S.; Netea, M.G.; Aaby, P. Randomized clinical trials of COVID-19 vaccines: Do adenovirus-vector vaccines have beneficial non-specific effects? *Iscience* **2023**, *26*, 106733. [CrossRef]

vaccines

MDPI

Article

Single Ferritin Nanocages Expressing SARS-CoV-2 Spike Variants to Receptor and Antibodies

Monikaben Padariya * and Umesh Kalathiya *

International Centre for Cancer Vaccine Science, University of Gdansk, ul. Kładki 24, 80-822 Gdansk, Poland
* Correspondence: monikaben.padariya@ug.edu.pl (M.P.); umesh.kalathiya@ug.edu.pl (U.K.)

Abstract: SARS-CoV-2 virus variants of concern (VOCs) have rapidly changed their transmissibility and pathogenicity primarily through mutations in the structural proteins. Herein, we present molecular details with dynamics of the ferritin nanocages stitched with synthetic chimeras displaying the Spike receptor binding domains (RBDs). Our findings demonstrated the potential usage of ferritin-based vaccines that may effectively inhibit viral entry by blocking the Spike–ACE2 network and may induce cross-protective antibody responses. Taking the nanocage constructs into consideration, we evaluated the effects of variants on the docked interface of the SARS-CoV-2 Spike RBD with the ACE2 (angiotensin-converting enzyme 2) host cell receptor and neutralizing antibodies (Abs). Investigating the VOCs revealed that most of the mutations reported a possibly reduced structural stability within the Spike RBD domain. Point mutations have moderate or no effect for VVH-72, CR3022, and S309 Abs when bound with the Spike RBD, whereas a significant effect was observed for B38, CB6, and m396 over the surface of the H-ferritin nanocage. In addition to providing useful therapeutic approaches against COVID-19 (coronavirus disease 2019), these structural details can also be used to fight future coronavirus outbreaks.

Keywords: antibodies; spike; host cell receptor; mutations; COVID-19; nanocages; ferritin; SARS-CoV-2

1. Introduction

Ferritin nanocages are known for their inherent cavity that varies in size, biocompatibility, and high water solubility, enabling potential applications in diverse disciplines such as medicine, food, nutrition, etc. Ferritin nanocages can vary in size (16-mer, 24-mer (a typical size), 48-mer, etc.), and among them, H-ferritins are well known for use in several applications [1,2]. The monodispersed architectures of these self-assembled ferritin nanocages generated by a small number of units have attracted researchers and are versatile nanoparticles among many types of nanocarriers such as liposomes, cyclodextrin, etc. [3–7]. The usage of ferritin molecules has been extensive for vaccine generation as they can be easily degraded and also have low toxicity and immunogenicity [8]. In oncology, these H-ferritin nanocages can also be used as a delivery system of indocyanine green (ICG) for fluorescence-guided surgery applications [9], alongside drug delivery in cancer therapies [10]. In addition to the drug molecules encapsulated within the nanocages, ferritins are often combined with different modifications to enhance their therapeutic effects [8]. They have been reported as an attractive molecule for vaccine development by displaying antigen molecules over its surface (in the active form) that could enhance immune response or modulating binding with the target gene [11–15].

Among the different SARS-CoV-2 structural proteins, the virus uses the glycosylated Spike to directly contact the host cell receptor through the ACE2 (angiotensin-converting enzyme 2). Individual subunits from the Spike homotrimer (a functional form) were found to gain different pre- and post-fusion conformations. In particular, the pre-fusion state or conformation of the Spike protein has been widely used to guide different therapeutics.

In our previous work [16], we investigated the dynamics of different ferritin (H and L) nanocages that can represent receptor binding domains (RBDs) from the SARS-CoV-2 Spike protein over its surface. Investigating differently sized linkers stitching ferritin and Spike RBD highlighted that a five amino acid (GGGGS) linker can be an optimal length to maintain the 'up' active conformations of RBDs [16,17]. These Spike RBDs forming direct interactions with the ACE2 host cell receptor [18–20] are potential therapeutic targets against SARS CoV 2 infection. The glycosylated homotrimer structure of the Spike protein has S1 and S2 subunits [21]; and the Spike RBD domain (329–521 amino acids; aa) belongs to the S1 subunits. Antibodies designed especially for these Spike RBDs can efficiently neutralize the infection [20]. The longevity of antibody response against the SARS-CoV-2 Spike protein from a dataset of vaccinated candidates revealed that it can be sustained up to 12 months [22]. Explicitly, we evaluated the behavior of the Spike RBD over the ferritin nanocages and their binding regions responsible for interacting with the host ACE2 receptor and different antibodies (Abs) such as VVH-72, B38, CB6, CR3066, m396, and S309 (Figure 1) [23–25]. These antibodies have a slight different interaction network or binding mechanism with the SARS-CoV-2 Spike RBD and ACE2 receptor [26–30]: (i) the VVH-72 and B38 Abs dock the Spike RBD, which eventually prevents its interaction with ACE2, (ii) m296 forms interactions with the Spike RBD without mimicking ACE2 (however, it can create allosteric effects that can block it with ACE2), (iii) CB6 mimics ACE2 binding to the Spike RBD, and (iv) S309 and CR3022 Abs interact with the Spike RBD domain without disrupting its interaction with ACE2. Alongside investigating dynamics and interaction patterns or patches of the Spike RBD over ferritin nanocages, using in silico techniques (Molecular Operating Environment, MOE; Chemical Computing Group Inc., Montreal, QC, Canada) [31], we studied its change in the binding affinity toward ACE2 or antibodies with respect to different mutations (variants of concerns; VOC) derived from the SARS-CoV-2 variants (Alpha, B.1.1.7; Beta, B.1.351; Delta, B.1.617.2 and B.1.617; Gamma, P.1; Lambda, C.37; and Omicron, B.1.1.529 (Figure 1) [32,33].

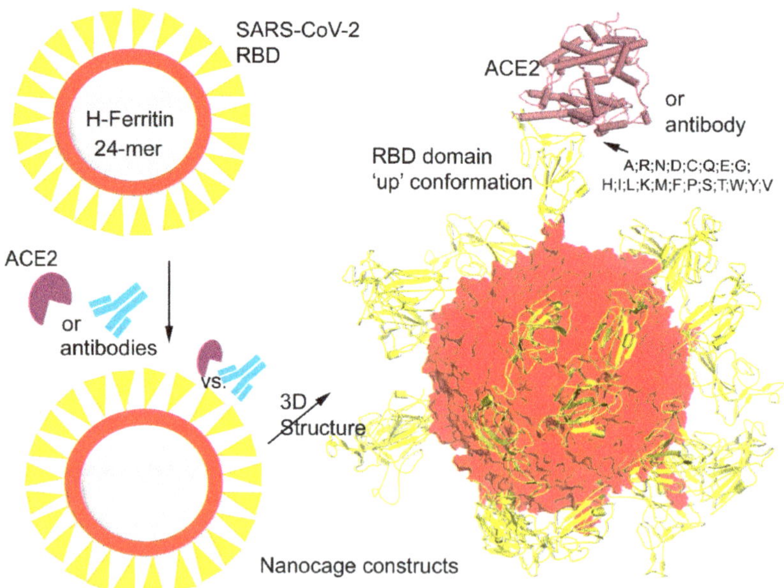

Figure 1. Diagram representing the model system of H-ferritin nanocage with SARS-CoV-2 Spike receptor binding domains (RBDs) docked with angiotensin-converting enzyme 2 (ACE2) host cell

receptor and different antibodies. The right panel demonstrates the 3D structure of the Spike RDB domain in the 'up' active conformation [16] stitched together with the ferritin nanocage, and these protein–protein or antibody (Abs) interfaces were considered to investigate the mutational landscape over the Spike RBD domain.

2. Materials and Methods

2.1. The Model Selection and Chimera Constructs of Ferritin–RBD–Receptor or Antibody Complexes

The constructs of H-ferritin connected by different sized linkers with the Spike RBD were designed in our previous work [16], which were generated based on the available structures from the PDB database (protein data bank; www.rcsb.org). The crystal structure of the Spike RBD domain (PDB ID: 6lzg [34]) in the 'up' active conformation docked with the ACE2 receptor was considered in this study. Implementing the nanocage generation module from the PDBePISA (proteins, interfaces, structures, and assemblies) [35], the 24-mer ferritin nanocage structure was built and was further optimized using molecular dynamics simulations (MDSs) [16]. The optimal five amino acids GGGGS linker that stabilizes the orientation in the 'up' active conformation of the Spike RBD domains over the H-ferritin nanocages was taken into consideration in our study. These ferritin–RBD–ACE2 or antibody systems were designed using different homology modeling pipelines and modules within the MOE package [16,18].

To investigate the binding or the docked interfaces of antibodies with the SARS-CoV-2 Spike RBD domain over the H-ferritin nanocages, the following structures were considered: (i) and (ii) VVH-72 (PDB ID: 6waq [30]) and B38 (PDB ID: 7bz5 [36]) forms an interaction with the Spike RDB where the ACE2 binds, (iii) m396 binds to the Spike RBD, preventing Spike–ACE2 docking (PDB ID: 2dd8 [26]), (iv) CB6 mimics the ACE2 interaction site over the Spike RBD (PDB ID: 7c01 [27]), (v) S309 (PDB ID: 6wps [28]) and (vi) CR3022 (PDB ID: 6w41 [29]) enable binding with the Spike RBD domain without disrupting its interaction with ACE2 [24]. The conformation or position of all six antibodies were sustained as retrieved from the PDB database, which were further considered to design homology models of the ferritin–linker–RBD (PDB ID: 6lzg [34]) complexes within the MOE package. Implementing the CHARMM27 forcefield [37], the constructed model systems over the ferritin–RBD–antibody were energy minimized. The MOE and BIOVIA Discovery Studio (DassaultSystèmes, BIOVIA Corp., San Diego, CA, USA) packages were used to represent proteins, antibodies, or nanocage structures.

2.2. The 'Residue Scan' Approach to Identify Change in the Binding Affinity

These ferritin–linker–RBD–receptor or antibody modeled structures were used to identify changes in the binding affinity or stability upon inserting point mutations retrieved from different SARS-CoV-2 variants: Alpha (B.1.1.7), Beta (B.1.351), Delta (B.1.617.2 and B.1.617), Gamma (P.1), Lambda (C.37), and Omicron (B.1.1.529) [32,33]. An optimized "residue scan" pipeline or module incorporated within the MOE packages was used to generate mutant models. Applying the concept of relative binding free energy ($\Delta\Delta G_{bind}$; thermostability), differences of wild-type and mutant energies were retrieved using the Boltzmann relative stability of the ensemble. Apart from the Spike RBD mutations that emerged from different SARS-CoV-2 variants, we further evaluated them with our pipelines, where a single residue can be mutated at a time with all possible amino acids: A, R, N, D, C, Q, E, G, H, I, L, K, M, F, P, S, T, W, Y, and V. For these mutations, the change in the binding affinity ($\Delta\Delta G$) of the Spike RBD–receptor or antibodies over the ferritin nanocage surface was measured using the LowModeMD ensemble (10k iterations) and CHARMM27 forcefield [16,38]. The negative ($\Delta\Delta G$) structural stability or binding affinity for a mutation induces the stability within the structure or protein–antibody energy, whereas a positive value shows contradictory results.

3. Results

Several studies have shown that the ferritin nanocages can explicitly display proteins or peptides over its surface [39–46]. In particular, the Spike RBD targeting vaccines and neutralizing antibodies can effectively block the viral entry by interrupting the binding between the ACE2 host cell receptor and SARS-CoV-2 Spike RBD domain [41–46]. Since this could provide useful therapeutic approaches against COVID-19 (coronavirus disease 2019), we investigated the mutational landscape of the Spike RBD with the ACE2 host–cell receptor or different antibodies displayed over the ferritin nanocages.

3.1. Influence of Mutational Landscape over the Spike RBD–ACE2 Interface

Mutations within the Spike RBD regions lead or have been correlated to the emergence of different SARS-CoV-2 variants such as Alpha (B.1.1.7), Beta (B.1.351), Delta (B.1.617.2 and B.1.617), Gamma (P.1), Lambda (C.37), and Omicron (B.1.1.529; Figure 2). Since these variants enhance the binding and infectivity of the virus compared to the wild type, we performed an analysis of their mutations by introducing them in an optimized Spike RBD over the H-ferritin (24 subunits) nanocage structures (Figures 2 and S1). These mutated SARS-CoV-2 Spike RBDs over the ferritin nanocage stitched by a five amino acids linker were reconstructed with the ACE2 receptor [34,47]. A comparative Spike RBD sequence variability from different SARS-CoV-2 variants guided the location of point mutations. The Spike RBD from the SARS-CoV-2 Omicron variant contains the highest number of mutations (15 amino acid changes) compared to the SARS-CoV-2 α, β, γ, and δ variants.

Such substitutions within the Spike RBD domain are crucial for SARS-CoV-2 infectivity, since they severely affect the binding of the Spike protein with the ACE2 host cell receptor. Subsequently, the potential influence of these mutations on properties like protein stability and binding affinity have been evaluated for the ferritin–RBD–ACE2 complexes (Figures 2 and S1). Replacing a specific mutated residue with every possible substitution (A, R, N, D, C, Q, E, G, H, I, L, K, M, F, P, S, T, W, Y, and V), the majority of the exchanges were reported to reduce the stability (positive values) of the Spike RBD domain (Figure S1). A set of mutations at positions 496, 498, and 501 were among the highest inducing (negative values) stability of the Spike RBD domain (Figure S1b). Investigating residues involved in the Spike RBD–ACE2 (protein–protein) interface were found mutated in different variants (Figure 2b), while a few substitutions at positions 446, 477, 478, 493, and 498 in the Spike RBD enhanced the affinity or binding of the RBD with the ACE2 receptor. In particular, regardless of the amino acids used for substitution, mutations at the 446 and 498 positions enhance ferritin–RBD affinity to the ACE2 receptor (Figure S1a).

The effect of a particular mutation was performed by applying the 'residue scan' approach on the Spike RBD–ACE2 complex over the H-ferritin nanocage. The changes in the binding affinity between the Spike RBD–ACE2 and stability upon inserting point mutations were characterized (Figures 2 and S1). Investigating the amino acid exchange found in selected mutations, K417N, K417T, L452R, L452Q, E484A, G496S, and N501Y have reduced the binding of Spike RBD to ACE2, whereas substitutions G446S, S477N, T478K, E484Q, Q493R, and Q498R have enhanced the binding affinity of Spike RBD–ACE2. A mutation-induced conformational switch was observed that could be responsible for increased (Q498R) or decreased (N501Y) binding affinity between Spike RBD and ACE2 (Figures 2 and S1).

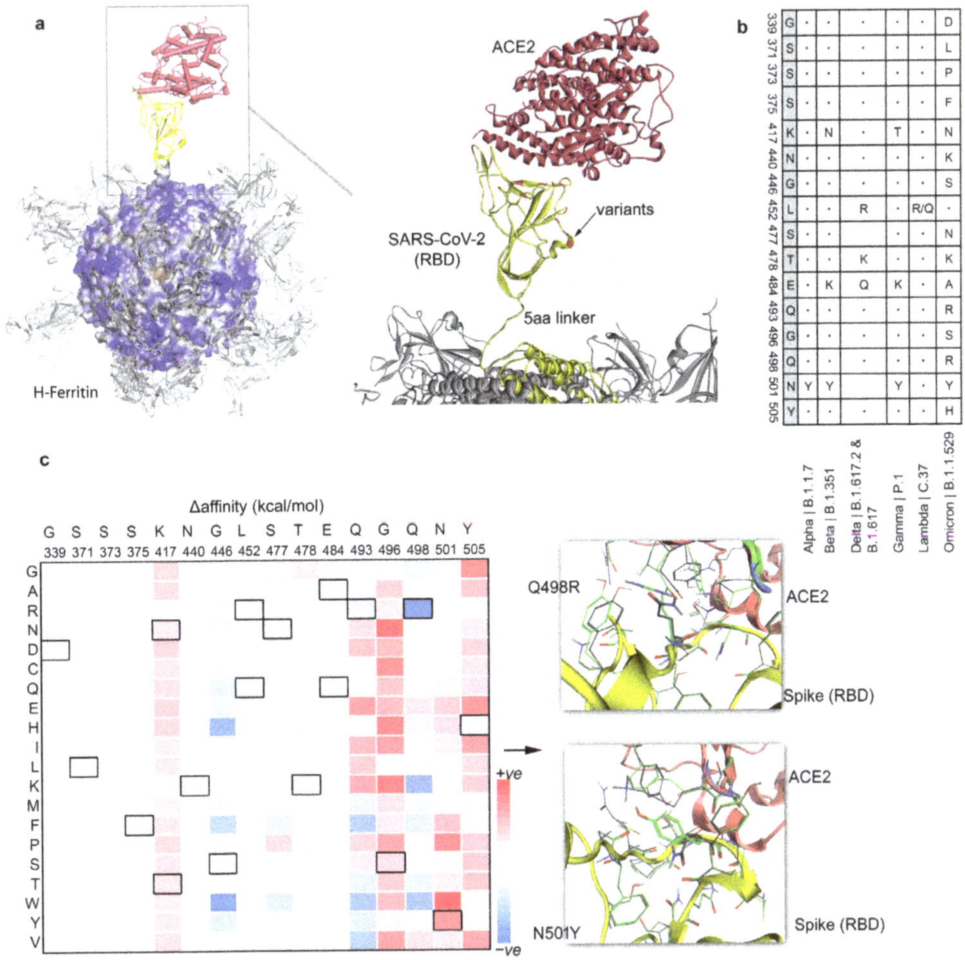

Figure 2. The SARS-CoV-2 Spike RBD–ACE2 interactions over the surface of the H-ferritin (24 subunits) nanocage. (**a**) The chimeric construct of the H-ferritin–GGGGS–Spike RBD investigated with the ACE2 host cell receptor. The right panel represents mutations derived from different SARS-CoV-2 variants within the Spike RBD domain (marked in red color): 24 subunits of Spike RBD (PDB ID: 6lzg [34]) presented over the H-ferritin (PDB ID: 2fha [47]). The outer and inner diameters of the H-ferritin cage are 12 nm and 8 nm, respectively. (**b**) Mutations from SARS-CoV-2 (Alpha, B.1.1.7), Beta (B.1.351), Delta (B.1.617.2 and B.1.617), Gamma (P.1), Lambda (C.37, and Omicron (B.1.1.529) [32,33] variants, residing within the RBD domain of the Spike protein. (**c**) Along with tracing change in the binding affinity upon inserting point mutation from different SARS-CoV-2 variants in the RBD domain with the ACE2 receptor, we investigated all different possible mutations at a particular site or residue. The heatmap represents change in the binding affinity (kcal/mol) between the Spike RBD and ACE2 receptor upon point mutations (A, R, N, D, C, Q, E, G, H, I, L, K, M, F, P, S, T, W, Y, and V). The right panel represents an example of a conformational switch of the residues upon mutation; Q498R (induced affinity) and N501Y (reduced affinity).

3.2. Binding of Spike RBD–Antibody Complex over Nanocages and Their Mutational Landscape

The Spike RBD, a very immunogenic and a major SARS-CoV neutralization determinant, can elicit effective neutralizing antibodies capable of outcompeting the ACE2 receptor. However, the structural basis of Spike RBD immunogenicity as well as Spike RBD-mediated neutralization remains limited [26]. We investigated different neutralizing antibodies such as VVH-72, B38, m396, CB6, S309, and CR3022 binding to the SARS-CoV-2 RBD domain over the H-ferritin nanocage constructs (Figures 3 and S2). In addition, the ferritin–RBD–antibody complex was analyzed with the mutations derived from different SARS-CoV-2 variants (Alpha, B.1.1.7; Beta, B.1.351; Delta, B.1.617.2 and B.1.617; Gamma, P.1; Lambda, C.37; and Omicron, B.1.1.529). The mutations identified in different SARS-CoV-2 variants were explored by replacing a specific mutated residue with every possible 20 substitution using the 'residue scan' technique. Our findings revealed that site-specific mutations at a specific amino acid position can influence the Spike RBD-binding affinity with different antibodies over the H-ferritin nanocage (Figures 3 and 4): VVH-72 (371, 373, and 375 Spike RBD amino acids; aa), B38 and CB6 (417, 477, 478, 484, 493, 496, 498, 501, and 505 aa), CR3022 (371 and 375 aa), S309 (339 and 440 aa), and M396 (375, 446, 493, 496, 498, 501, and 505 aa).

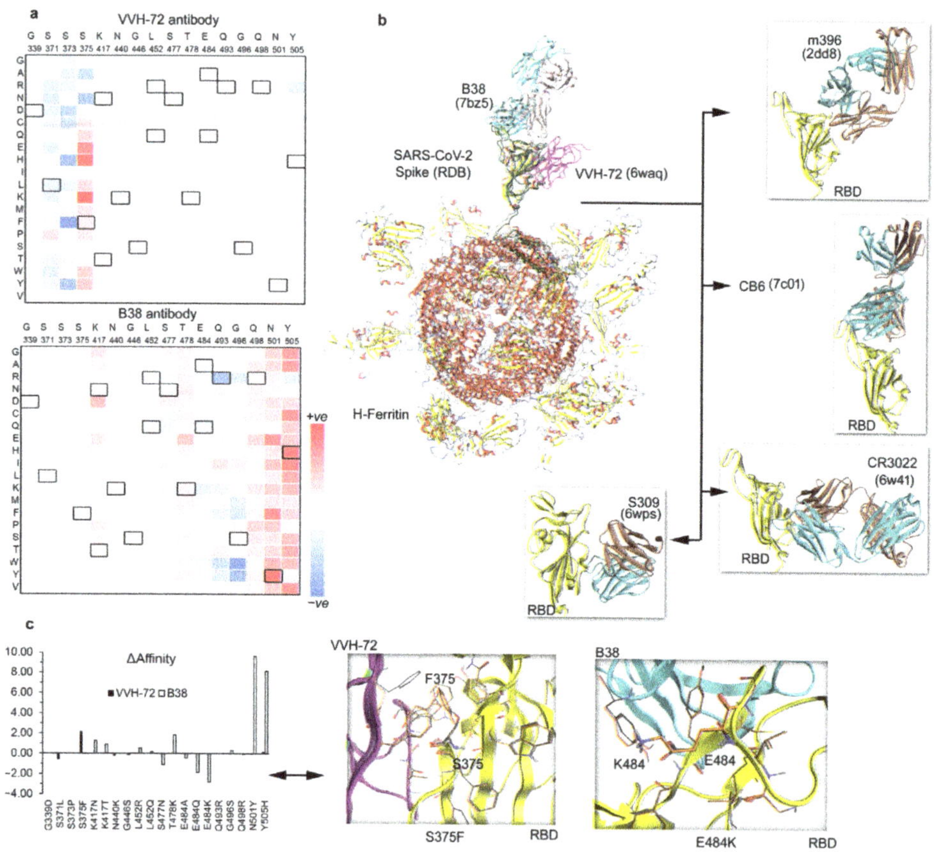

Figure 3. Ferritin nanocage constructs of the SARS-CoV-2 RBD domain with different antibodies. (**a**) Individual VVH-72 and B38 antibodies were built over the H-ferritin nanocage binding the Spike RBD domain, and the changes in the binding affinity were traced upon inserting point mutations. Mutations from SARS-CoV-2 virus variants (Alpha, B.1.1.7; Beta, B.1.351; Delta, B.1.617.2 and B.1.617; Gamma, P.1; Lambda, C.37; and Omicron, B.1.1.529) were further investigated by 20 different possible

substitutions using the 'residue scan' approach. The heatmap represents a change in the binding affinity upon inserting mutations in the Spike RBD domains over the ferritin nanocage. (**b**) Investigating the antibodies binding with the SARS-CoV-2 RBD domain over the H-ferritin nanocage constructs. The VVH-72 (PDB ID: 6waq [30]) and B38 (PDB ID: 7bz5 [36]) imitates ACE2 binding to the interface on the RBD of SARS-CoV, m396 binds to the RBD of SARS-CoV without functionally mimicking ACE2, preventing the RBD from binding to ACE2 (PDB ID: 2dd8 [26]), CB6 functionally mimics ACE2 binding to the interface on the RBD of SARS-CoV-2 (PDB ID: 7c01 [27]), and S309 binds to the RBD of SARS-CoV-2 without blocking the binding of RBD to ACE2 (PDB ID: 6wps) [24,28]. In addition, the SARS-CoV specific CR3022 binds to the RBD of SARS-CoV-2 without blocking the binding of RBD of SARS-CoV-2 to ACE2 (PDB ID: 6w41) [24,29]. (**c**) The change in the binding affinity within the Spike RBD–antibody complexes upon inserting SARS-CoV-2 virus variants in the RBD domain. Individual effects of mutations describe a contrary dynamic in the presence of VVH-72 or B38. The left panel represents the change in the binding affinity within the Spike RBD antibodies upon inserting mutations in the SARS-CoV-2 RBD domain. The right panel describes the conformational switch of the S375F and E484K mutations with VVH-72 and B38 antibody, respectively.

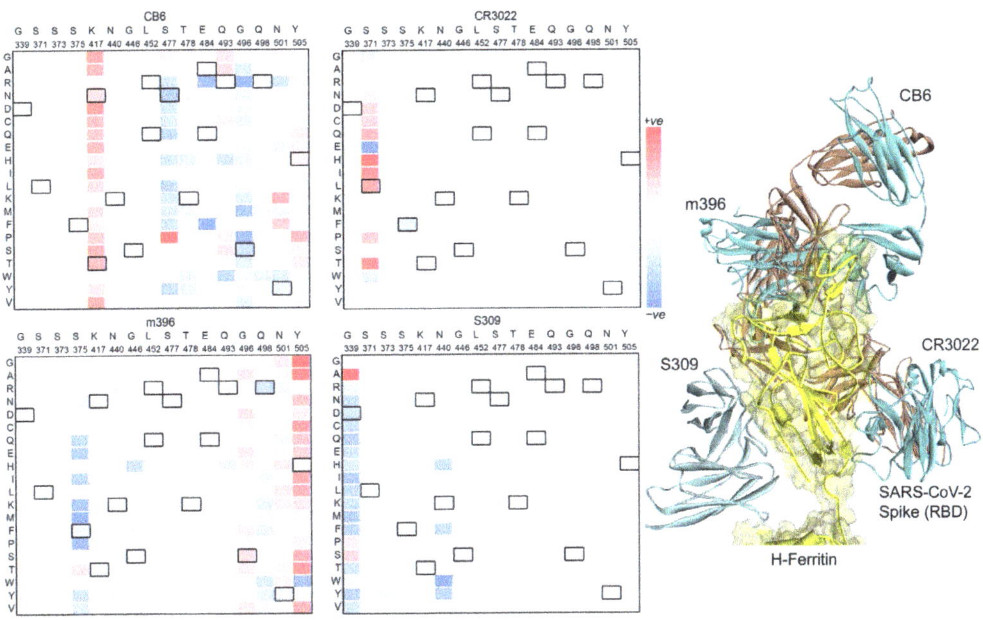

Figure 4. Investigating the CB6, CR3066, m396, and S309 antibodies binding with the SARS-CoV-2 Spike RBD over the H-ferritin nanocage. The left panel represents the heatmap of the affinity change upon the insertion of point mutations over the Spike RBD domain. The right panel describes the positioning or the location of all four antibodies over the ferritin–Spike RBD complex.

Mutations from different SARS-CoV-2 variants (Alpha, Beta, Delta, Gamma, and Omicron) were analyzed with VVH-72, B38, CB6, CR3066, m396, and S309 antibodies, and the mutation-induced changes in their binding affinity between Spike RBD were predicted (Figure 3c). In the ferritin–RBD–VVH-72 complex, the substitutions at S371L, N440K, and G446S positions have improved the binding energy, whereas mutations S375F and Y505H reduced the Spike RBD–antibody binding affinity. For the ferritin–RBD–B38 complex, the S477N, E484A, E484Q, E484K, and Q498R mutations gained the binding affinity, whereas K417N, K417T, L452R, L452Q, T478K, G496S, N501Y, and Y505H lowered the binding between Spike RBD and Ab (Figure 3c). Overall, the binding affinity of VVH-72, CR3022, and S309 antibodies with the Spike RBD demonstrated an unstirred effect upon most point mutations, although there were moderate binding affinities changes for a small sets of residues (Figures S2b and S3). The Spike RBD mutated in the presence of m396 (which binds to the RBD of SARS-CoV without functionally mimicking ACE2, preventing the RBD from binding to ACE2) and CB6 (functionally mimics ACE2 binding to the interface on RBD) has a higher influence in the protein–Ab binding affinities (Figure 4).

4. Discussion

Our findings and different studies revealed that the SARS-CoV-2 Spike RBD domain can be an attractive target for the development of RBD-based vaccines against different SARS-CoV-2 variants. In order to adapt distinct variants, a chimeric Spike RBD-dimer vaccine construct has been reported which stitches two RBD domains (Delta–Omicron or prototype–Beta conjugates) together originating from similar or distinct SARS-CoV-2 variants [44]. Implementing the surface plasmon resonance (SPR) assays, the binding of such Spike RBD-dimer vaccines with ACE2 was evaluated. Such chimeric-designed vaccine-treated mice showed an enhanced protection or neutralization of SARS-CoV-2 variants [44]. In addition, cryo-electron microscopy (cryo-EM) revealed that such Spike RBD-dimer vaccines, in particular prototype-Beta, can bind with CB6 mAb at 11.5–11.6 Å resolution [44]. Furthermore, the genetic fusion of the Spike RBD domains stitched over the ferritin nanocages subunits, making synthetic chimeras, may generate moderate to high levels of immune responses (Figures 2 and 3), similar to that described in several studies [41–46].

The SARS-CoV-2 Spike expressed over the ferritin nanocages surface and their binding with different monoclonal antibodies were evaluated and demonstrated by the cryo-EM technique [41]. A single-dose vaccination of Spike presented over the ferritin nanocages enhances the stimulation of neutralizing antibodies, and a twofold increase (>convalescent plasma) in neutralizing antibody titers was reported upon single immunization with Spike–ferritin particles to mice [41]. Expressing the Spike RBD domain over ferritin nanocages in the eukaryotic expression system (293i cells) and immunizing rhesus monkeys (20 μg) with such constructs (Spike RBD–ferritin) induced the humoral immunity and T-cell response. In addition, cross-neutralizing antibodies have been reported against different SARS-CoV-2 strains [42]. Over the self-assembled ferritin nanocages with the Spike RBD domain, the Spike RBD-HR (heptad repeat) subunit was reported to be displayed that enhances the immune responses (B and T cells) along with the production of neutralizing antibodies [45]. In such a promising vaccination approach, the Spike RBD-specific antibodies blocked the interaction with the ACE2 host cell receptor [45].

Additionally, implementing the SpyTag-SpyCatcher system, different strategies have been applied to develop Spike RBD-based vaccine candidates, where the Spike RBD domain is conjugated with 24-mer ferritin, 60-mer mi3, and 120-mer I53–50 nanoparticles [46]. Immunizing mice with such a Spike RBD displayed over different nanoparticles induced a 8–120 fold greater neutralizing activity compared to monomeric Spike RBD treatment [46]. In addition, the mice immunized sera revealed that such Spike RBD-conjected nanoparticles can inhibit the binding activity of the Spike RBD domain with the ACE2 receptor [46]. Along with the expression of the Spike RBD domain over ferritin, the Spike protein has been found to be present over the Dps nanoparticles, and the RBD-S-Dps construct induced a neutralizing antibody response in mice [43]. The immunization of a single round with such a Spike RBD-S-Dps treatment to mice resulted in a reduced level of the virus in the lungs upon infection [43]. Moreover, combining different approaches (gene fusion, chemical conjugation, and SpyTag/SpyCatcher), nanoparticles were extracted from the turnip mosaic virus (TuMV; a crucial tool for diagnostics and immunodetection) that could represent a functional Spike RBD and enhance antibody sensing [48]. Ferritin nanoparticles have been reported to induce RFP (red fluorescence protein)-specific cytotoxic CD8+ T cell response as well as in live mice inhibiting tumor (melanoma) growth [39]. Falvo et al. reported the combination of ferritin nanoparticles stitched together with the antibody drug conjugate can enhance therapeutic indexes in melanoma tumors [40].

In our studies, we made use of the MD simulations, which can help to understand the structural folding or properties of a gene (structural or nonstructural) at an atomic scale along with predicting the possible variability that can emerge from a viral protein. Such techniques allow investigating model systems prior to validation along with selecting the most feasible domains of the target protein or a linker to be presented over the ferritin surface [16,49]. Intermolecular interactions between proteins over the simulation time from MDS can be considered to design SARS-CoV-2 S self-derived peptides [38] emerging within the viral components, and these can be displayed over the ferritin nanocages as potential blockers or inhibitors of the target protein. Considering the existing knowledge from the literature, the modeling techniques can predict the possible epitopes of new emerging viruses that can dock with the host cell receptors or ribosomal components [50]. Herein, our study we implemented MD simulation to find the most suitable linker for the ferritin–RBD constructs, and proposed that it may have the potential to induce a cross-protective antibody response. Such Spike RBD-targeting vaccines and neutralizing antibodies can effectively block the viral entry by interrupting the binding between Spike–ACE2 networks. Since this could provide useful therapeutic approaches against the current COVID-19 pandemic as well as future such infections, we optimized the structure of the H-ferritin–GGGGS–RBD complex which was further evaluated with the ACE2 host cell receptor or antibodies (Figures 1–3).

5. Conclusions

In the field of nanomaterials, great progress has been reported, and ferritin nanocages with monodisperse architectures have been widely used in a number of disciplines, including vaccine development and generation. In our current work, we demonstrated the structural dynamics of ferritin nanocages stitched together with synthetic chimeras displaying the Spike RBD domains in the 'up' active conformations. Based on our findings, we postulated that such nanocage constructs may be an effective tool to induce cross-protective antibody responses. Taking the H-ferritin nanocage constructs into consideration, we evaluated the effects of variants on the binding of the SARS-CoV-2 Spike RBD to the host receptor ACE2 and different neutralizing antibodies. Our data predicted that these Spike RBD-targeting ferritin-based vaccines and neutralizing antibodies shall effectively block the viral entry by interrupting the binding between Spike and ACE2. Our in silico findings can, however, be validated by characterizing the morphology of the Spike RBD–ferritin nanocages and performing biochemical assays to evaluate their binding to ACE2.

Variants of concern have rapidly changed the transmissibility and pathogenicity of the SARS-CoV-2 virus and occurred mainly due to mutations in the main structural proteins. Variants within the Spike RBD regions lead or have been correlated to the emergence of novel SARS-CoV-2 variants such as Alpha (B.1.1.7), Beta (B.1.351), Delta (B.1.617.2 and B.1.617), Gamma (P.1), Lambda (C.37), and Omicron (B.1.1.529). The Spike RBD domain in the SARS-CoV-2 Omicron variant contains the highest number of mutations compared to other variants (α, β, γ, and δ). The effect of a particular mutation was performed by applying the 'residue scan' approach on the Spike RBD–ACE2/antibody complex over the H-ferritin nanocage. Changes in the binding affinity or structural stability between the Spike RBD antibody and stability upon inserting point mutations were characterized. Investigating the VOCs revealed that most of the variants reported a clearly reduced stability of the Spike RBD domain. Mutations have a moderate effect over the binding affinity for VVH-72, CR3022, and S309 Abs with the Spike RBD, whereas for the B38, CB6 or m396 Abs, they had a significant influence when evaluated over the H-ferritin nanocages. In particular, some mutations that induced conformational switches were observed that could be responsible for increased (Q498R) or decreased (N501Y) binding affinity between Spike RBD and ACE2. We believe these structural details can provide useful therapeutic approaches against SARS-CoV-2. With the undergoing grand challenges of designing vaccines against the current mutating SARS-CoV-2 and any future virus infections, we propose possible protein-based vaccine strategies along with evaluating their VOC profile.

Supplementary Materials: The following supporting information can be downloaded at: https://www.mdpi.com/article/10.3390/vaccines12050446/s1, Figure S1: The complex of SARS-CoV-2 Spike RBD-ACE2 was constructed over the H-ferritin nanocage; Figure S2: Constructing dataset of mutations in the SARS-CoV-2 Spike RBD structures in the presence of different antibodies; Figure S3: Change in binding affinity with the CB6, CR3066, m396, and S309 antibodies and stability upon inserting point mutations in the SARS-CoV-2 Spike RBD over the H-Ferritin nanocage.

Author Contributions: Conceptualization, U.K.; Methodology, M.P. and U.K.; Software, U.K.; Formal analysis, M.P. and U.K.; Investigation, M.P.; Data curation, U.K.; Writing—original draft, M.P. and U.K; Visualization, U.K. All authors have read and agreed to the published version of the manuscript.

Funding: The International Centre for Cancer Vaccine Science project is carried out within the International Research Agendas programme of the Foundation for Polish Science co-financed by the European Union under the European Regional Development Fund. We gratefully acknowledge Poland's high-performance computing infrastructure PLGrid (HPC Centers:) for providing computer facilities and support within computational grant no. PLG/2019/012567.

Institutional Review Board Statement: Not applicable.

Informed Consent Statement: Not applicable.

Data Availability Statement: Data is contained within the article or supplementary material.

Conflicts of Interest: The authors declare no conflicts of interest.

References

1. Wong, F.; Sen, A. Progress toward Light-Harvesting Self-Electrophoretic Motors: Highly Efficient Bimetallic Nanomotors and Micropumps in Halogen Media. *ACS Nano* **2016**, *10*, 7172–7179. [CrossRef] [PubMed]
2. Cosottini, L.; Zineddu, S.; Massai, L.; Ghini, V.; Turano, P. 19F: A Small Probe for a Giant Protein. *J. Inorg. Biochem.* **2023**, *244*, 112236. [CrossRef] [PubMed]
3. Kanekiyo, M.; Wei, C.-J.; Yassine, H.M.; McTamney, P.M.; Boyington, J.C.; Whittle, J.R.R.; Rao, S.S.; Kong, W.-P.; Wang, L.; Nabel, G.J. Self-Assembling Influenza Nanoparticle Vaccines Elicit Broadly Neutralizing H1N1 Antibodies. *Nature* **2013**, *499*, 102–106. [CrossRef] [PubMed]
4. Zhang, J.; Cheng, D.; He, J.; Hong, J.; Yuan, C.; Liang, M. Cargo loading within ferritin nanocages in preparation for tumor-targeted delivery. *Nat. Protoc.* **2021**, *16*, 4878–4896. [CrossRef]
5. Zhang, C.; Zhang, X.; Zhao, G. Ferritin Nanocage: A Versatile Nanocarrier Utilized in the Field of Food, Nutrition, and Medicine. *Nanomaterials* **2020**, *10*, 1894. [CrossRef] [PubMed]
6. Pieters, B.J.G.E.; van Eldijk, M.B.; Nolte, R.J.M.; Mecinović, J. Natural Supramolecular Protein Assemblies. *Chem. Soc. Rev.* **2016**, *45*, 24–39. [CrossRef] [PubMed]
7. Jutz, G.; van Rijn, P.; Santos Miranda, B.; Böker, A. Ferritin: A Versatile Building Block for Bionanotechnology. *Chem. Rev.* **2015**, *115*, 1653–1701. [CrossRef]
8. Stanley, S. Biological Nanoparticles and Their Influence on Organisms. *Curr. Opin. Biotechnol.* **2014**, *28*, 69–74. [CrossRef]
9. Sevieri, M.; Sottani, C.; Chesi, A.; Bonizzi, A.; Sitia, L.; Robustelli Della Cuna, F.S.; Grignani, E.; Corsi, F.; Mazzucchelli, S. Deciphering the Role of H-Ferritin Nanocages in Improving Tumor-Targeted Delivery of Indocyanine Green: Combined Analysis of Murine Tissue Homogenates with UHPLC–MS/MS and Fluorescence. *ACS Omega* **2023**, *8*, 48735–48741. [CrossRef]
10. Sitia, L.; Galbiati, V.; Bonizzi, A.; Sevieri, M.; Truffi, M.; Pinori, M.; Corsini, E.; Marinovich, M.; Corsi, F.; Mazzucchelli, S. In Vitro Immunoreactivity Evaluation of H-Ferritin-Based Nanodrugs. *Bioconjug. Chem.* **2023**, *34*, 845–855. [CrossRef]
11. Dong, Y.; Ma, Y.; Li, X.; Wang, F.; Zhang, Y. ERK-Peptide-Inhibitor-Modified Ferritin Enhanced the Therapeutic Effects of Paclitaxel in Cancer Cells and Spheroids. *Mol. Pharm.* **2021**, *18*, 3365–3377. [CrossRef] [PubMed]
12. Steinmetz, N.F.; Lim, S.; Sainsbury, F. Protein Cages and Virus-like Particles: From Fundamental Insight to Biomimetic Therapeutics. *Biomater. Sci.* **2020**, *8*, 2771–2777. [CrossRef] [PubMed]
13. Chattopadhyay, S.; Chen, J.-Y.; Chen, H.-W.; Hu, C.-M.J. Nanoparticle Vaccines Adopting Virus-like Features for Enhanced Immune Potentiation. *Nanotheranostics* **2017**, *1*, 244–260. [CrossRef] [PubMed]
14. Wang, Z.; Xu, L.; Yu, H.; Lv, P.; Lei, Z.; Zeng, Y.; Liu, G.; Cheng, T. Ferritin Nanocage-Based Antigen Delivery Nanoplatforms: Epitope Engineering for Peptide Vaccine Design. *Biomater. Sci.* **2019**, *7*, 1794–1800. [CrossRef] [PubMed]
15. Kim, S.; Jeon, J.-O.; Jun, E.; Jee, J.; Jung, H.-K.; Lee, B.-H.; Kim, I.-S.; Kim, S. Designing Peptide Bunches on Nanocage for Bispecific or Superaffinity Targeting. *Biomacromolecules* **2016**, *17*, 1150–1159. [CrossRef] [PubMed]
16. Kalathiya, U.; Padariya, M.; Fahraeus, R.; Chakraborti, S.; Hupp, T.R. Multivalent Display of SARS-CoV-2 Spike (RBD Domain) of COVID-19 to Nanomaterial, Protein Ferritin Nanocages. *Biomolecules* **2021**, *11*, 297. [CrossRef] [PubMed]

17. Bjelkmar, P.; Larsson, P.; Cuendet, M.A.; Hess, B.; Lindahl, E. Implementation of the CHARMM Force Field in GROMACS: Analysis of Protein Stability Effects from Correction Maps, Virtual Interaction Sites, and Water Models. *J. Chem. Theory Comput.* **2010**, *6*, 459–466. [CrossRef] [PubMed]
18. Kitchen, D.B.; Decornez, H.; Furr, J.R.; Bajorath, J. Docking and Scoring in Virtual Screening for Drug Discovery: Methods and Applications. *Nat. Rev. Drug Discov.* **2004**, *3*, 935–949. [CrossRef] [PubMed]
19. Wrapp, D.; Wang, N.; Corbett, K.S.; Goldsmith, J.A.; Hsieh, C.-L.; Abiona, O.; Graham, B.S.; McLellan, J.S. Cryo-EM Structure of the 2019-nCoV Spike in the Prefusion Conformation. *Science* **2020**, *367*, 1260–1263. [CrossRef]
20. Shang, J.; Ye, G.; Shi, K.; Wan, Y.; Luo, C.; Aihara, H.; Geng, Q.; Auerbach, A.; Li, F. Structural Basis of Receptor Recognition by SARS-CoV-2. *Nature* **2020**, *581*, 221–224. [CrossRef]
21. Du, L.; He, Y.; Zhou, Y.; Liu, S.; Zheng, B.-J.; Jiang, S. The Spike Protein of SARS-CoV—A Target for Vaccine and Therapeutic Development. *Nat. Rev. Microbiol.* **2009**, *7*, 226–236. [CrossRef] [PubMed]
22. Pasev, M.; Trifonova, A.; Velichkov, A.; Terzieva, V. Duration of Antibody Response to the Receptor Binding Domain of SARS-CoV-2 in Infected or Vaccinated Individuals—A One Year Retrospective Cohort Study. *Int. Immunopharmacol.* **2024**, *133*, 112084. [CrossRef] [PubMed]
23. Yu, F.; Xiang, R.; Deng, X.; Wang, L.; Yu, Z.; Tian, S.; Liang, R.; Li, Y.; Ying, T.; Jiang, S. Receptor-Binding Domain-Specific Human Neutralizing Monoclonal Antibodies against SARS-CoV and SARS-CoV-2. *Signal Transduct. Target. Ther.* **2020**, *5*, 212. [CrossRef] [PubMed]
24. Sun, J.; Yang, Z.-D.; Xie, X.; Li, L.; Zeng, H.-S.; Gong, B.; Xu, J.-Q.; Wu, J.-H.; Qu, B.-B.; Song, G.-W. Clinical Application of SARS-CoV-2 Antibody Detection and Monoclonal Antibody Therapies against COVID-19. *World J. Clin. Cases* **2023**, *11*, 2168–2180. [CrossRef] [PubMed]
25. Krissinel, E.; Henrick, K. Inference of Macromolecular Assemblies from Crystalline State. *J. Mol. Biol.* **2007**, *372*, 774–797. [CrossRef] [PubMed]
26. Prabakaran, P.; Gan, J.; Feng, Y.; Zhu, Z.; Choudhry, V.; Xiao, X.; Ji, X.; Dimitrov, D.S. Structure of Severe Acute Respiratory Syndrome Coronavirus Receptor-Binding Domain Complexed with Neutralizing Antibody. *J. Biol. Chem.* **2006**, *281*, 15829–15836. [CrossRef] [PubMed]
27. Shi, R.; Shan, C.; Duan, X.; Chen, Z.; Liu, P.; Song, J.; Song, T.; Bi, X.; Han, C.; Wu, L.; et al. A Human Neutralizing Antibody Targets the Receptor-Binding Site of SARS-CoV-2. *Nature* **2020**, *584*, 120–124. [CrossRef]
28. Pinto, D.; Park, Y.-J.; Beltramello, M.; Walls, A.C.; Tortorici, M.A.; Bianchi, S.; Jaconi, S.; Culap, K.; Zatta, F.; De Marco, A.; et al. Cross-Neutralization of SARS-CoV-2 by a Human Monoclonal SARS-CoV Antibody. *Nature* **2020**, *583*, 290–295. [CrossRef] [PubMed]
29. Yuan, M.; Wu, N.C.; Zhu, X.; Lee, C.-C.D.; So, R.T.Y.; Lv, H.; Mok, C.K.P.; Wilson, I.A. A Highly Conserved Cryptic Epitope in the Receptor Binding Domains of SARS-CoV-2 and SARS-CoV. *Science* **2020**, *368*, 630–633. [CrossRef]
30. Wrapp, D.; De Vlieger, D.; Corbett, K.S.; Torres, G.M.; Wang, N.; Van Breedam, W.; Roose, K.; van Schie, L.; Hoffmann, M.; Pöhlmann, S.; et al. Structural Basis for Potent Neutralization of Betacoronaviruses by Single-Domain Camelid Antibodies. *Cell* **2020**, *181*, 1436–1441. [CrossRef]
31. Vijay, A.; Shenoy, S.; Sindgikar, S.P. Neonatal Arterial Thrombosis: An Arcane COVID Sequelae. *BMJ Case Rep.* **2024**, *17*, e256793. [CrossRef] [PubMed]
32. Where Proteins and Innovation Advance Biomedicine. Available online: https://acrobiosystems.com.cn (accessed on 1 January 2023).
33. Zhang, L.; Cui, Z.; Li, Q.; Wang, B.; Yu, Y.; Wu, J.; Nie, J.; Ding, R.; Wang, H.; Zhang, Y.; et al. Ten Emerging SARS-CoV-2 Spike Variants Exhibit Variable Infectivity, Animal Tropism, and Antibody Neutralization. *Commun. Biol.* **2021**, *4*, 1196. [CrossRef] [PubMed]
34. Wang, Q.; Zhang, Y.; Wu, L.; Niu, S.; Song, C.; Zhang, Z.; Lu, G.; Qiao, C.; Hu, Y.; Yuen, K.-Y.; et al. Structural and Functional Basis of SARS-CoV-2 Entry by Using Human ACE2. *Cell* **2020**, *181*, 894–904.e9. [CrossRef] [PubMed]
35. Li, Y.; Wang, J.; Liang, S.; Zhang, Y.; Feng, Z.; Cai, G. Clinical Phenotype of AAV, Anti-GBM Disease and Double-Positive Patients after SARS-CoV-2 Vaccination. *Autoimmun. Rev.* **2024**, *23*, 103521. [CrossRef] [PubMed]
36. Wu, Y.; Wang, F.; Shen, C.; Peng, W.; Li, D.; Zhao, C.; Li, Z.; Li, S.; Bi, Y.; Yang, Y.; et al. A Noncompeting Pair of Human Neutralizing Antibodies Block COVID-19 Virus Binding to Its Receptor ACE2. *Science* **2020**, *368*, 1274–1278. [CrossRef] [PubMed]
37. Akcay, S.N.; Saylan, C.C.; Tekin, A.; Baday, S. Optimization of CHARMM Force Field Parameters for Ryanodine Receptor Inhibitory Drug Dantrolene Using FFTK and FFParam. *J. Mol. Model.* **2024**, *30*, 46. [CrossRef]
38. Padariya, M.; Daniels, A.; Tait-Burkard, C.; Hupp, T.; Kalathiya, U. Self-Derived Peptides from the SARS-CoV-2 Spike Glycoprotein Disrupting Shaping and Stability of the Homotrimer Unit. *Biomed. Pharmacother.* **2022**, *151*, 113190. [CrossRef] [PubMed]
39. Lee, B.-R.; Ko, H.K.; Ryu, J.H.; Ahn, K.Y.; Lee, Y.-H.; Oh, S.J.; Na, J.H.; Kim, T.W.; Byun, Y.; Kwon, I.C.; et al. Engineered Human Ferritin Nanoparticles for Direct Delivery of Tumor Antigens to Lymph Node and Cancer Immunotherapy. *Sci. Rep.* **2016**, *6*, 35182. [CrossRef]
40. Falvo, E.; Tremante, E.; Fraioli, R.; Leonetti, C.; Zamparelli, C.; Boffi, A.; Morea, V.; Ceci, P.; Giacomini, P. Antibody–Drug Conjugates: Targeting Melanoma with Cisplatin Encapsulated in Protein-Cage Nanoparticles Based on Human Ferritin. *Nanoscale* **2013**, *5*, 12278. [CrossRef]

41. Powell, A.E.; Zhang, K.; Sanyal, M.; Tang, S.; Weidenbacher, P.A.; Li, S.; Pham, T.D.; Pak, J.E.; Chiu, W.; Kim, P.S. A Single Immunization with Spike-Functionalized Ferritin Vaccines Elicits Neutralizing Antibody Responses against SARS-CoV-2 in Mice. *ACS Cent. Sci.* **2021**, *7*, 183–199. [CrossRef]
42. Li, H.; Guo, L.; Zheng, H.; Li, J.; Zhao, X.; Li, J.; Liang, Y.; Yang, F.; Zhao, Y.; Yang, J.; et al. Self-Assembling Nanoparticle Vaccines Displaying the Receptor Binding Domain of SARS-CoV-2 Elicit Robust Protective Immune Responses in Rhesus Monkeys. *Bioconjug. Chem.* **2021**, *32*, 1034–1046. [CrossRef] [PubMed]
43. Salzer, R.; Clark, J.J.; Vaysburd, M.; Chang, V.T.; Albecka, A.; Kiss, L.; Sharma, P.; Gonzalez Llamazares, A.; Kipar, A.; Hiscox, J.A.; et al. Single-dose Immunisation with a Multimerised SARS-CoV-2 Receptor Binding Domain (RBD) Induces an Enhanced and Protective Response in Mice. *FEBS Lett.* **2021**, *595*, 2323–2340. [CrossRef] [PubMed]
44. Xu, K.; Gao, P.; Liu, S.; Lu, S.; Lei, W.; Zheng, T.; Liu, X.; Xie, Y.; Zhao, Z.; Guo, S.; et al. Protective Prototype-Beta and Delta-Omicron Chimeric RBD-Dimer Vaccines against SARS-CoV-2. *Cell* **2022**, *185*, 2265–2278. [CrossRef] [PubMed]
45. Ma, X.; Zou, F.; Yu, F.; Li, R.; Yuan, Y.; Zhang, Y.; Zhang, X.; Deng, J.; Chen, T.; Song, Z.; et al. Nanoparticle Vaccines Based on the Receptor Binding Domain (RBD) and Heptad Repeat (HR) of SARS-CoV-2 Elicit Robust Protective Immune Responses. *Immunity* **2020**, *53*, 1315–1330.e9. [CrossRef] [PubMed]
46. Kang, Y.-F.; Sun, C.; Zhuang, Z.; Yuan, R.-Y.; Zheng, Q.; Li, J.-P.; Zhou, P.-P.; Chen, X.-C.; Liu, Z.; Zhang, X.; et al. Rapid Development of SARS-CoV-2 Spike Protein Receptor-Binding Domain Self-Assembled Nanoparticle Vaccine Candidates. *ACS Nano* **2021**, *15*, 2738–2752. [CrossRef] [PubMed]
47. Hempstead, P.D.; Yewdall, S.J.; Fernie, A.R.; Lawson, D.M.; Artymiuk, P.J.; Rice, D.W.; Ford, G.C.; Harrison, P.M. Comparison of the Three-Dimensional Structures of Recombinant Human H and Horse L Ferritins at High Resolution 1. *J. Mol. Biol.* **1997**, *268*, 424–448. [CrossRef] [PubMed]
48. Medrano-Arranz, C.; Rincón, S.; Zurita, L.; Ponz, F.; Truchado, D.A. Antigen-Functionalized Turnip Mosaic Virus Nanoparticles Increase Antibody Sensing in Saliva. A Case Study with SARS-CoV-2 RBD. *Diagn. Microbiol. Infect. Dis.* **2024**, *109*, 116298. [CrossRef]
49. Chakraborti, S.; Chakrabarti, P. Self-Assembly of Ferritin: Structure, Biological Function and Potential Applications in Nanotechnology. In *Advances in Experimental Medicine and Biology*; Springer: Singapore, 2019; pp. 313–329, ISBN 9789811397905.
50. Schubert, K.; Karousis, E.D.; Jomaa, A.; Scaiola, A.; Echeverria, B.; Gurzeler, L.-A.; Leibundgut, M.; Thiel, V.; Mühlemann, O.; Ban, N. SARS-CoV-2 Nsp1 Binds the Ribosomal mRNA Channel to Inhibit Translation. *Nat. Struct. Mol. Biol.* **2020**, *27*, 959–966. [CrossRef]

vaccines

MDPI

Article

Hybrid Immunity and the Incidence of SARS-CoV-2 Reinfections during the Omicron Era in Frontline Healthcare Workers

Carmen-Daniela Chivu [1,2], Maria-Dorina Crăciun [1,2,*], Daniela Pițigoi [1,3,†], Victoria Aramă [3,4], Monica Luminița Luminos [3,5], Gheorghiță Jugulete [3,5], Viorela Gabriela Nițescu [2,6], Andreea Lescaie [2,6], Cătălin Gabriel Apostolescu [3,4] and Adrian Streinu Cercel [3,4,†]

1 Department of Epidemiology 1, Carol Davila University of Medicine and Pharmacy, 050474 Bucharest, Romania; carmen-daniela.chivu@drd.umfcd.ro (C.-D.C.); daniela.pitigoi@umfcd.ro (D.P.)
2 Emergency Clinical Hospital for Children "Grigore Alexandrescu", 011743 Bucharest, Romania; viorela.nitescu@umfcd.ro (V.G.N.); andreea.lescaie@drd.umfcd.ro (A.L.)
3 National Institute for Infectious Diseases "Prof. Dr. Matei Balș", 021105 Bucharest, Romania; victoria.arama@umfcd.ro (V.A.); luminita.luminos@umfcd.ro (M.L.L.); gheorghita.jugulete@umfcd.ro (G.J.); catalin-gabriel.apostolescu@drd.umfcd.ro (C.G.A.); adrian.streinucercel@umfcd.ro (A.S.C.)
4 Department of Infectious Diseases 1, Carol Davila University of Medicine and Pharmacy, 020021 Bucharest, Romania
5 Department of Infectious Diseases 3, Carol Davila University of Medicine and Pharmacy, 020021 Bucharest, Romania
6 Department of Pediatrics, Carol Davila University of Medicine and Pharmacy, 020021 Bucharest, Romania
* Correspondence: maria.craciun@umfcd.ro
† These authors contributed equally to this work.

Abstract: During the coronavirus disease (COVID-19) pandemic healthcare workers (HCWs) acquired immunity by vaccination or exposure to multiple variants of severe acute respiratory syndrome coronavirus 2 (SARS-CoV-2). Our study is a comparative analysis between subgroups of HCWs constructed based on the number of SARS-CoV-2 infections, vaccination, and the dominant variant of SARS-CoV-2 in the population. We collected and analyzed data using the χ^2 test and density incidence of reinfections in Microsoft Excel for Mac, Version 16.84, and MedCalc®, 22.026. Of the 829 HCWs, 70.1% (581) had only one SARS-CoV-2 infection and 29.9% (248) had two infections. Of the subjects with two infections, 77.4% (192) worked in high-risk departments and 93.2% (231) of the second infections were registered during Omicron dominance. The density incidence of reinfections was higher in HCWs vaccinated with the primary schedule than those vaccinated with the first booster, and the incidence ratio was 2.8 (95% CI: 1.2; 6.7). The probability of reinfection was five times lower (95% CI: 2.9; 9.2) in HCWs vaccinated with the primary schedule if the first infection was acquired during Omicron dominance. The subjects vaccinated with the first booster had a density incidence of reinfection three times lower (95% CI: 1.9; 5.8) if the first infection was during Omicron. The incidence ratio in subgroups constructed based on characteristics such as gender, age group, job category, and department also registered significant differences in density incidence. The history of SARS-CoV-2 infection by variant is important when interpreting and understanding public health data and the results of studies related to vaccine efficacy for hybrid immunity subgroup populations.

Keywords: SARS-CoV-2; reinfection; healthcare workers; vaccines protection; variant of concern

1. Introduction

The COVID-19 pandemic was declared by the World Health Organization (WHO) to be a public health emergency of international concern (PHEIC) on 30 January 2020, based on International Health Regulations (IHR) [1,2]. The meeting of the IHR Emergency Committee on the COVID-19 pandemic on 4 May 2023 acknowledged that this public health emergency was an established and ongoing health issue [3,4]. During the time interval when COVID-19 was PHEIC, almost 7 million deaths and over 750 million confirmed cases were reported [5].

Due to the potential evolution of SARS-CoV-2, the WHO has recommended a long-term strategic attitude consisting of calibrated measures regarding research, public health interventions, and continuous collaborative surveillance [6,7]. Studies and public health indicators have shown a waning immunity against evolving variants of SARS-CoV-2, thus the WHO recommended vaccination and revaccination for priority groups [8]. The effectiveness of prevention and control strategies has also been proposed for monitoring [8].

Genomic surveillance of SARS-CoV-2 showed an important genetic diversity, with an impact on transmission, case severity, and immunity escape of the virus. The variants of SARS-CoV-2 were named variants of concern (VOC) if important genetic mutations with an impact on transmission, severity, or immunity escape were acquired, or variants of interest and variants under monitoring in cases of minor mutations.

The laboratory testing of suspected cases and genome sequencing were guided through methodologies, also reporting the data [9–12]. The Romanian National Institute of Public Health (NIPH) released methodological criteria for the genomic surveillance of SARS-CoV-2 [11]. Changes in the epidemiological, laboratory, and representativeness of the selection criteria are summarized in Supplemental Data S1. Reports regarding genomic surveillance were published weekly by the Romanian NIPH, starting from February 2021 [13]. Summarized data regarding the positive cases of SARS-CoV-2 VOC are presented in Supplemental Data S2.

In Romania, SARS-CoV-2 evolved from the ancestral variant (hCoV-19/Wuhan/WIV04/2019) to Alpha (B1.1.7 lineage), Delta (B1.1617.2), and Omicron variants [13,14]. The Alpha variant (B1.1.7 lineage) was characterized by an increase in the severity of the cases and the transmission, with no impact on immunity escape. The Delta variant (B1.1617.2) exhibited an impact on immunity escape and a rise in the transmission and severity of cases. All Omicron variants for which evidence-based data existed were characterized by an increase in transmission, a decrease in the severity of the cases, and an impact on immunity protection after vaccination [15,16]. The mutation registered in the Omicron variants involved the spike protein and receptor binding domain. These mutations have affected the transmission dynamics and the targets of the neutralizing antibodies, resulting in a lower efficiency of the previous vaccination. Updated vaccines have been developed to address the decreasing immunity against new Omicron variants. Although the originally authorized vaccines continue to be efficient in preventing hospitalization, severe illness, and death, protection against mild and moderate clinical outcomes is low.

During the COVID-19 pandemic, HCWs acquired immunity induced by vaccination, SARS-CoV-2 infection, or both. Recommendations for the use of updated vaccines for primary vaccination and re-vaccination have been made for risk groups [8,17]. In populations with hybrid immunity, the SARS-CoV-2 VOC, which determined the prior infection, may play an important role in individual protection and in the incidence of reinfections.

The current study continues and complements previous research on the risk of COVID-19 in HCWs in a designated hospital for treating COVID-19 patients in Bucharest, Romania. The previously published research evaluated the clinical outcome in relation to nonpharmacological protective measures, vaccination, and individual risk [18,19]. Data showed that risk factors associated with the severity of the first SARS-CoV-2 infection were exposure to COVID-19 confirmed cases, age, obesity and anemia [18]. The risk of COVID-19 across all clinical events was lower in HCWs with the first booster administered compared with the risk in HCWs with the primary schedule or who were nonvaccinated [19].

The current study aims to compare the transmission dynamics of SARS-CoV-2 in HCWs vaccinated with the primary schedule and the first booster by estimating the density incidence of reinfections during the Omicron variant circulation in Romania. The study also considers the circulating variant of SARS-CoV-2 during the first infection of HCWs.

2. Materials and Methods

2.1. Hospital Setting, Participants, and Definitions

During the COVID-19 pandemic in Romania, the National Institute for Infectious Diseases (INBI) "Professor Dr. Matei Balș" in Bucharest admitted multiple COVID-19 cases covering all pandemic waves. HCWs were actively surveyed, and epidemiological investigations were performed on a case-by-case basis, to establish risk factors related to work or individuals.

This retrospective cohort study included HCWs with previously confirmed SARS-CoV-2 infection. The cases were identified and tested according to the national methodology and testing protocol [11]. Cases were suspected if the clinical criteria from the case definition were met, or if there was an identified high risk of exposure in the community or hospital. Laboratory criteria consisted of positive reverse transcription–polymerase chain reaction (RT–PCR) or rapid antigen test (RAT).

Protection of HCWs during medical activities was provided through personal protective equipment (PPE) and vaccination campaigns when vaccines became available. HCWs were trained in the proper use of PPE as a specific regulation of the hospital. The vaccination campaign for the primary schedule started on 27 December 2020, and from September 2021 booster shots were administered. A vaccination center was established at the hospital level and HCWs were prioritized for vaccination.

The HCWs were included in the study based on their professional activity at INBI "Prof. Dr. Matei Balș", as confirmed by their employment contract, and the history of previous SARS-CoV-2 infection detected according to national methodology [11]. The exclusion criteria were undetermined professional role, unknown infection status before vaccination, and uninfected HCWs. Reinfections were defined as confirmed cases by methodological laboratory testing at least 90 days apart from a previous infection. HCWs with more than two infections were registered; however, they did not meet all the study protocol criteria and were excluded from the analysis.

The HCWs were considered vaccinated with the primary schedule after 14 days from the last dose administered had elapsed. HCWs vaccinated with the first booster were represented by persons who received an additional dose of the vaccine at least six months after receiving the primary schedule. High-risk departments were defined as wards where there were identified possibilities for direct and indirect transmission by contact with suspected or confirmed COVID-19 cases or their contaminated environments. The healthcare auxiliary role was defined as employees who participated in activities related to the environment of the patients, but without performing any procedures (e.g., cleaning staff).

Hybrid immunity was defined as the immune protection of vaccinated individuals who had experienced at least one SARS-CoV-2 infection before or after the initiation of vaccination [20]. The history of SARS-CoV-2 infection by variant was assumed based on the circulant variant reported by the NIPH in Romania, with Omicron being dominant from January 2022 (Supplemental Datas S1 and S2) [13]. The study workflow and timeline of the surveyed events are shown in Figure 1.

2.2. Study Period

We analyzed the reinfection in HCWs from January 2022 to the end of May 2023, when SARS-CoV-2 Omicron variants were dominant in Romania.

2.3. Data Sources and Collection

The primary data source was the register of HCWs constructed by the Infection Prevention and Control (IPC) team prospectively with data regarding age, gender, professional role, department of activity, laboratory tests, vaccination, and recommendations. Vaccination status was verified retrospectively from the National Electronic Registry of Vaccinations, along with information regarding the date of vaccination [21].

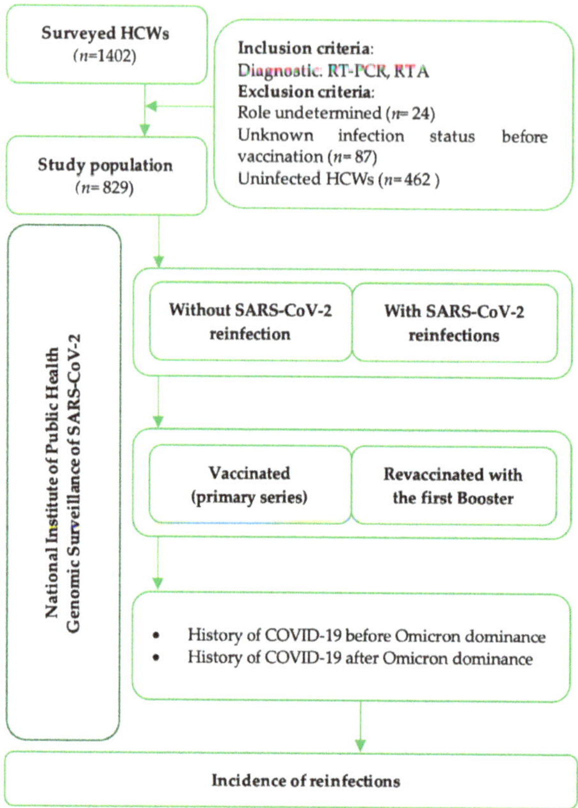

Figure 1. The workflow diagram of the HCWs study in the National Institute for Infectious Diseases "Professor Dr. Matei Balș", Bucharest, Romania, January 2022–May 2023.

2.4. Statistical Analysis

The comparison groups were independently constructed based on the number of SARS-CoV-2 infections, primary vaccination schedule, first booster shot, and history of the first SARS-CoV-2 infections during the Omicron era. A descriptive analysis of the study group and the infections and reinfections during SARS-CoV-2 VOC in HCWs was performed.

The comparative analysis used groups of HCWs without SARS-CoV-2 reinfection and HCWs with reinfections and characteristics such as age, gender, professional role, department, and vaccination status. We also compared groups of HCWs with the first SARS-CoV-2 infection acquired before or after the dominance of SARS-CoV-2 Omicron variants in Romania. We evaluated and compared the density incidence of reinfections in HCWs vaccinated with the primary schedule and those vaccinated with the first booster.

Continuous and categorical variables were presented in mean, median, interquartile ranges (IQR), numbers, and percentages. Differences between the proportions of categorical variables were assessed using χ^2 tests in MedCalc® 22.026 Software by Ostend, Belgium (https://www.medcalc.org; accessed on 1 March 2024). Density incidence was calculated based on the number of events in different groups of HCWs reported as the number of person-days of HCWs at risk [22]. The results are expressed in values per 10,000 person-days with 95% confidence intervals (95% CI). The comparison of the density incidence was made using the incidence ratio, with a threshold for significance of p-value < 0.05. Visualization of data was performed using Microsoft® Excel for Mac, Version 16.84.

2.5. Ethics Approval

The Institutional Bioethics Committee approved the study protocol with the registration numbers C02648/16.03.2022 and C08784/27.07.2023. Due to the retrospective nature of the study, only standard informed consent was required from the participants. Access to data was limited to the IPC team and study investigators, ensuring confidentiality.

3. Results

We included 829 participants with documented SARS-CoV-2 first infection, of which 70.1% (581) had no reinfection and 29.9% (248) had SARS-CoV-2 reinfection. The study group was composed of 84.3% (699) females with a median age of 44 years, with an interquartile range (IQR) of 36 to 51. Of the female participants, 41.5% (344) were nurses and 71.4% (592) worked in high-risk departments. Comparing the group of HCWs without SARS-CoV-2 reinfection and the group of HCWs with SARS-CoV-2 reinfection, we found statistically significant differences regarding the frequency of the cases by department. In high-risk departments, we identified 77.4% (192) reinfections ($p = 0.012$). Detailed data regarding the descriptive demographics of HCWs from the study and comparison between groups are presented in Table 1.

Table 1. Descriptive characteristics of the study group and comparative analysis between HCWs without reinfections and HCWs with reinfection during the study period.

Characteristics	Study Participants	Without SARS-CoV-2 Reinfection	With SARS-CoV-2 Reinfection	*p*-Value
	829 (%)	581 (70.1)	248 (29.9)	
Gender				
Female	699 (84.3)	491 (84.5)	208 (83.9)	0.828
Male	130 (15.7)	90 (15.5)	40 (16.1)	
Age				
Mean (SD)	43 (9.9)	43 (10.2)	43 (9.14)	
Median age (years), IQR	44 (36–51)	44 (35–44)	44 (36–50)	
≤29	78 (9.4)	61 (10.5)	17 (6.9)	0.105
30–39	196 (23.6)	136 (23.4)	60 (24.2)	0.804
40–49	293 (35.3)	200 (34.4)	93 (37.5)	0.393
≥50	262 (31.6)	184 (31.7)	78 (31.5)	0.955
Job category				
Nurses	344 (41.5)	236 (40.6)	108 (43.5)	0.438
Physicians	156 (18.8)	111 (19.1)	45 (18.1)	0.736
Healthcare auxiliary activities	203 (24.5)	143 (24.6)	60 (24.2)	0.903
Other categories	126 (15.2)	91 (15.7)	35 (14.1)	0.557
Department				
High Risk [1]	592 (71.4)	400 (68.8)	192 (77.4)	0.012
Low risk [2]	237 (28.6)	181 (31.2)	56 (22.6)	

[1] ICU, emergency, COVID-19 wards; [2] nonCOVID-19 wards, laboratory; SD, standard deviation; IQR, interquartile range.

Regarding vaccination status, the study group had 737 (88.9%) HCWs vaccinated with the primary schedule, 301 (36.7%) vaccinated with the first booster, and 92 (11.1%) HCWs were unvaccinated. Among HCWs vaccinated with the first booster, only one person had an updated vaccine formula. The second booster was identified in 21 (6.9%) persons, of whom 9 (42.9%) were vaccinated with originally authorized vaccines and 12 (57%) had boosters with bivalent vaccines.

Descriptive data regarding the first SARS-CoV-2 infection and the reinfections in different periods of the COVID-19 pandemic defined by the dominance of SARS-CoV-2 variants in Romania, also correlated with data regarding vaccination, are presented in Table 2.

Table 2. Descriptive analysis of the first and second SARS-CoV-2 infection of the HCWs from INBI" Prof. Dr. Matei Balș" by pandemic wave corresponding to the predominant transmission period of main SARS-CoV-2 variants.

Characteristics of COVID-19 Cases in the Study Group	First SARS-CoV-2 Infection		Second SARS-CoV-2 Infection	
	829	%	248	29.9 * (%)
hCoV-19/Wuhan/WIV04/2019 (February 2020–February 2021)				
Total	**378**	**45.6**	**5**	**2.0**
Nonvaccinated HCWs	378	45.6	5	100.0
HCWs vaccinated with the primary series	0	0.0	0	0.0
HCWs vaccinated with the first booster dose	0	0.0	0	0.0
Alpha (March 2021–June 2021)				
Total	**20**	**2.4**	**0**	**0.0**
Nonvaccinated HCWs	14	70.0	0	0.0
HCWs vaccinated with the primary series	6	30.0	0	0.0
Median number of days since immunization (IQR)	44.5 (36–52)	-	-	-
HCWs vaccinated with the first booster dose	0	0.0	0	0.0
Delta (June 2021–December 2021)				
Total	**123**	**14.8**	**12**	**4.8**
Nonvaccinated HCWs	38	30.9	6	50.0
HCWs vaccinated with the primary series	85	69.1	6	50.0
Median number of days since immunization (IQR)	240 (218–257)	-	203 (169–301)	-
HCWs vaccinated with the first booster dose	0	0.0	0	0.0
Omicron (January 2022–May 2023)				
Total	**308**	**37.2**	**231**	**93.2**
Nonvaccinated HCWs	30	9.7	29	12.5
HCWs vaccinated with the primary series	139	45.1	130	56.3
Median number of days since immunization (IQR)	352 (241–384)	-	365 (238–519)	-
HCWs vaccinated with the first booster dose	139	45.1	72	31.2
Median number of days since revaccination (IQR)	127 (98–257)	-	169 (99–361)	-

SD, standard deviation; IQR, interquartile range; * percent of reinfections.

The data indicated that 45.6% (378) of the first SARS-CoV-2 infections were registered during the dominance of the ancestral variant of SARS-CoV-2 and 37.2% (308) during the Omicron variants. There were 248 (29.9%) reinfections, of which 93.2% (231) were detected during the Omicron dominance period. Of the SARS-CoV-2 reinfections during the Omicron period, 56.3% (130) were registered in HCWs vaccinated with the primary series and 31.2% (72) in HCWs who received the first booster. The reinfected HCWs had a median number of days since the last vaccine shot of 365 days (IQR: 238–519) if they were vaccinated with the primary schedule and 169 days (IQR: 99–361) if they acquired the first booster shot.

The vaccination campaign for HCWs commenced on 27 December 2020. The HCWs' option regarding vaccination with the primary schedule continued until April 2022. The administration of booster shots started in September 2021, and the HCWs' option regarding the first booster continued until September 2022.

Cumulative data regarding the first and second SARS-CoV-2 infections, vaccination status, and booster are represented graphically in Figure 2. The temporal representation of both the first and second SARS-CoV-2 infections pointed out a dramatic rise in the number of cases starting at the end of 2021, corresponding with the detection of Omicron variant BA.1 of SARS-CoV-2 in the community; in January 2022, the variant becoming dominant.

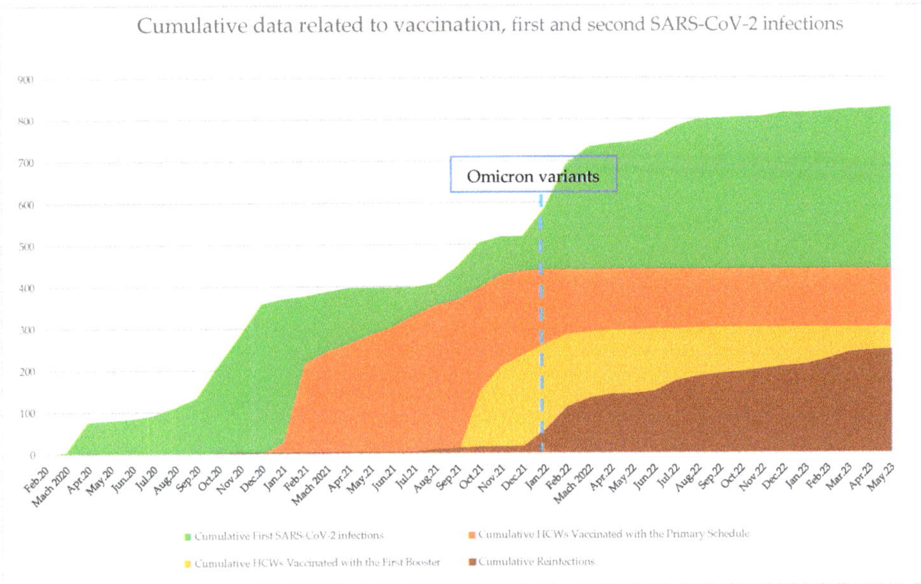

Figure 2. Graphical representation of cumulative data regarding vaccination status, first and second SARS-CoV-2 infections in HCWs included in the study.

3.1. Reinfections during Omicron in Vaccinated HCWs

Comparing the density of incidence of SARS-CoV-2 reinfections of HCWs vaccinated with the primary series and those vaccinated with the first booster showed that the male HCWs vaccinated with the primary series had a density of incidence of 2.8 (95% CI: 1.2; 6.7) times higher than that of HCWs vaccinated with the first booster. Other groups also registered differences, but with no statistical significance indicated by a p-value > 0.05 or 95% confidence interval including a value of 1. Detailed data are presented in Table 3.

Table 3. The incidence density of SARS-CoV-2 reinfection, in those vaccinated with the primary schedule and vaccinated with the first booster HCWs by demographic characteristics.

Characteristics	Reinfections during Omicron in HCWs Vaccinated with the Primary Schedule			Reinfections during Omicron in HCWs Vaccinated with the First Booster			Incidence Rate Ratio (95% CI)	p-Value
	N	P-d	Rate × 10,000 (95% CI)	N	P-d	Rate × 10,000 (95% CI)		
Total	130	179,208	7.3 (6.1; 8.6)	72	130,371	5.5 (4.3; 6.9)	0.8 (0.6; 1.0)	0.062
Gender								
Female	105	154,864	6.8 (5.5; 8.2)	63	106,242	5.9 (4.6; 7.6)	1.1 (0.8; 1.6)	0.402
Male	25	24,344	10.3 (6.7; 15.2)	9	24,129	3.7 (1.7; 7.1)	2.8 (1.2; 6.7)	0.006
Age								
≤29	6	16,179	3.7 (1.4; 8.1)	8	15,398	5.2 (2.2; 10.2)	0.7 (0.2; 2.3)	0.545
30–39	36	41,502	8.7 (6.1; 12.0)	17	31,329	5.4 (3.2; 8.7)	1.6 (0.9; 3.0)	0.108
40–49	49	68,750	7.1 (5.3; 9.4)	23	41,592	5.5 (5.5; 8.3)	1.3 (0.7; 2.4)	0.405
≥50	39	52,777	7.4 (5.3; 10.1)	24	42,052	5.7 (3.7; 8.5)	1.3 (0.8; 2.2)	0.322

Table 3. *Cont.*

Characteristics	Reinfections during Omicron in HCWs Vaccinated with the Primary Schedule			Reinfections during Omicron in HCWs Vaccinated with the First Booster			Incidence Rate Ratio (95% CI)	p-Value
	N	P-d	Rate × 10,000 (95% CI)	N	P-d	Rate × 10,000 (95% CI)		
Job category								
Nurses	60	79,950	7.5 (5.7; 9.7)	24	45,965	5.2 (3.3; 7.8)	1.4 (0.9; 2.4)	0.129
Physicians	15	16,179	9.3 (5.2; 15.3)	28	45,984	6.1 (4.0; 8.8)	1.5 (0.8; 2.9)	0.197
Healthcare auxiliary activities	36	51,822	6.9 (4.9; 9.6)	14	24,181	5.8 (3.2; 9.7)	1.2 (0.6; 2.4)	0.576
Other categories	19	31,257	6.1 (3.7; 9.5)	6	14,241	4.2 (1.5; 9.2)	1.4 (0.6; 4.4)	0.448
Department								
High Risk [1]	102	119,918	8.5 (6.9; 10.3)	63	103,558	6.1 (4.7; 7.8)	1.4 (1.0; 1.9)	0.035
Low risk [2]	28	59,290	4.7 (3.1; 6.8)	9	26,813	3.4 (1.5; 6.4)	1.4 (0.6; 3.4)	0.381

[1] ICU, emergency, COVID-19 wards; [2] nonCOVID-19 wards, laboratory, other departments.

3.2. Reinfections in HCWs Vaccinated with the Primary Series by the History of SARS-CoV-2 Infection

Overall, there were fewer COVID-19 cases in the group with a history of infection after January 2022. The incidence density of reinfections in HCWs vaccinated with the primary schedule registered significant differences between groups constructed based on the history of infection before and after January 2022. HCWs with a history of COVID-19 before Omicron variant dominance had an incidence density 5.0 (95% CI 2.9; 9.2) times higher than HCWs with a history of COVID-19 after Omicron became dominant in Romania. Subgroups that had significant differences were females, with an incidence density in the group with a history of first COVID-19 before January 2022 that was 6.1 (95% CI 3.2; 13.1) times higher than in the group with a history of first infection after January 2022.

The incidence density by age groups indicated significant differences between age groups above 30 years, with a lower incidence density in the group with a history of infection after January 2022. The job category presented significant differences only for density incidence in the healthcare auxiliary and other categories. In both high-risk and low-risk departments, there were registered differences with lower values in the group of HCWs with a history of infection after January 2022. The data are presented in Table 4.

Table 4. The incidence density of SARS-CoV-2 reinfection in HCWs vaccinated with the primary schedule by history of infection before and after the Omicron era.

Characteristics	History of Infection before January 2022			History of Infection after January 2022			Incidence Rate Ratio (95% CI)	p-Value
	N	P-d	Rate × 10,000 (95% CI)	N	P-d	Rate × 10,000 (95% CI)		
HCWs Vaccinated with the Primary Schedule	115	108,570	10.6 (8.7; 12.7)	15	70,638	2.1 (1.2; 3.5)	5.0 (2.9; 9.2)	<0.001
Gender								
Female	95	94,359	10.1 (8.2; 12.3)	10	60,505	1.7 (0.8; 3.0)	6.1 (3.2; 13.1)	<0.001
Male	20	14,211	14.1 (8.6; 21.7)	5	10,133	4.9 (1.6; 11.5)	2.9 (1.0; 9.7)	0.026

Table 4. *Cont.*

Characteristics	History of Infection before January 2022			History of Infection after January 2022			Incidence Rate Ratio (95% CI)	*p*-Value
	N	P-d	Rate × 10,000 (95% CI)	N	P-d	Rate × 10,000 (95% CI)		
Age								
≤29	5	7180	7.0 (2.3; 16.3)	1	8999	1.1 (0.0; 6.2)	6.3 (0.7; 296.4)	0.073
30–39	32	23,366	13.7 (9.4; 19.3)	4	18,136	2.2 (0.6; 5.6)	6.2 (2.2; 24.2)	<0.001
40–49	43	43,875	9.8 (7.1; 13.2)	6	24,875	2.4 (0.9; 5.3)	6.1 (2.2; 23.4)	<0.001
≥50	35	34,149	10.3 (7.1; 14.3)	4	18,628	2.1 (0.6; 5.5)	7.2 (2.7; 27.5)	<0.001
Job category								
Nurses	53	49,520	10.7 (8.0; 14.0)	7	30,430	2.3 (0.9; 4.7)	6.3 (0.7; 296.4)	0.073
Physicians	12	8863	13.5 (7.0; 23.7)	3	7316	4.1 (0.8; 12.0)	3.3 (0.9; 18.2)	0.051
Healthcare auxiliary activities	33	33,053	10.0 (6.9; 14.0)	3	18,769	1.6 (0.3; 4.7)	6.2 (2.0; 31.8)	<0.001
Other categories	17	17,134	9.9 (5.8; 15.9)	2	14,123	1.4 (0.2; 5.1)	7.0(1.7; 62.5)	0.002
Department								
High Risk [1]	91	71,816	12.7 (10.2; 15.6)	11	48,102	2.3 (1.1; 4.1)	5.5 (3.0; 11.5)	<0.0001
Low risk [2]	24	36,754	6.5 (4.2; 9.7)	4	22,536	1.8 (0.5; 4.5)	3.7 (1.3; 14.6)	0.0072

[1] ICU, emergency, COVID-19 wards; [2] nonCOVID-19 wards, laboratory, other departments.

3.3. *Reinfections in HCWs Vaccinated with the First Booster and the History of SARS-CoV-2 Infection*

Overall, there were fewer COVID-19 cases in the group with a history of infection after January 2022. The incidence density of reinfections in HCWs was significantly different between subgroups of females, age groups over 30 years, nurses, physicians, healthcare auxiliary personnel, and high-risk departments. All mentioned subgroups had a lower incidence density if the participants had a history of SARS-CoV-2 infection after January 2022. Detailed data are presented in Table 5.

Table 5. The incidence density of SARS-CoV-2 reinfection in HCWs vaccinated with the first booster by history of infection before and after the Omicron era.

Characteristics	History of Infection before January 2022			History of Infection after January 2022			Incidence Rate Ratio (95% CI)	*p*-Value
	N	P-d	Rate × 10,000 (95% CI)	N	P-d	Rate × 10,000 (95% CI)		
HCWs Vaccinated with the First Booster	**53**	**60,438**	8.8 (6.6; 11.5)	**19**	**69,933**	2.7 (1.6; 4.2)	3.2 (1.9; 5.8)	<0.001
Gender								
Female	45	51,578	8.7 (6.4; 11.7)	18	54,664	3.3 (2.0; 5.2)	2.6 (1.5; 4.9)	<0.001
Male	8	8860	9.0 (3.9; 17.8)	1	15,269	0.7 (0.0; 3.6)	13.8 (1.8; 611.8)	0.002
Age								
≤29	5	6155	8.1 (2.6; 19.0)	3	9243	3.2 (0.7; 9.5)	2.5 (0.5; 16.1)	0.223
30–39	13	11,646	11.2 (5.9; 19.1)	4	19,683	2.0 (0.6; 5.2)	5.5 (1.7; 23.1)	0.002
40–49	15	16,973	8.8 (4.9; 14.6)	8	24,619	3.3 (1.4; 6.4)	2.7 (1.1; 7.4)	0.021
≥50	20	25,664	7.8 (4.8; 12.0)	4	16,388	2.4 (0.7; 6.2)	3.2 (1.1; 12.8)	0.022

Table 5. *Cont.*

Characteristics	History of Infection before January 2022			History of Infection after January 2022			Incidence Rate Ratio (95% CI)	*p*-Value
	N	P-d	Rate × 10,000 (95% CI)	N	P-d	Rate × 10,000 (95% CI)		
Job category								
Nurses	19	23,464	8.1 (4.9; 12.6)	5	22,501	2.2 (0.7; 5.2)	3.6 (1.3; 12.5)	0.006
Physicians	17	18,213	9.3 (5.4; 14.9)	11	27,771	4.0 (2.0; 7.1)	2.4 (1.0; 5.6)	0.027
Healthcare auxiliary activities	11	12,760	8.6 (4.3; 15.4)	3	11,421	2.6 (0.5; 7.7)	3.3 (0.9; 18.3)	0.056
Other categories	6	6001	10.0 (3.7; 21.8)	0	8240	0 (0;0)	0 (0;0)	-
Department								
High Risk [1]	46	45,773	10.1 (7.4; 13.4)	17	57,785	2.9 (1.7; 4.7)	3.4 (1.9; 6.4)	<0.001
Low risk [2]	7	14,665	4.8 (1.9; 9.8)	2	12,148	1.6 (0.2; 5.9)	2.9 (0.6; 28.6)	0.182

[1] ICU, emergency, COVID-19 wards; [2] nonCOVID-19 wards, laboratory, other departments.

4. Discussion

The present study identified aspects related to the dynamics of SARS-CoV-2 transmission in HCWs, considering specific characteristics of the participants such as gender, age, occupational category, department of activity, vaccination status, and history of prior SARS-CoV-2 infection before or during Omicron dominance in Romania.

The first objective of this study was to compare groups to identify differences between HCWs without reinfection versus HCWs with reinfection during the study period. The current study showed that the characteristics represented by gender, age, and occupational category did not indicate statistically significant differences in the comparison of HCWs groups. Reinfections were more common in HCWs from high-risk departments. Our study detected a higher rate of reinfections in HCWs than other studies as the current study comprised a much longer time period and implied multiple variants of Omicron [23–31]. Also, in the studies performed during Omicron circulation the populations received multiple vaccine doses after the primary schedule [25,26,30,31].

We considered the circulation of SARS-CoV-2 in the community by establishing periods of dominance of VOC strains according to weekly reports from the Romanian NIPH. Thus, we had four periods: the initial variant of SARS-CoV-2 dominance (hCoV-19/Wuhan/WIV04/2019), and the dominance of VOC Alpha, Delta, and Omicron [13,14].

The dominance periods of SARS-CoV-2 VOC strains varied in length, with a shorter period of dominance circulation of the Alpha and Delta VOC, accounting for almost four months and six months, respectively, during 2021 [13,14]. In Romania, the initial variant of SARS-CoV-2 (hCoV-19/Wuhan/WIV04/2019) circulated for approximately one year, and Omicron variants became dominant at the beginning of 2022. During the Omicron dominance, there was an increase in the number of COVID-19 cases, primary infections, and reinfections in HCWs, although most of the HCWs were vaccinated with the primary schedule, and some also had the first booster administered. The assumption that the high number of infections could be explained by the increased transmissibility of Omicron variants has been demonstrated in multiple studies worldwide [15,16,32].

The time elapsed from vaccination to infection or reinfection is an important indicator for tailoring public health measures regarding the administration of booster shots [33–35]. In our study, the average time elapsed from the primary vaccination to reinfection was almost one year. Although a significant proportion of the participants received boosters, there were several reinfections in this category as well. Notably, the boosters used were not adapted to the circulating variants.

Natural and artificial immunity has been assessed by evaluating the dynamics of protective antibodies over time or by using epidemiological indicators from surveillance data. Both types of study have shown that natural and artificial immunity both wane over time and have led to the adaptation of recommendations regarding vaccination schedules [8,17,19,27,35–42]. Common epidemiological indicators of frequency in other studies showed increases in the number of reinfections and primo-infections in the Omicron era, similar to our study [25,26,43,44]. The previously published study on the first SARS-CoV-2 infection, on the same population of HCWs, showed a higher severity of the cases registered in HCWs from the high-risk departments [18].

The demographic characteristics of HCWs, such as age, gender, profession, and department, are important in identifying differences between subgroups. These characteristics have been studied and reported in surveillance data throughout the COVID-19 pandemic, providing information on potential protective measures or additional monitoring of these categories [25,26].

The incidence density of reinfections during Omicron in the male gender and in HCWs from high-risk departments was higher in HCWs vaccinated with the primary schedule than in HCWs vaccinated with the first booster.

A study from the United States of America (USA) conducted in 2020–2021 on a cohort of 62,310 people in the general population also reported a higher frequency of COVID-19 cases in the male gender [45]. Other studies have reported more frequent reinfections in males [46,47].

The higher frequency of infections and reinfections during Omicron circulation reported in other studies has been explained by changes in the transmissibility of Omicron variants and vaccine effectiveness [16,43,44,48]. Although during the study period the HCWs wore PPE in healthcare activities, in the community they were exposed to asymptomatic or suspected COVID-19 cases, as restrictions were fewer during Omicron compared to other waves. The proper use of PPE was assessed for the first COVID-19 confirmed cases in a previously published study using a WHO standardized questionnaire, and a high risk of exposure was identified in 6.8% of HCWs [18].

In terms of disease history, published studies have supported the importance of hybrid immunity [19,39,49]. The study ORCHESTRA compared subjects re-vaccinated with the first booster and a history of SARS-CoV-2 infection with subjects with no prior infection, and the relative risk ratio was 0.11 (95% CI: 0.05–0.25). A cohort retrospective study of HCWs showed a rate of reinfection of 16.2% (95% CI: 13.5–19.3%) in the hybrid immunity group compared with HCWs with no prior infection, which registered a rate of reinfection of 41.7% (95% CI: 40.3–43.0%). In our cohort, surveillance data demonstrated an advantage in terms of protection in individuals with hybrid immunity compared with HCWs vaccinated with the primary schedule and no prior infection, with a hazard ratio (HR) across all COVID-19 events of 0.6 (95% CI: 0.47–0.77) [19]. The HCWs with hybrid immunity and first booster compared to HCWs vaccinated with the primary schedule and no prior infection had a HR of 0.42 (95% CI: 0.30–0.58) [19].

The incidence density of reinfection in different subgroups of HCWs vaccinated with the primary schedule had higher values if there was a history of the first SARS-CoV-2 infection before Omicron compared to HCWs with a history of disease after Omicron dominant circulation. The low likelihood of developing reinfections in this subgroup of HCWs with the first SARS-CoV-2 infection during Omicron emphasizes the importance of the circulating variants when interpreting the hybrid immunity.

Comparing the incidence density of HCWs vaccinated with the primary schedule and the first booster, it was found that those with a history of primoinfection during Omicron were three times less likely to develop a reinfection compared to those who had a history of reinfection before Omicron, but the incidence of reinfections in HCWs vaccinated with the primary schedule versus HCWs vaccinated with the first booster showed no significant differences. This suggests the need for adapted boosters and the importance of recent infections in interpreting vaccine efficacy in populations with hybrid immunity [15,16,50–53].

Studies demonstrating complex mechanisms or correlating antibody levels and their dynamics postvaccination or post-SARS-CoV-2 infection are extremely useful for understanding the pathological phenomenon. In a hybrid immunity population, the infection-induced and the vaccine-induced antibodies cannot be differentiated, but the duration of persistence of the antibodies is very useful for establishing vaccination programs and the optimal timing for boosters [15,16,20,53–55]. As the current study shows, indicators like density incidence are useful for evaluating the effectiveness of control measures in specific subgroups of the population in specific SARS-CoV-2 VOC circulation periods.

The strengths of this study are represented by the quality of data obtained through active surveillance of HCWs by a specialized team in field epidemiology. In addition, the data (comprised of multiple sources) were both manually and automatically validated.

However, our study had some limitations. In particular, we did not consider transition periods where two SARS-CoV-2 variants of concern were co-circulating, and we only took into account the moment when a VOC of SARS-CoV-2 became dominant, a situation imposed given the reduced circulation as a time period of Alpha and Delta variants. However, the objective was to assess the incidence of pre-Omicron disease and post-Omicron disease in HCWs, but not for each strain. In addition, we did not have data to compare non-adapted boosters with adapted boosters, as our cohort had administered only a few adapted boosters.

5. Conclusions

The presence of a history of illness during the Omicron circulation period influenced the incidence density of reinfections in HCWs, including in subgroups based on demographic characteristics. Thus, our study highlights the importance of considering the history of SARS-CoV-2 infection when interpreting and understanding the public health data and the results of studies related to the evaluation of vaccine efficacy in hybrid immunity subgroup populations.

Supplementary Materials: The following supporting information can be downloaded at: https://www.mdpi.com/article/10.3390/vaccines12060682/s1. Supplemental Data S1 (Table S1: Changes in National Methodology for COVID-19 surveillance, regarding Genomic Surveillance; Table S2: Criteria for selecting cases for testing in the surveillance system, from April 2021 to July 2021; Table S3: Criteria for selecting cases for testing in the surveillance system, from August 2021 to January 2022; Table S4: Criteria for selecting cases for testing in the surveillance system, from July 2022 to May 2023). Supplemental Data S2 (Table S5: Summarised surveillance data regarding sequencing, from reports of the Romanian National Institute of Public Health; Figure S1: Weekly positive sequenced samples according to reports of the Romanian National Institute of Public Health).

Author Contributions: Conceptualization, C.-D.C., A.S.C., V.A., M.L.L., G.J. and D.P.; methodology, C.-D.C., C.G.A., V.G.N., A.L., M.-D.C., D.P. and A.S.C.; software, C.-D.C. and A.L.; validation, C.-D.C. and V.G.N.; formal analysis, C.-D.C., V.G.N., M.-D.C. and A.L.; data curation, C.-D.C.; writing—original draft preparation, C.-D.C.; writing—review and editing, C.-D.C., M.-D.C., D.P., V.A., M.L.L., G.J., V.G.N., A.L., C.G.A. and A.S.C.; visualization, C.-D.C.; supervision, M.-D.C., D.P., V.A., M.L.L., G.J. and A.S.C. All authors have read and agreed to the published version of the manuscript.

Funding: This research received no external funding.

Institutional Review Board Statement: The study was conducted following the Declaration of Helsinki, and the Institutional Bioethics Committee of the National Institute for Infectious Diseases "Professor Dr. Matei Balș", Bucharest, Romania, approved this study (protocol C08784/27 July 2023).

Informed Consent Statement: Informed consent was obtained from all subjects involved in the study.

Data Availability Statement: The datasets generated and analyzed during the current study are available from the corresponding author upon reasonable request.

Acknowledgments: The authors thank the Infection Control Department and the participants. Publication of this paper was supported by the University of Medicine and Pharmacy "Carol Davila" through the institutional program Publish not Perish.

Conflicts of Interest: The authors declare no conflicts of interest.

References

1. WHO. COVID-19 Public Health Emergency of International Concern (PHEIC) Global Research and Innovation Forum. Available online: https://www.who.int/publications/m/item/covid-19-public-health-emergency-of-international-concern-(pheic)-global-research-and-innovation-forum (accessed on 7 May 2024).
2. WHO. International Health Regulations. Available online: https://www.who.int/health-topics/international-health-regulations (accessed on 7 May 2024).
3. WHO. Statement on the Fifteenth Meeting of the IHR (2005) Emergency Committee on the COVID-19 Pandemic. Available online: https://www.who.int/news/item/05-05-2023-statement-on-the-fifteenth-meeting-of-the-international-health-regulations-(2005)-emergency-committee-regarding-the-coronavirus-disease-(covid-19)-pandemic (accessed on 9 December 2023).
4. European Medicines Agency. COVID-19 Public Health Emergency of International Concern (2020–23). Available online: https://www.ema.europa.eu/en/human-regulatory-overview/public-health-threats/coronavirus-disease-covid-19/covid-19-public-health-emergency-international-concern-2020-23#external-links-19865 (accessed on 7 May 2024).
5. WHO. COVID-19 Cases | WHO COVID-19 Dashboard. Available online: https://data.who.int/dashboards/covid19/cases (accessed on 7 May 2024).
6. WHO. From Emergency Response to Long-Term COVID-19 Disease Management: Sustaining Gains Made during the COVID-19 Pandemic. Available online: https://www.who.int/publications-detail-redirect/WHO-WHE-SPP-2023.1 (accessed on 7 May 2024).
7. WHO. Standing Recommendations for COVID-19 Issued by the Director-General of the World Health Organization (WHO) in Accordance with the International Health Regulations (2005) (IHR). Available online: https://www.who.int/publications/m/item/standing-recommendations-for-covid-19-issued-by-the-director-general-of-the-world-health-organization-(who)-in-accordance-with-the-international-health-regulations-(2005)-(ihr) (accessed on 7 May 2024).
8. WHO. WHO SAGE Roadmap for Prioritizing Uses of COVID-19 Vaccines: An Approach to Optimize the Global Impact of COVID-19 Vaccines, Based on Public Health Goals, Global and National Equity, and Vaccine Access and Coverage Scenarios. Available online: https://www.who.int/publications-detail-redirect/WHO-2019-nCoV-Vaccines-SAGE-Prioritization-2023.1 (accessed on 7 May 2024).
9. WHO. Laboratory Testing for 2019 Novel Coronavirus (2019-nCoV) in Suspected Human Cases. Available online: https://www.who.int/publications-detail-redirect/10665-331501 (accessed on 20 May 2024).
10. ECDC. Guidance for Representative and Targeted Genomic SARS-CoV-2 Monitoring. Available online: https://www.ecdc.europa.eu/sites/default/files/documents/Guidance-for-representative-and-targeted-genomic-SARS-CoV-2-monitoring-updated-with%20erratum-20-May-2021.pdf (accessed on 20 May 2024).
11. INSP. Metodologii—Institutul Național de Sănătate Publică. Available online: https://insp.gov.ro/centrul-national-de-supraveghere-si-control-al-bolilor-transmisibile-cnscbt/metodologii/ (accessed on 20 May 2024).
12. Enciu, B.G.; Tănase, A.A.; Drăgănescu, A.C.; Aramă, V.; Pițigoi, D.; Crăciun, M.-D. The COVID-19 Pandemic in Romania: A Comparative Description with Its Border Countries. *Healthcare* **2022**, *10*, 1223. [CrossRef]
13. INSP. Centrul Național de Supraveghere şi Control al Bolilor Transmisibile—Analiză Cazuri Confirmate COVID19. Available online: https://www.cnscbt.ro/index.php/analiza-cazuri-confirmate-covid19 (accessed on 9 December 2023).
14. GISAID. GISAID-hCov19 Variants. Available online: https://gisaid.org/hcov19-variants/ (accessed on 7 May 2024).
15. Manathunga, S.S.; Abeyagunawardena, I.A.; Dharmaratne, S.D. A comparison of transmissibility of SARS-CoV-2 variants of concern. *Virol. J.* **2023**, *20*, 59. [CrossRef]
16. ECDC. SARS-CoV-2 Variants of Concern as of 26 April 2024. Available online: https://www.ecdc.europa.eu/en/covid-19/variants-concern (accessed on 7 May 2024).
17. EMA. EMA and ECDC Statement on Updating COVID-19 Vaccines to Target New SARS-CoV-2 Virus Variants | European Medicines Agency. Available online: https://www.ema.europa.eu/en/news/ema-and-ecdc-statement-updating-covid-19-vaccines-target-new-sars-cov-2-virus-variants (accessed on 20 May 2024).
18. Chivu, C.-D.; Crăciun, M.-D.; Pițigoi, D.; Aramă, V.; Luminos, M.L.; Jugulete, G.; Apostolescu, C.G.; Streinu Cercel, A. Vaccination and Factors Related to the Clinical Outcome of COVID-19 in Healthcare Workers—A Romanian Front-Line Hospital's Experience. *Vaccines* **2023**, *11*, 899. [CrossRef]
19. Chivu, C.-D.; Crăciun, M.-D.; Pițigoi, D.; Aramă, V.; Luminos, M.L.; Jugulete, G.; Constantin, C.; Apostolescu, C.G.; Streinu Cercel, A. The Dynamic Risk of COVID-19-Related Events in Vaccinated Healthcare Workers (HCWs) from a Tertiary Hospital in Bucharest, Romania: A Study Based on Active Surveillance Data. *Vaccines* **2024**, *12*, 182. [CrossRef]
20. WHO. Interim Statement on Hybrid Immunity and Increasing Population Seroprevalence Rates. Available online: https://www.who.int/news/item/01-06-2022-interim-statement-on-hybrid-immunity-and-increasing-population-seroprevalence-rates (accessed on 12 June 2024).

21. Enciu, B.G.; Pițigoi, D.; Zaharia, A.; Popescu, R.; Niculcea, A.; Crăciun, M.-D.; Pistol, A. COVID-19 Vaccination in Romania and the Benefits of the National Electronic Registry of Vaccinations. *Vaccines* **2023**, *11*, 370. [CrossRef]
22. Celentano, D. *Gordis Epidemiology*, 6th ed.; Elsevier: Amsterdam, The Netherlands, 2018.
23. Deng, L.; Li, P.; Zhang, X.; Jiang, Q.; Turner, D.; Zhou, C.; Gao, Y.; Qian, F.; Zhang, C.; Lu, H.; et al. Risk of SARS-CoV-2 reinfection: A systematic review and meta-analysis. *Sci. Rep.* **2022**, *12*, 20763. [CrossRef]
24. Rivelli, A.; Fitzpatrick, V.; Blair, C.; Copeland, K.; Richards, J. Incidence of COVID-19 reinfection among Midwestern healthcare employees. *PLoS ONE* **2022**, *17*, e0262164. [CrossRef]
25. Cegolon, L.; Negro, C.; Mastrangelo, G.; Filon, F.L. Primary SARS-CoV-2 Infections, Re-infections and Vaccine Effectiveness during the Omicron Transmission Period in Healthcare Workers of Trieste and Gorizia (Northeast Italy), 1 December 2021–31 May 2022. *Viruses* **2022**, *14*, 2688. [CrossRef]
26. Cegolon, L.; Magnano, G.; Negro, C.; Filon, F.L.; ORCHESTRA Working Group. SARS-CoV-2 Reinfections in Health-Care Workers, 1 March 2020–31 January 2023. *Viruses* **2023**, *15*, 1551. [CrossRef]
27. Guedes, A.R.; Oliveira, M.S.; Tavares, B.M.; Luna-Muschi, A.; Lazari, C.D.S.; Montal, A.C.; de Faria, E.; Maia, F.L.; Barboza, A.D.S.; Leme, M.D.; et al. Reinfection rate in a cohort of healthcare workers over 2 years of the COVID-19 pandemic. *Sci. Rep.* **2023**, *13*, 712. [CrossRef]
28. Nieto, M.A.; Caballero, N.; Remolina, C.I.; Moreno, S.; Vega, D.; Quintero, J. Incidence and risk factors related to SARS-CoV-2 infection, reinfection, and seroconversion: Analysis of a healthcare workers cohort from a university hospital in Colombia. *IJID Reg.* **2023**, *9*, 63–71. [CrossRef]
29. Karimi, Y.; Abdollahi, A.; Ahmadi, S.A.Y.; Riahi, T.; Kalantari, S.; Nafissi, N.; Shokri, S.; Baradaran, H.R.; Goodarzi, A. COVID-19 Reinfection in Healthcare Workers: An Original Comprehensive Longitudinal Study. 14 November 2023, PREPRINT (Version 1) Available at Research Square. Available online: https://www.researchsquare.com/article/rs-3596390/v1 (accessed on 7 May 2024).
30. Zhang, C.; Guo, T.; Zhang, L.; Gu, A.; Ye, J.; Lin, M.; Chu, M.; Zhu, F.; Zhu, L. The Infection of Healthcare Workers and the Reinfection of Patients by Omicron Variant—Jiangsu Province, China, December 2022 to January 2023. *China CDC Wkly.* **2023**, *5*, 402–406. [CrossRef]
31. Ma, X.; Wang, Z.; Chen, Y.; Li, Z. The symptoms and interval of Omicron SARS-CoV-2 reinfection among healthcare workers in a hospital of Southern China: A cross-sectional study. *BMC Infect. Dis.* **2024**, *24*, 354. [CrossRef]
32. Niu, Y.; Luo, L.; Yang, S.; Abudurusuli, G.; Wang, X.; Zhao, Z.; Rui, J.; Li, Z.; Deng, B.; Liu, W.; et al. Comparison of epidemiological characteristics and transmissibility of different strains of COVID-19 based on the incidence data of all local outbreaks in China as of March 1, 2022. *Front. Public Health* **2022**, *10*, 949594. [CrossRef] [PubMed]
33. Malhotra, S.; Mani, K.; Lodha, R.; Bakhshi, S.; Mathur, V.P.; Gupta, P.; Kedia, S.; Sankar, M.J.; Kumar, P.; Kumar, A.; et al. COVID-19 infection, and reinfection, and vaccine effectiveness against symptomatic infection among health care workers in the setting of omicron variant transmission in New Delhi, India. *Lancet Reg. Health Southeast Asia* **2022**, *3*, 100023. [CrossRef]
34. Lanièce Delaunay, C.; Martínez-Baz, I.; Sève, N.; Domegan, L.; Mazagatos, C.; Buda, S.; Meijer, A.; Kislaya, I.; Pascu, C.; Carnahan, A.; et al. COVID-19 vaccine effectiveness against symptomatic infection with SARS-CoV-2 BA.1/BA.2 lineages among adults and adolescents in a multicentre primary care study, Europe, December 2021 to June 2022. *Eurosurveillance* **2024**, *29*, 2300403. [CrossRef]
35. Hönning, A.; Tomczyk, S.; Hermes, J.; Grossegesse, M.; Hofmann, N.; Michel, J.; Neumann, M.; Nitsche, A.; Hoppe, B.; Eckmanns, T.; et al. Follow-up SARS-CoV-2 serological study of a health care worker cohort following COVID-19 booster vaccination. *BMC Infect. Dis.* **2024**, *24*, 436. [CrossRef]
36. Long, Q.Y.; Zheng, Y.L.; Gao, Z.C. Analysis of the clinical characteristics of COVID-19 reinfection cases. *Zhonghua Jie He He Hu Xi Za Zhi Zhonghua Jiehe He Huxi Zazhi Chin. J. Tuberc. Respir. Dis.* **2021**, *44*, 793–799. [CrossRef]
37. Pilz, S.; Theiler-Schwetz, V.; Trummer, C.; Krause, R.; Ioannidis, J.P.A. SARS-CoV-2 reinfections: Overview of efficacy and duration of natural and hybrid immunity. *Environ. Res.* **2022**, *209*, 112911. [CrossRef]
38. Goldberg, Y.; Mandel, M.; Bar-On, Y.M.; Bodenheimer, O.; Freedman, L.S.; Ash, N.; Alroy-Preis, S.; Huppert, A.; Milo, R. Protection and Waning of Natural and Hybrid Immunity to SARS-CoV-2. *N. Engl. J. Med.* **2022**, *386*, 2201–2212. [CrossRef]
39. Porru, S.; Monaco, M.G.L.; Spiteri, G.; Carta, A.; Caliskan, G.; Violán, C.; Torán-Monserrat, P.; Vimercati, L.; Tafuri, S.; Boffetta, P.; et al. Incidence and Determinants of Symptomatic and Asymptomatic SARS-CoV-2 Breakthrough Infections After Booster Dose in a Large European Multicentric Cohort of Health Workers-ORCHESTRA Project. *J. Epidemiol. Glob. Health* **2023**, *13*, 577–588. [CrossRef]
40. Spiteri, G.; D'Agostini, M.; Abedini, M.; Ditano, G.; Collatuzzo, G.; Boffetta, P.; Vimercati, L.; Sansone, E.; De Palma, G.; Modenese, A.; et al. Protective role of SARS-CoV-2 anti-S IgG against breakthrough infections among European healthcare workers during pre and post-Omicron surge-ORCHESTRA project. *Infection* **2024**. [CrossRef]
41. Martín Pérez, C.; Aguilar, R.; Jiménez, A.; Salmerón, G.; Canyelles, M.; Rubio, R.; Vidal, M.; Cuamba, I.; Barrios, D.; Díaz, N.; et al. Correlates of protection and determinants of SARS-CoV-2 breakthrough infections 1 year after third dose vaccination. *BMC Med.* **2024**, *22*, 103. [CrossRef]
42. Kurra, N.C.; Sriram, K.; Gandrakota, N.; Nagarajan, J.S.; Khasnavis, S.; Ramakrishnan, M.; Dalal, S.; Irfan, S.A.; Khan, S.; Jk, H.; et al. Frontliners on the Move: A Quantitative Analysis of the Prevalence of COVID-19 Reinfection Among Healthcare Workers. *Cureus* **2022**, *14*, e24652. [CrossRef]

43. Ibanes-Gutierrez, C.; Martínez-Rivera, N.; Martin-Onraet, A.; Rivera-Buendia, F.; Piñeirua-Menendez, A.; Villaseñor-Echavarri, R.; Serrano-Ortega, J.; Vilar-Compte, D. SARS-CoV-2 infection in health care workers during the first 2-years of the pandemic at a cancer hospital in Mexico. *Am. J. Infect. Control* **2024**, *52*, 517–524. [CrossRef]
44. Yu, W.; Guo, Y.; Hu, T.; Liu, Y.; Fan, Q.; Guo, L.; Zheng, B.; Kong, Y.; Zhu, H.; Yu, J.; et al. Incidence and severity of SARS-CoV-2 reinfection, a multicenter cohort study in Shanghai, China. *J. Med. Virol.* **2023**, *95*, e28997. [CrossRef]
45. Kharroubi, S.A.; Diab-El-Harake, M. Sex-differences in COVID-19 diagnosis, risk factors and disease comorbidities: A large US-based cohort study. *Front. Public Health* **2022**, *10*, 1029190. [CrossRef]
46. Nisha, B.; Dakshinamoorthy, K.; Padmanaban, P.; Jain, T.; Neelavarnan, M. Infection, reinfection, and postvaccination incidence of SARS-CoV-2 and associated risks in healthcare workers in Tamil Nadu: A retrospective cohort study. *J. Fam. Community Med.* **2022**, *29*, 49–55. [CrossRef]
47. Tavakoli, A.; Lotfi, F.; Lotfi, M.; Bayati, M.; Seif, M.; Salesi, M.; Emadi, M.; Keshavarz, K.; Delavari, S. COVID-19 Reinfection Rate and Related Risk Factors in Fars Province, Iran: A Retrospective Cohort Study. *Iran. J. Med. Sci.* **2023**, *48*, 302–312. [CrossRef]
48. Medić, S.; Anastassopoulou, C.; Lozanov-Crvenković, Z.; Vuković, V.; Dragnić, N.; Petrović, V.; Ristić, M.; Pustahija, T.; Gojković, Z.; Tsakris, A.; et al. Risk and severity of SARS-CoV-2 reinfections during 2020–2022 in Vojvodina, Serbia: A population-level observational study. *Lancet Reg. Health Eur.* **2022**, *20*, 100453. [CrossRef]
49. Jacobson, M.A.; Blanc, P.D.; Tulsky, J.; Tilly, M.; Meister, R.; Huen, W.; McNicholas, J.E., Jr. Risk of subsequent SARS-CoV-2 infection among vaccinated employees with or without hybrid immunity acquired early in the Omicron-predominant era of the COVID-19 pandemic. *Am. J. Ind. Med.* **2024**, *67*, 334–340. [CrossRef]
50. Jacot, D.; von Rotz, U.; Pellaton, C.; Blondet, F.; Aebischer, O.; Perreau, M.; De Rham, M.; Pantaleo, G.; Marchetti, O.; Greub, G. SARS-CoV-2 neutralizing antibody response in vaccinated and non-vaccinated hospital healthcare workers with or without history of infection. *Microbes Infect.* **2023**, *25*, 105077. [CrossRef]
51. Chin, E.T.; Leidner, D.; Lamson, L.; Lucas, K.; Studdert, D.M.; Goldhaber-Fiebert, J.D.; Andrews, J.R.; Salomon, J.A. Protection against Omicron from Vaccination and Previous Infection in a Prison System. *N. Engl. J. Med.* **2022**, *387*, 1770–1782. [CrossRef]
52. Kahn, F.; Bonander, C.; Moghaddassi, M.; Christiansen, C.B.; Bennet, L.; Malmqvist, U.; Inghammar, M.; Björk, J. Previous SARS-CoV-2 infections and their impact on the protection from reinfection during the Omicron BA.5 wave—A nested case-control study among vaccinated adults in Sweden. *IJID Reg.* **2024**, *10*, 235–239. [CrossRef]
53. Tan, C.Y.; Chiew, C.J.; Pang, D.; Lee, V.J.; Ong, B.; Lye, D.C.; Tan, K.B. Protective immunity of SARS-CoV-2 infection and vaccines against medically attended symptomatic omicron BA.4, BA.5, and XBB reinfections in Singapore: A national cohort study. *Lancet Infect. Dis.* **2023**, *23*, 799–805. [CrossRef]
54. Beaudoin-Bussières, G.; Tauzin, A.; Dionne, K.; Gendron-Lepage, G.; Medjahed, H.; Perreault, J.; Levade, I.; Alfadhli, L.; Bo, Y.; Bazin, R.; et al. A Recent SARS-CoV-2 Infection Enhances Antibody-Dependent Cellular Cytotoxicity against Several Omicron Subvariants following a Fourth mRNA Vaccine Dose. *Viruses* **2023**, *15*, 1274. [CrossRef]
55. Vargas-De-León, C.; Cureño-Díaz, M.A.; Salazar, M.I.; Cruz-Cruz, C.; Loyola-Cruz, M.Á.; Durán-Manuel, E.M.; Zamora-Pacheco, E.R.; Bravata-Alcántara, J.C.; Lugo-Zamudio, G.E.; Fernández-Sánchez, V.; et al. Neutralizing Antibodies against SARS-CoV-2: Importance of Comorbidities in Health Personnel against Reinfections. *Viruses* **2023**, *15*, 2354. [CrossRef]

vaccines

MDPI

Article

Risk Factors for Impaired Cellular or Humoral Immunity after Three Doses of SARS-CoV-2 Vaccine in Healthy and Immunocompromised Individuals

Jae-Hoon Ko [1,†], Choon-Mee Kim [2,†], Mi-Seon Bang [3], Da-Yeon Lee [3], Da-Young Kim [3], Jun-Won Seo [3], Na-Ra Yun [3], Jin-Young Yang [1], Kyong-Ran Peck [1], Kyo-Won Lee [4], Sung-Hoon Jung [5], Hyun-Jin Bang [5], Woo-Kyun Bae [5], Tae-Jong Kim [6,‡], Kyeong-Hwan Byeon [7], Sung-Han Kim [8] and Dong-Min Kim [3,*,‡]

1 Division of Infectious Diseases, Department of Medicine, Samsung Medical Center, Sungkyunkwan University School of Medicine, Seoul 06351, Republic of Korea; jaehoon.ko@gmail.com (J.-H.K.); jinyoung89.yang@samsung.com (J.-Y.Y.); kr.peck@samsung.com (K.-R.P.)
2 Department of Premedical Science, College of Medicine, Chosun University, Gwangju 61452, Republic of Korea; choonmeekim@chosun.ac.kr
3 Department of Internal Medicine, College of Medicine, Chosun University, Gwangju 61452, Republic of Korea; ktandms@gmail.com (M.-S.B.); barody222@gmail.com (D.-Y.L.); dayz02@hanmail.net (D.-Y.K.); kaist-105@hanmail.net (J.-W.S.); shine@chosun.ac.kr (N.-R.Y.)
4 Division of Transplantation, Department of Surgery, Samsung Medical Center, Sungkyunkwan University School of Medicine, Seoul 06351, Republic of Korea; kw1980.lee@samsung.com
5 Department of Internal Medicine, Chonnam National University Medical School and Hwasun Hospital, Hwasun 58128, Republic of Korea; shglory@hanmail.net (S.-H.J.); daunjin@gmail.com (H.-J.B.); drwookyun@gmail.com (W.-K.B.)
6 Department of Rheumatology, Chonnam National University Medical School, Gwangju 61469, Republic of Korea; ktj1562@jnu.ac.kr
7 Department of Parasitology and Tropical Medicine, Chonnam National University Medical School, Gwangju 61469, Republic of Korea; eidanus@naver.com
8 Department of Infectious Diseases, Asan Medical Center, University of Ulsan College of Medicine, Seoul 05505, Republic of Korea; kimsunghanmd@hotmail.com
* Correspondence: drongkim@chosun.ac.kr
† These authors contributed equally to this work.
‡ These authors contributed equally to this work.

Abstract: Background: We aimed to identify the risk factors for impaired cellular and humoral immunity after three doses of the SARS-CoV-2 vaccine. **Methods:** Six months after the third vaccine dose, T-cell immunity was evaluated using interferon-gamma release assays (IGRAs) in 60 healthy and 139 immunocompromised (IC) individuals, including patients with hematologic malignancy (HM), solid malignancy (SM), rheumatic disease (RD), and kidney transplantation (KT). Neutralizing antibody titers were measured using the plaque reduction neutralization test (PRNT) and surrogate virus neutralization test (sVNT). **Results:** T-cell immunity results showed that the percentages of IGRA-positive results using wild-type/alpha spike protein (SP) and beta/gamma SP were 85% (51/60) and 75% (45/60), respectively, in healthy individuals and 45.6% (62/136) and 40.4% (55/136), respectively, in IC individuals. IC with SM or KT showed a high percentage of IGRA-negative results. The underlying disease poses a risk for impaired cellular immune response to wild-type SP. The risk was low when all doses were administered as mRNA vaccines. The risk factors for an impaired cellular immune response to beta/gamma SP were underlying disease and monocyte%. In the sVNT using wild-type SP, 12 of 191 (6.3%) individuals tested negative. In the PRNT of 46 random samples, 6 (13%) individuals tested negative for the wild-type virus, and 19 (41.3%) tested negative with omicrons. KT poses a risk for an impaired humoral immune response. **Conclusions:** Underlying disease poses a risk for impaired cellular immune response after the third dose of the SARS-CoV-2 vaccine; KT poses a risk for impaired humoral immune response, emphasizing the requirement of precautions in patients.

Keywords: COVID-19 vaccine; immunosuppressed host; interferon-gamma release tests; neutralizing antibody; omicron variant

1. Introduction

Coronavirus disease (COVID-19) is a communicable infectious disease of the respiratory system caused by the Severe Acute Respiratory Syndrome coronavirus 2 (SARS-CoV-2) that caused a global pandemic [1]. Vaccines to prevent SARS-CoV-2 infection are considered the most effective means of suppressing its spread and to prevent severe forms of disease. After SARS-CoV-2 infection, most patients produce neutralizing antibodies and antibodies against the receptor binding domain (RBD) of the viral spike protein (SP) [2]. Among non-survivors of severe COVID-19 disease, there was attenuated IgG response, compromised Fcγ receptor binding, and Fc effector activity [3].

Patients who have recovered from COVID-19 and individuals who have received a COVID-19 vaccination develop $CD4^+$ and $CD8^+$ T-cell immune responses specific to SARS-CoV-2, suggesting the possibility of durable T-cell immune responses [4,5].

In a study involving 3593 individuals who had received COVID-19 vaccinations from Pfizer BionNTech (BNT162b2), Moderna (mRNA-1273), Sinovac (CoronaVac), and Sinopharm (BBIBP-CorV), those with and without an antibody response to SARS-CoV-2 SP were compared [6]. Seroconversion against the SARS-CoV-2 RBD of the SP was observed in 84% of individuals, while a poor immune response was associated with male sex, age $\geq$65 years, and recent chemotherapy [6].

The immunogenicity and efficacy of COVID-19 vaccines are lower in immunocompromised (IC) individuals compared to the general population. The proportion of immune non-responders were higher among those with solid organ transplant recipients (18–100%), hematological malignancy (14–61%), those with cancers (2–36%), and those on hemodialysis (2–30%) [7]. In patients with chronic kidney disease or those with kidney transplants, the mean antibody concentration levels were lower than healthy individuals after vaccination with two doses of the mRNA-1273 COVID-19 vaccine [8]. Based on the data of patients with cancers having received three or four doses of the mRNA vaccine, those with three doses of the vaccine had lower antibody levels than those with four doses and an overall lower cell-mediated response [9].

However, few studies have investigated the risk factors for impaired humoral or cellular immune responses [3,6,10,11]. Therefore, this study aimed to identify the risk factors for impaired humoral and cellular immune responses in healthy individuals and patients with IC.

2. Materials and Methods

2.1. Study Subjects

This multicenter observational study was conducted with the approval of the institutional review board of each center. The study subjects included 123 healthy subjects and 233 subjects with solid malignancy (SM), hematologic malignancy (HM), or rheumatic disease (RD) and patients who underwent kidney transplantation (KT) who had received three homologous or heterologous doses with mRNA (Pfizer, Pfizer and BioNTech, Puurs Belgium, Cambridge, MA, USA), adenovirus (AstraZeneca, AstraZeneca, Cambridge, UK), or other (Janssen, Janssen Biotech, Raritan, NJ, USA) vaccines.

2.2. Sample Collection

Blood samples were collected from both healthy individuals and IC patients 3–6 months after the third dose of the SARS-CoV-2 vaccine.

2.3. Interferon-Gamma Releasing Assay

To investigate the cellular immune responses in both healthy and IC patients after the third dose of the anti-SARS-CoV-2 vaccine, an interferon-gamma (IFN-γ) releasing assay (IGRA) was performed using an enzyme-linked immunosorbent assay (ELISA; Covi-FERON ELISA, SD Biosensor, Suwon-si, Gyeonggi-do, Republic of Korea). The IFN-γ levels induced by SARS-CoV-2 wild-type/alpha SP and SARS-CoV-2 beta/gamma SP have been measured [10]. Based on the 0.25 U/mL cutoff recommended by the manufacturer, participants were categorized into positive and negative groups, and the risk factors were analyzed by comparing participants' characteristics.

2.4. Neutralizing Antibody Assay

To assess the neutralizing antibody titer against SARS-CoV-2 in both healthy and IC after three doses of the vaccine, a plaque reduction neutralization test (PRNT) was performed using Vero E6 cells (*Cercopithecus aethiops* kidney epithelial cells, CRL-1586, ATCC). The neutralizing antibody titer was measured against the SARS-CoV-2 wild-type (V clade [B lineage], isolated hCoV-19/South Korea/KUMC01/2020, GISAID accession no. EPI_ISL_413017) and omicrons (GR clade [B.1.1.529 lineage]), and isolated hCoV-19/Korea/KDCA447321/2021, Accession no. NCCP43408) was purchased from the Korea Disease Control and Prevention Agency. $PRNT_{50}$, the level at which SARS-CoV-2 viral growth is suppressed by 50%, was defined as the neutralizing antibody titer [12]. Participants were categorized into positive and negative groups using a cutoff of 1:8, and risk factors were analyzed by comparing participants' characteristics [13].

2.5. Neutralizing Antibody Titer Analysis Using the GenBody Rapid Kit

For the surrogate virus neutralizing test (sVNT), the GenBody fluorescence immunoassay (FIA) COVID-19 NAb kit (GenBody, Cheonan-si, Chungcheongnam-do, Republic of Korea) was used. The GenBody sVNT is an FIA used to measure the inhibition of RBD-ACE2 binding based on the antibody-mediated blockage of the interaction between ACE2 and wild-type SARS-CoV-2 SP. Following the manufacturer's guideline, a cutoff $\geq$30% (GenBody) was applied.

2.6. Statistical Analysis

Six months after the third dose of the SARS-CoV-2 vaccine, healthy and IC individuals were categorized into positive and negative groups based on their $PRNT_{50}$, sVNT, and IFN-γ responses against the viral SP (original and variant strains). The χ^2 test was used to analyze the results, accounting for factors such as sex, vaccine type, underlying disease, median age, body mass index (BMI), and laboratory test results.

To analyze the risk factors, odds ratios (ORs; 95% confidence interval [CI]) and *p*-values were calculated based on binary logistic regression analysis for $PRNT_{50}$, sVNT, and IFN-γ responses against viral SP (original and variants). Subsequently, a multivariate logistic regression analysis was applied to items with a significant *p*-value in the binary logistic regression analysis to estimate the OR (95% CI) and *p*-value. The level of significance was set at $p < 0.05$. Prism version 8.0.1 (Graphpad Software, San Diego, CA, USA) and SPSS version 26 (IBM, Amonk, NY, USA) were used to analyze the collected data.

3. Results

The initial number of participants included 123 healthy individuals and 223 IC individuals before receiving the third dose of the SARS-CoV-2 vaccine. The final number of participants who underwent the sVNT test 3–6 months after the third dose was 60 in the healthy group and 141 in the IC group (41 HM, 49 SM, 23 RD, and 28 KT), accounting for losses to follow up. Among these participants, cellular immune responses were measured using IGRA in all 60 healthy individuals and 139 of the 141 IC individuals (n = 199 in total). A total of 3 of the 139 IC individuals had indeterminable results; therefore, the data of 136 participants were analyzed (n = 196 in total, including healthy individuals).

The results of T-cell immune responses in healthy and IC individuals showed that 83 of 196 (42.3%) participants tested negative in the IGRA using the tube coated with wild-type/alpha SP, whereas 96 of 196 (49%) participants tested negative in the IGRA using beta/gamma SP. Individuals with a negative IGRA to wild-type/alpha SP tended to be older on average, and most had underlying diseases (diabetes, hypertension, cancer, and chronic kidney disease; Table 1). In the comparison between healthy and IC individuals, 85% of healthy individuals and 45.6% of IC patients were IGRA-positive. The percentage of

IGRA-negative results was higher in patients who underwent SM ($p = 0.01$) or KT ($p < 0.001$; Table 1). Regarding the vaccine type, the rate of IGRA (wild-type/alpha SP) positivity was higher in individuals who received an mRNA/mRNA/mRNA vaccine than in those who received an adenovirus vector/adenovirus vector/mRNA vaccine (Ad/Ad/mRNA; $p = 0.002$; Table 1). In the univariate analysis of the risk factors for negative IGRA results, the OR in patients with underlying diseases, such as diabetes, hypertension, cancer, and chronic kidney disease, was 5.883 (95% CI 2.929–11.819; $p < 0.001$; Table 2). The OR of IGRA-negative results was 0.148 in healthy individuals and 6.8 (3.085–14.826) in IC individuals ($p < 0.001$). The OR was 2.38 in patients who underwent SM ($p = 0.001$) and 6.04 in patients with KT ($p < 0.001$). Furthermore, the OR increased 2.7-fold in the adenovirus vector/adenovirus vector/mRNA vaccine group but decreased 0.4-fold in the mRNA/mRNA/mRNA vaccine group ($p = 0.002$; Table 2). In the multivariate analysis, which included variables with a $p < 0.1$ in the univariate analysis, the OR for IGRA-negative results was 4.7 in patients with an underlying disease ($p = 0.045$), while it decreased to 0.4 in the mRNA/mRNA/mRNA vaccine group ($p = 0.045$; Table 2).

Table 1. Comparison of the IGRA-positive and -negative groups against SARS-CoV-2 wild-type/alpha SP and beta/gamma SP in both healthy individuals and IC individuals.

Characteristics	IGRA Using Wild-Type/Alpha		*p* Value	IGRA Using Beta/Gamma		*p* Value
	Negative (n = 83)	Positive (n = 113)		Negative (n = 96)	Positive (n = 100)	
Male gender, N (%)	50 (60.2%)	66 (58.4%)	0.796	58 (60.4%)	58 (58.0%)	0.731
Age, median (IQR)	56.0 (49.0–67.0)	51.0 (39.0–60.5)	0.024	55.5 (48.0–65.0)	52.0 (38.25–62.0)	0.115
BMI, median (IQR)	22.9 (20.31–25.79)	23.14 (21.14–25.08)	0.574	23.15 (20.5–25.54)	22.86 (21.04–25.27)	0.701
Underlying diseases, N (%)	70 (56.5%)	54 (43.5%)	<0.001	73 (58.9%)	51 (41.1%)	<0.001
Cardiovascular disease, N (%)	9 (42.9%)	12 (57.1%)	0.960	10 (47.6%)	11 (52.4%)	0.895
Diabetes mellitus, N (%)	24 (58.5%)	17 (41.5%)	0.018	23 (56.1%)	18 (43.9%)	0.305
Hypertension, N (%)	40 (64.5%)	22 (35.5%)	<0.001	40 (64.5%)	22 (35.5%)	0.003
Chronic lung disease, N (%)	4 (80.0%)	1 (20.0%)	0.084	4 (80.0%)	1 (20.0%)	0.160
Cancer, N (%)	47 (53.4%)	41 (46.6%)	0.005	51 (58.0%)	37 (42.0%)	0.023
Chronic kidney disease, N (%)	21 (70.0%)	9 (30.0%)	0.001	20 (66.7%)	10 (33.3%)	0.035
Disease status			<0.001			<0.001
Healthy, N (%)	9 (15.0%)	51 (85.0)	<0.001	15 (25.0%)	45 (75.0%)	<0.001
IC, N (%)	74 (54.4%)	62 (45.6%)	<0.001	81 (59.6%)	55 (40.4%)	<0.001
Hematologic malignancy, N (%)	20 (48.8%)	51 (51.2%)	0.348	22 (53.7%)	19 (46.3%)	0.500
Solid malignancy, N (%)	27 (58.7%)	19 (41.3%)	0.010	29 (63.0%)	17 (37.0%)	0.029
Rheumatic disease, N (%)	6 (27.3%)	16 (72.7%)	0.129	11 (50.0%)	11 (50.0%)	0.919
Kidney transplantation, N (%)	21 (77.8%)	6 (22.2%)	<0.001	19 (70.4%)	8 (29.6%)	0.017
Vaccine type (1st/2nd/3rd)			0.002			0.043
Ad/Ad/mRNA, N (%)	35 (59.3%)	24 (40.7%)	0.002	35 (59.3%)	24 (40.7%)	0.057
mRNA/mRNA/mRNA, N (%)	28 (30.8%)	63 (69.2%)	0.002	36 (39.6%)	55 (60.4%)	0.014
Other, N (%)	20 (43.5%)	26 (56.5%)	0.859	25 (54.3%)	21 (45.7%)	0.405
CBC						
WBC (10^3/mL)	5.5 (4.28–6.73)	5.7 (4.93–7.08)	0.407	5.5 (4.3–6.85)	5.7 (5.05–7.0)	0.250
Neutrophils (%)	55.55 (49.5–63.0)	54.05 (46.83–63.83)	0.426	55.5 (49.55–63.45)	54.0 (47.05–61.6)	0.563
Lymphocytes (%)	31.8 (23.85–39.75)	32.95 (24.65–39.78)	0.927	30.7 (23.7–39.8)	33.6 (25.7–39.55)	0.894
Monocyte (%)	8.4 (6.1–11.33)	8.45 (6.63–12.3)	0.103	8.3 (6.15–11.25)	8.5 (6.85–12.8)	0.060
Eosinophil (%)	2.0 (1.08–3.7)	2.25 (1.3–3.63)	0.551	2.0 (1.2–3.7)	2.2 (1.0–3.75)	0.871
Platelet (10^3/μL)	217.0 (162.25–276.25)	230.0 (172.5–286.5)	0.644	218.0 (163.5–273.5)	231.0 (159.5–291.5)	0.492

Cf. IGRA (interferon-gamma release assay), IQR (interquartile range), BMI (body mass index), IC (immunocompromised host), CBC (complete blood cell), WBC (white blood cell).

Table 2. Risk factor analysis of the IGRA-negative results against SARS-CoV-2 wild-type/alpha SP and beta/gamma SP in both healthy individuals and IC individuals.

Characteristics	IGRA Using Wild-Type/Alpha				IGRA Using Beta/Gamma			
	Univariate Analysis		Multivariate Analysis		Univariate Analysis		Multivariate Analysis	
	Odds Ratio (95% CI)	*p* Value	Odds Ratio (95% CI)	*p* Value	Odds Ratio (95% CI)	*p* Value	Odds Ratio (95% CI)	*p* Value
Male gender, N (%)	1.079 (0.606–1.922)	0.796			1.105 (0.625–1.955)	0.731		
Age, median (IQR)	1.023 (1.003–1.043)	0.025	0.992 (0.967–1.018)	0.544	1.015 (0.996–1.035)	0.116		
BMI, median (IQR)	0.976 (0.899–1.060)	0.572			0.984 (0.907–1.067)	0.699		
Underlying disease total, N (%)	5.883 (2.929–11.819)	<0.001	4.712 (1.586–14.003)	0.005	3.049 (1.655–5.618)	<0.001	3.582 (1.031–12.441)	0.045

Table 2. *Cont.*

Characteristics	IGRA Using Wild-Type/Alpha				IGRA Using Beta/Gamma			
	Univariate Analysis		Multivariate Analysis		Univariate Analysis		Multivariate Analysis	
	Odds Ratio (95% CI)	*p* Value	Odds Ratio (95% CI)	*p* Value	Odds Ratio (95% CI)	*p* Value	Odds Ratio (95% CI)	*p* Value
Cardiovascular disease, N (%)	1.024 (0.410–2.555)	0.960			0.941 (0.380–2.328)	0.895		
Diabetes mellitus, N (%)	2.297 (1.140–4.630)	0.020			1.435 (0.718–2.869)	0.307		
Hypertension, N (%)	3.848 (2.041–7.255)	<0.001			2.532 (1.358–4.723)	0.003		
Chronic lung disease, N (%)	5.671 (0.622–51.702)	0.124			4.304 (0.472–39.222)	0.195		
Cancer, N (%)	2.293 (1.285–4.092)	0.005			1.930 (1.091–3.414)	0.024		
Chronic kidney disease, N (%)	3.914 (1.687–9.083)	0.001			2.368 (0.045–5.368)	0.039		
Disease status								
Healthy, N (%)	0.148 (0.067–0.324)	<0.001			0.226 (0.115–0.446)	<0.001		
IC, N (%)	6.763 (3.085–14.826)	<0.001	2.193 (0.763–6.303)	0.145	4.418 (2.244–8.697)	<0.001	1.758 (0.530–5.830)	0.357
Hematologic malignancy, N (%)	1.391 (0.697–2.776)	0.350			1.267 (0.636–2.527)	0.501		
Solid malignancy, N (%)	2.385 (1.216–4.679)	0.011			2.113 (1.071–4.170)	0.031		
Rheumatic disease, N (%)	0.472 (0.176–1.265)	0.136			1.047 (0.431–2.542)	0.919		
Kidney transplantation, N (%)	6.040 (2.313–15.771)	<0.001			2.838 (1.177–6.840)	0.020		
Vaccine type (1st/2nd/3rd)								
Ad/Ad/mRNA, N (%)	2.704 (1.445–5.061)	0.002	0.790 (0.278–2.245)	0.659	1.817 (0.978–3.375)	0.059	0.766 (0.234–2.513)	0.660
mRNA/mRNA/mRNA, N (%)	0.404 (0.225–0.727)	0.002	0.380 (0.148–0.981)	0.045	0.491 (0.277–0.869)	0.015	0.500 (0.164–1.524)	0.223
Other, N (%)	1.062 (0.545–2.070)	0.859			1.325 (0.683–2.570)	0.406		
CBC								
WBC (10^3/mL)	0.939 (0.811–1.088)	0.405			0.918 (0.792–1.063)	0.252		
Neutrophils (%)	1.011 (0.984–1.039)	0.424			1.008 (0.981–1.036)	0.560		
Lymphocytes (%)	0.999 (0.970–1.028)	0.926			1.002 (0.973–1.032)	0.893		
Monocyte (%)	0.935 (0.861–1.015)	0.109			0.927 (0.855–1.006)	0.068	0.867 (0.779–0.964)	0.008
Eosinophil (%)	0.942 (0.777–1.144)	0.548			1.016 (0.838–1.232)	0.870		
Platelet (10^3/μL)	0.999 (0.995–1.003)	0.641			0.998 (0.997–1.003)	0.489		

Cf. IGRA (interferon-gamma release assay), IQR (interquartile range), BMI (body mass index), IC (immunocompromised host), CBC (complete blood cell), WBC (white blood cell).

In the univariate analysis of IGRA-positive results for beta/gamma SP, underlying disease (hypertension, cancer, and chronic kidney disease), current status (healthy or IC), and vaccine type were identified as factors influencing the rate of IGRA positivity (Table 2). The OR of negative IGRA (beta/gamma SP) was 3.6 in patients with an underlying disease ($p = 0.045$). Furthermore, a 1% increase in the monocyte% led to a 0.87-fold decrease in the rate of negative IGRA results ($p = 0.008$; Table 2).

The sVNT, conducted using the GenBody rapid kit and wild-type SP, showed that only 12 of 191 (6.3%) individuals tested negative (Table 3). In the univariate analysis of risk factors for the lack of neutralizing antibodies, underlying diseases, such as chronic kidney disease, and current status (healthy or IC) were identified as influencing factors. The OR for sVNT-negative results increased to 11 in patients with KT ($p < 0.001$) and to 3.4 in the adenovirus vector/adenovirus vector/mRNA vaccine group ($p = 0.043$). In the multivariate analysis, using variables with $p < 0.1$ from the univariate analysis, the OR of sVNT-negative results increased to 14 in patients with KT ($p = 0.01$; Table 4).

Table 3. Comparison of the surrogate virus neutralizing test-positive and -negative groups.

Characteristics	Surrogate Virus Neutralizing Test		p Value
	Negative (n = 12)	Positive (n = 189)	
Male gender, N (%)	10 (83.3%)	107 (56.6%)	0.069
Age, median (IQR)	56.5 (37.25–70.25)	54.0 (44.5–64.0)	0.874
BMI, median (IQR)	21.57 (19.41–24.94)	23.0 (20.91–25.41)	0.207
Underlying disease total, N (%)	11 (8.6%)	113 (91.4%)	0.035
Cardiovascular disease, N (%)	2 (9.5%)	19 (90.5%)	0.468
Diabetes mellitus, N (%)	2 (4.8%)	40 (95.2%)	0.710
Hypertension, N (%)	7 (10.9%)	57 (89.1%)	0.042
Chronic lung disease, N (%)	0 (0%)	6 (100%)	0.531
Cancer, N (%)	5 (5.5%)	86 (94.5%)	0.796
Chronic kidney disease, N (%)	6 (18.8%)	26 (81.3%)	0.001
Disease status			<0.001
Healthy, N (%)	0 (0.0%)	60 (100%)	0.020
IC, N (%)	12 (8.5%)	129 (91.5%)	0.020
Hematologic malignancy, N (%)	2 (4.9%)	39 (95.1%)	0.741
Solid malignancy, N (%)	3 (6.1%)	46 (93.9%)	0.959
Rheumatoid disease, N (%)	0 (0%)	23 (100%)	0.199
Kidney transplantation, N (%)	7 (25%)	21 (75%)	<0.001
Vaccine type (1st/2nd/3rd)			0.102
Ad/Ad/mRNA, N (%)	7 (11.3%)	55 (88.7%)	0.033
mRNA/mRNA/mRNA, N (%)	3 (3.3%)	88 (96.7%)	0.146
Other, N (%)	2 (4.2%)	46 (95.8%)	0.546
CBC			
WBC (10^3/mL)	5.45 (5.15–8.93)	5.65 (4.48–6.9)	0.376
Neutrophils (%)	53.95 (41.28–75.0)	54.9 (48.7–62.1)	0.801
Lymphocytes (%)	28.0 (19.63–43.65)	32.85 (24.58–39.93)	0.717
Monocyte (%)	10.35 (6.58–13.35)	8.4 (6.5–11.33)	0.318
Eosinophil (%)	1.2 (0.08–2.93)	2.2 (1.2–3.73)	0.083
Platelet (10^3/μL)	168.0 (152.5–236.5)	225.5 (164.25–282.0)	0.283

Cf. IQR (interquartile range), BMI (body mass index), IC (immunocompromised host), CBC (complete blood cell), WBC (white blood cell).

A risk factor analysis using $PRNT_{50}$ was performed on 46 random samples. A total of 6 (13%) individuals tested negative when the wild-type virus was used, and 19 (41.3%) individuals tested negative when the omicron virus was used.

Regarding PRNT with the wild-type virus, a negative PRNT result of <1:8 was found in 33.3% of patients with chronic kidney disease (p = 0.015) and 36.4% of patients with KT (p = 0.01; Table 5). In the univariate analysis, the OR for the risk of PRNT-negative results increased 8-fold in patients with chronic kidney disease and 9.4-fold in patients who underwent KT ($p < 0.05$). In the multivariate analysis, the OR for PRNT-negative results was 8.7-fold higher in patients with KT (p = 0.049; Table 6). Regarding PRNT with the omicron virus, the OR for PRNT-negative results was higher in patients with underlying diseases, such as hypertension, chronic kidney disease, and KT. Furthermore, the OR was higher in the adenovirus vector/adenovirus vector/mRNA vaccine group than in the mRNA/mRNA/mRNA vaccine group (p = 0.035; Table 6). In the multivariate analysis, which included variables with a $p < 0.1$ in the univariate analysis, the OR for PRNT-negative results for the omicron virus increased 8.2-fold in patients who underwent KT (p = 0.039).

Table 4. Risk factor analysis of the surrogate virus neutralizing test-negative group.

Characteristics	Univariate Analysis		Multivariate Analysis	
	Odds Ratio (95% CI)	p Value	Odds Ratio (95% CI)	p Value
Male gender, N (%)	3.832 (0.817–17.967)	0.088	1.928 (0.319–11.670)	0.475
Age, median (IQR)	1.003 (0.965–1.043)	0.874		
BMI, median (IQR)	0.886 (0.735–1.069)	0.206		
Underlying disease total, N (%)	6.769 (0.856–53.541)	0.070	1.263 (0.101–15.791)	0.856
Cardiovascular disease, N (%)	1.789 (0.365–8.779)	0.473		
Diabetes mellitus, N (%)	0.745 (0.157–3.537)	0.711		
Hypertension, N (%)	3.242 (0.987–10.646)	0.053		
Chronic lung disease, N (%)	0.0 (0.0-)	0.999		
Cancer, N (%)	0.855 (0.262–2.792)	0.796		
Chronic kidney disease, N (%)	6.269 (1.879–20.917)	0.003		
Disease status				
Healthy, N (%)	0.0 (0.0-)	0.997		
IC, N (%)	4.418 (2.244–8.697)	<0.001		
Hematologic malignancy, N (%)	0.769 (0.162–3.655)	0.741		
Solid malignancy, N (%)	1.036 (0.269–3.990)	0.959		
Rheumatoid disease, N (%)	0.0 (0.0-)	0.998		
Kidney transplantation, N (%)	11.2 (3.260–38.473)	<0.001	13.777 (1.852–102.499)	0.010
Vaccine type (1st/2nd/3rd)				
Ad/Ad/mRNA, N (%)	3.411 (1.038–11.210)	0.043	5.521 (0.780–39.087)	0.087
mRNA/mRNA/mRNA, N (%)	0.383 (0.10–1.457)	0.159		
Other, N (%)	0.622 (0.131–2.941)	0.549		
CBC				
WBC (10^3/mL)	1.132 (0.861–1.489)	0.375		
Neutrophils (%)	1.008 (0.949–1.071)	0.799		
Lymphocytes (%)	0.988 (0.925–1.055)	0.715		
Monocyte (%)	1.068 (0.937–1.218)	0.322		
Eosinophil (%)	0.588 (0.314–1.099)	0.096	0.635 (0.310–1.302)	0.216
Platelet (10^3/μL)	0.993 (0.981–1.006)	0.283		

Cf. IQR (interquartile range), BMI (body mass index), IC (immunocompromised host), CBC (complete blood cell), WBC (white blood cell).

Table 5. Comparison of the plaque reduction neutralization test ($PRNT_{50}$)-positive and -negative groups against the SARS-CoV-2 wild-type (V clade (B lineage)) or omicron (GR clade (B.1.1.529 lineage)).

Characteristics	PRNT Using WT		p Value	PRNT Using Omicron		p Value
	Negative (n = 6)	Positive (n = 40)		Negative (n = 19)	Positive (n = 27)	
Male gender, N (%)	3 (50%)	19 (47.5%)	0.909	10 (52.6%)	12 (44.4%)	0.584
Age, median (IQR)	51.0 (45.0–74.0)	58.0 (51.5–70.5)	0.495	57.0 (52.0–72.0)	58.0 (47.0–71.0)	0.904
BMI, median (IQR)	21.12 (18.88–23.18)	23.25 (21.01–26.62)	0.217	22.9 (20.92–26.61)	22.66 (20.76–26.62)	0.899
Underlying diseases, N (%)	6 (17.1%)	29 (82.9%)	0.160	17 (48.6%)	18 (51.4%)	0.107
Cardiovascular disease, N (%)	0 (0%)	8 (100%)	0.228	3 (37.5%)	5 (62.5%)	0.810
Diabetes mellitus, N (%)	2 (15.4%)	11 (84.6%)	0.767	7 (53.8%)	6 (46.2%)	0.278
Hypertension, N (%)	5 (20.8%)	19 (79.2%)	0.101	14 (58.3%)	10 (41.7%)	0.014
Chronic lung disease, N (%)	0 (0%)	0 (0%)		0 (0%)	0 (0%)	
Cancer, N (%)	2 (10.0%)	18 (90.0%)	0.591	7 (35.0%)	13 (65.0%)	0.446
Chronic kidney disease, N (%)	4 (33.3%)	8 (66.7%)	0.015	8 (66.7%)	4 (33.3%)	0.038
Disease status			0.065			0.078
Healthy, N (%)	0 (0%)	9 (100%)	0.221	1 (12.5%)	7 (87.5%)	0.061
IC, N (%)	6 (16.2%)	31 (83.9%)	0.195	18 (48.6%)	19 (51.4%)	0.040
Hematologic malignancy, N (%)	2 (16.7%)	10 (83.3%)	0.692	4 (33.3%)	8 (66.7%)	0.467
Solid malignancy, N (%)	0 (0%)	8 (100%)	0.221	3 (37.5%)	5 (62.5%)	0.766
Rheumatic disease, N (%)	0 (0%)	6 (100%)	0.302	3 (50.0%)	3 (50.0%)	0.679
Kidney transplantation, N (%)	4 (36.4%)	7 (63.6%)	0.010	8 (72.7%)	3 (27.3%)	0.018
Vaccine type (1st, 2nd, 3rd)			0.810			0.035
Ad/Ad/mRNA, N (%)	2 (13.3%)	13 (86.7%)	0.968	9 (60.0%)	6 (40.0%)	0.073
mRNA/mRNA/mRNA, N (%)	2 (18.2%)	18 (90.0%)	0591	4 (20%)	16 (80.0%)	0.010
Other, N (%)	2 (10.0%)	9 (81.8%)	0.586	6 (54.5%)	5 (45.5%)	0.341
CBC						
WBC (10^3/mL)	7.0 (5.85–9.95)	5.2 (4.4–6.3)	0.044	5.9 (4.83–7.98)	5.15 (4.48–6.2)	0.110
Neutrophils (%)	54.9 (38.2–66.2)	54.9 (51.2–69.6)	0.417	53.95 (48.03–68.75)	56.05 (52.2–69.38)	0.807
Lymphocytes (%)	36.0 (21.5–49.85)	30.6 (22.8–36.0)	0.321	34.0 (20.18–68.75)	30.35 (23.28–35.05)	0.493
Monocyte (%)	8.0 (6.95–12.1)	8.7 (6.3–12.1)	0.817	8.0 (5.38–10.95)	8.75 (7.0–13.15)	0.529
Eosinophil (%)	1.5 (1.1–2.95)	1.5 (0.9–4.1)	0.735	1.25 (0.83–3.33)	1.75 (1.2–4.18)	0.232
Platelet (10^3/μL)	191.0 (184.0-)	207.0 (143.75–256.0)	0.743	198.0 (184.0–223.0)	208.0 (134.5–274.0)	0.790

Cf. IQR (interquartile range), BMI (body mass index), IC (immunocompromised host), CBC (complete blood cell), WBC (white blood cell).

Table 6. Risk factor analysis of the plaque reduction neutralization test ($PRNT_{50}$)-negative group against the SARS-CoV-2 wild-type (V clade (B lineage)) or omicron (GR clade (B.1.1.529 lineage)).

Characteristics	PRNT Using WT				PRNT Using Omicron			
	Univariate Analysis		Multivariate Analysis		Univariate Analysis		Multivariate Analysis	
	Odds Ratio (95% CI)	*p* Value	Odds Ratio (95% CI)	*p* Value	Odds Ratio (95% CI)	*p* Value	Odds Ratio (95% CI)	*p* Value
Male gender, N (%)	1.105 (0.199–6.150)	0.909			1.003 (0.960–1.047)	0.901		
Age, median (IQR)	0.977 (0.917–1.042)	0.488			1.389 (0.428–4.510)	0.585		
BMI, median (IQR)	0.851 (0.657–1.102)	0.220			0.989 (0.842–1.163)	0.897		
Underlying disease total, N (%)	334,236,182.8 (0.0-)	0.999			4.250 (0.801–22.563)	0.089	2.573 (0.284–23.344)	0.401
Cardiovascular disease, N (%)	0.0 (0.0-)	0.999			0.825 (0.172–3.964)	0.810		
Diabetes mellitus, N (%)	1.318 (0.211–8.249)	0.768			2.042 (0.556–7.497)	0.282		
Hypertension, N (%)	5.526 (0.591–51.647)	0.134			4.760 (1.316–17.216)	0.017		
Chronic lung disease, N (%)								
Cancer, N (%)	0.611 (0.100–3.727)	0.593			0.628 (0.189–2.085)	0.447		
Chronic kidney disease, N (%)	8.00 (1.238–51.690)	0.029			4.182 (1.032–16.939)	0.045		
Disease status								
Healthy, N (%)	0.0 (0.0-)	0.999			0.132 (0.015–1.163)	0.068		
IC, N (%)	312,672,558.7 (0.0-)	0.999			7.579 (0.860–66.813)	0.068		
Hematologic malignancy, N (%)	1.500 (0.238–9.465)	0.666			0.633 (0.160–2.512)	0.516		
Solid malignancy, N (%)	0.0 (0.0-)	0.999			0.825 (0.172–3.964)	0.810		
Rheumatic disease, N (%)	0.0 (0.0-)	0.999			1.500 (0.268–8.383)	0.644		
Kidney transplantation, N (%)	9.429 (1.434–61.986)	0.020	8.679 (1.009–74.659)	0.049	5.818 (1.290–26.249)	0.022	8.217 (1.107–6.966)	0.039
Vaccine type (1st/2nd/3rd)								
Ad/Ad/mRNA, N (%)	1.038 (0.168–6.421)	0.968			3.150 (0.877–11.311)	0.079	1.297 (0.153–10.966)	0.811
mRNA/ mRNA/mRNA, N (%)	0.611 (0.100–3.727)	0.593			0.183 (0.048–0.703)	0.013	0.129 (0.016–1.070)	0.058
Other, N (%)	1.722 (0.270–10.981)	0.565			2.031 (0.516–7.997)	0.311		
CBC								
WBC (10^3/mL)	1.422 (0.981–2.062)	0.063	1.363 (0.887–2.094)	0.158	1.274 (0.936–1.732)	0.123		
Neutrophils (%)	0.966 (0.891–1.048)	0.410			0.993 (0.943–1.047)	0.801		
Lymphocytes (%)	1.043 (0.960–1.133)	0.317			1.020 (0.966–1.077)	0.483		
Monocyte (%)	0.972 (0.770–1.227)	0.811			0.950 (0.813–1.111)	0.520		
Eosinophil (%)	0.896 (0.483–1.661)	0.727			0.770 (0.503–1.179)	0.229		0.770 (0.503–1.179)
Platelet (10^3/μL)	0.997 (0.977–1.016)	0.733			0.999 (0.990–1.008)	0.813		0.999 (0.990–1.008)

Cf. IQR (interquartile range), BMI (body mass index), IC (immunocompromised host), CBC (complete blood cell), WBC (white blood cell).

4. Discussion

During the COVID-19 pandemic, the reported COVID-19-related mortality rate in IC individuals with conditions such as solid organ transplantation, those on immunosuppressant medication, and those with HIV or congenital immunodeficiency ranged between 20 and 29% [14,15]. Reduced immune responses to SARS-CoV-2 after vaccination were associated with higher mortality or higher proportions of intensive care admissions in IC individuals with SM, HM, solid organ transplantation, or immunosuppressant use [3,16].

In a study involving patients with organ transplantation, antibodies were not produced in 80% of patients after two doses of the SARS-CoV-2 vaccine, and even after the third booster shot, 53% of patients remained antibody-negative [17]. Among those KT patients, non-seroconversion after the mRNA-1273 SARS-CoV-2 vaccine (Moderna) based on anti-spike IgG was 43.1% after the second dose and 25.6% after the third dose [11].

Patients with kidney failure are known to be at increased risk for SARS-CoV-2 infection, highlighting the critical need for effective vaccinations [18]. The humoral immune response is adequate in patients undergoing hemodialysis or peritoneal dialysis, but non-responders have been reported in some cases [7,19]. In a study involving 281 patients enrolled from five dialysis centers in northern Poland, cellular immunity was higher in patients with a pre-vaccination history of SARS-CoV-2 infection. The positive cellular response to vaccination was a positive factor to reduce all-cause mortality [16]. Therefore, assessing patient-related risk factors is critical for a lack of cellular or humoral immune responses.

In the present study, IC patients more frequently exhibited a lack of cellular immune response. Specifically, patients with SM or KT showed a greater percentage of IGRA-negative results. This finding is consistent with a study among 209 patients after two doses of the mRNA vaccine where positive IGRA was documented in 89.3% on peritoneal dialysis, 77.6% on hemodialysis, 61.3% of KT patients more than 1 year post-transplant, and only 36% in those transplanted within past 12 months [20]. Patients with malignancy of the lung, breast, colon, bladder, head–neck, prostate, rectum, and esophagus were found to have lower percentage of $CD4^+$ and $CD8^+$ T cells compared to those who had received four doses of the mRNA vaccine or those patients on hemodialysis [9].

GenBody rapid kit-based sVNT using wild-type SP showed that only 12 of 191 (6.3%) individuals tested negative, indicating that most individuals developed neutralizing antibodies against the wild-type virus. This is similar to a study among healthy individuals based on sVNT in Thailand where receiving two or three heterologous boosters with DNA- and/or mRNA vaccines was highly effective against Wuhan Hu-1 strain but had significant variations against the omicron variant [21]. However, those receiving three booster doses had higher levels of the neutralizing antibody than those who had received only two booster doses [21].

In our study, the PRNT was not performed for all patients, as it is a labor-intensive test. Only 6 of 46 (13%) individuals tested negative for the wild-type virus, whereas 19 (41.3%) individuals tested negative for the omicron virus on PRNT. These results suggested a significantly lower neutralizing antibody titer against the omicron variant than against the wild-type virus. This is similar to a study among IC individuals with cancer or hemodialysis, where the overall $PRNT_{50}$ titer against omicron was lower than that against the Wuhan strain ($p < 0.0001$) [9]. Cancer patients with lung, breast, colon, bladder, head–neck, prostate, rectum, and stomach malignancies who had only three doses of the vaccine had a lower $PRNT_{50}$ titer against omicron compared to those on hemodialysis, but there was no difference among those cancer patients who had received four doses when compared to those on hemodialysis [9].

Three to six months after vaccination, 22.2–29.6% of the KT patients in this study exhibited a cellular immune response. The percentage of PRNT-positive results was 63.6% against the wild-type virus but only 27.3% against the omicron virus, indicating that KT is a critical risk factor for impaired cellular or humoral immunity.

The risk factors associated with an impaired cellular immune response to beta/gamma SP were monocyte% and underlying diseases (hypertension, cancer, and chronic kidney disease). During acute SARS-CoV-2 infection, the number and function of immune cells, including T cells, natural killer cells, monocytes, and dendritic cells, decrease significantly [22,23]. Specifically, patients with COVID-19 experience a substantial reduction in monocyte counts compared to controls [22]. Peripheral blood monocytes are thought to contribute to immune responses against viral pathogens and select monocyte subsets may be related to disease outcomes [23,24]. However, further studies are required to investigate the impact of monocytes on the cellular immune response in the context of immunization via COVID-19 vaccination as monocytes exposed to inactivated SARS-CoV-2 were found to secrete higher levels of IL-6, TNF-α, CXCL10, CXCL9, and CXCL11 upon restimulation [25].

According to a previous study, a more durable humoral response could be achieved when a third heterologous vaccination using a viral vector vaccine was administered after two doses of an mRNA vaccine compared to a homologous mRNA vaccine [26]. However, this study showed that the third heterologous vaccination using an mRNA vaccine after two doses of the viral vector vaccine resulted in a 40% PRNT-positive rate against the omicron virus, while three homologous doses of mRNA vaccines led to an 80% PRNT-positive rate. These findings suggest that homologous vaccination with mRNA may be more effective at eliciting humoral immunity. Based on the IGRA using the wild-type/alpha SP, analyzing risk factors for impaired cellular immune response revealed that the risk of impaired cellular immunity was higher with homologous doses of mRNA vaccines than with the heterologous third dose of an mRNA vaccine after two doses of viral vector vaccines. Thus, it can be hypothesized that homologous doses of mRNA vaccines might be more effective in patients with risk factors for an impaired cellular immune response, although further randomized controlled trials should be conducted as other studies suggest no differences in neutralizing antibody or T-cell response [21].

This study has several limitations. First, the neutralizing antibody titer using $PRNT_{50}$ was not analyzed in all patients; instead, an indirect test using sVNT was conducted. However, both $PRNT_{50}$ and sVNT identified KT as a critical risk factor for the lack of neutralizing antibody induction. Another limitation is that only the wild-type SARS-CoV-2 SP was used in the sVNT without testing the response to the omicron viral SP. In the IGRA, only the antigens of wild-type SARS-CoV-2 and the alpha, beta, and gamma variants were tested without evaluating the cellular immune response against the omicron virus.

5. Conclusions

In summary, this study showed that underlying diseases, such as hypertension, cancer, and chronic kidney disease, are risk factors for an impaired cellular immune response after the third dose of the SARS-CoV-2 vaccine. Furthermore, KT has been identified as a risk factor for impaired humoral immune response. Overall, these results suggest the requirement of precautions against impaired immune responses in patients with an underlying disease or a history of KT.

Author Contributions: Conceptualization, D.-M.K. and J.-H.K.; methodology, M.-S.B., D.-Y.L. and C.-M.K.; formal analysis, D.-Y.K., J.-W.S., N.-R.Y., J.-Y.Y., K.-R.P., K.-W.L., S.-H.J., H.-J.B., W.-K.B., T.-J.K., K.-H.B., S.-H.K. and D.-M.K.; investigation, D.-Y.K., J.-W.S., N.-R.Y., J.-Y.Y., K.-R.P., K.-W.L., S.-H.J., H.-J.B., W.-K.B., T.-J.K., K.-H.B., S.-H.K. and D.-M.K.; writing—original draft preparation, D.-M.K. and J.-H.K.; writing—review and editing, J.-H.K., J.-W.S., N.-R.Y., J.-Y.Y., K.-R.P., K.-W.L., S.-H.J., H.-J.B., W.-K.B., T.-J.K., K.-H.B., S.-H.K. and D.-M.K.; supervision, D.-M.K.; funding acquisition, D.-M.K. All authors have read and agreed to the published version of the manuscript.

Funding: This study was supported by research fund from Chosun University 2022. The funding organizations had no involvement in data collection, analysis, interpretation, trial design, patient recruitment, any aspect pertinent to the study, nor in the writing of the manuscript or the decision to submit it for publication.

Institutional Review Board Statement: The study was conducted in accordance with the Declaration of Helsinki, and approved by the Institutional Review Board (or Ethics Committee) of Chosun University Hospital, Gwangju, Republic of Korea(protocol code 2021-10-018 and date of approval 28 January 2022).

Informed Consent Statement: Informed consent was obtained from all subjects involved in the study.

Data Availability Statement: The data presented in this study are available on request from the corresponding author due to (Ethical reasons).

Acknowledgments: We acknowledge Thinley Dorji from the Central Regional Referral Hospital in Bhutan for his contributions in reviewing this article.

Conflicts of Interest: J.-H.K. serves as a member of the medical advisory committee of SD Biosensor. D.-M.K. serves as a member of the medical advisory committee of GenBody Inc. All authors have read and understood the journal's policies, and we believe that neither the manuscript nor the study violates any of them.

References

1. To, K.K.-W.; Tsang, O.T.-Y.; Leung, W.-S.; Tam, A.R.; Wu, T.-C.; Lung, D.C.; Yip, C.C.-Y.; Cai, J.-P.; Chan, J.M.-C.; Chik, T.S.-H.; et al. Temporal profiles of viral load in posterior oropharyngeal saliva samples and serum antibody responses during infection by SARS-CoV-2: An observational cohort study. *Lancet Infect. Dis.* **2020**, *20*, 565–574. [CrossRef]
2. Wölfel, R.; Corman, V.M.; Guggemos, W.; Seilmaier, M.; Zange, S.; Müller, M.A.; Niemeyer, D.; Jones, T.C.; Vollmar, P.; Rothe, C.; et al. Virological assessment of hospitalized patients with COVID-2019. *Nature* **2020**, *581*, 465–469. [CrossRef] [PubMed]
3. Zohar, T.; Loos, C.; Fischinger, S.; Atyeo, C.; Wang, C.; Slein, M.D.; Burke, J.; Yu, J.; Feldman, J.; Hauser, B.M.; et al. Compromised Humoral Functional Evolution Tracks with SARS-CoV-2 Mortality. *Cell* **2020**, *183*, 1508–1519.e12. [CrossRef]
4. Dan, J.M.; Mateus, J.; Kato, Y.; Hastie, K.M.; Yu, E.D.; Faliti, C.E.; Grifoni, A.; Ramirez, S.I.; Haupt, S.; Frazier, A.; et al. Immunological memory to SARS-CoV-2 assessed for up to 8 months after infection. *Science* **2021**, *371*, 6529. [CrossRef]
5. Cui, Z.; Luo, W.; Chen, R.; Li, Y.; Wang, Z.; Liu, Y.; Liu, S.; Feng, L.; Jia, Z.; Cheng, R.; et al. Comparing T- and B-cell responses to COVID-19 vaccines across varied immune backgrounds. *Signal. Transduct. Target. Ther.* **2023**, *8*, 179. [CrossRef]
6. Wankhede, D.; Grover, S.; Hofman, P. Determinants of humoral immune response to SARS-CoV-2 vaccines in solid cancer patients: A systematic review and meta-analysis. *Vaccine* **2023**, *41*, 1791–1798. [CrossRef]
7. Galmiche, S.; Luong Nguyen, L.B.; Tartour, E.; de Lamballerie, X.; Wittkop, L.; Loubet, P.; Launay, O. Immunological and clinical efficacy of COVID-19 vaccines in immunocompromised populations: A systematic review. *Clin. Microbiol. Infect.* **2022**, *28*, 163–177. [CrossRef]
8. Sanders, J.-S.F.; Bemelman, F.J.; Messchendorp, A.L.; Baan, C.C.; van Baarle, D.; van Binnendijk, R.; Diavatopoulos, D.A.; Frölke, S.C.; Geers, D.; GeurtsvanKessel, C.H.; et al. The RECOVAC Immune-response Study: The Immunogenicity, Tolerability, and Safety of COVID-19 Vaccination in Patients With Chronic Kidney Disease, on Dialysis, or Living With a Kidney Transplant. *Transplantation* **2022**, *106*, 821–834. [CrossRef]
9. Campagna, R.; Dominelli, F.; Zingaropoli, M.A.; Ciurluini, F.; Grilli, G.; Amoroso, A.; De Domenico, A.; Amatore, D.; Lia, M.S.; Cortesi, E.; et al. COVID-19 vaccination in cancer patients: Immune responses one year after the third dose. *Vaccine* **2024**, *42*, 2687–2694. [CrossRef]
10. Yang, J.; Lee, K.W.; Baek, J.Y.; Bae, S.; Lee, Y.H.; Kim, H.; Huh, K.; Cho, S.Y.; Kang, C.-I.; Chung, D.R.; et al. Augmented humoral and cellular immunity against severe acute respiratory syndrome coronavirus 2 after breakthrough infection in kidney transplant recipients who received 3 doses of coronavirus disease 2019 vaccine. *Am. J. Transplant.* **2023**, *23*, 565–572. [CrossRef]
11. Frölke, S.C.; Bouwmans, P.; Messchendorp, A.L.; Geerlings, S.E.; Hemmelder, M.H.; Gansevoort, R.T.; Hilbrands, L.B.; Reinders, M.E.J.; Sanders, J.-S.F.; Bemelman, F.J.; et al. Predictors of Nonseroconversion to SARS-CoV-2 Vaccination in Kidney Transplant Recipients. *Transpl. Direct* **2022**, *8*, e1397. [CrossRef]
12. Cohen, B.J.; Audet, S.; Andrews, N.; Beeler, J. Plaque reduction neutralization test for measles antibodies: Description of a standardised laboratory method for use in immunogenicity studies of aerosol vaccination. *Vaccine* **2007**, *26*, 59–66. [CrossRef]
13. Lee, B.; Ko, J.-H.; Lee, K.H.; Kim, Y.C.; Song, Y.G.; Park, Y.S.; Baek, Y.J.; Ahn, J.Y.; Choi, J.Y.; Song, K.H.; et al. Estimation of SARS-CoV-2 Neutralizing Activity and Protective Immunity in Different Vaccine Types Using Three Surrogate Virus Neutralization Test Assays and Two Semiquantitative Binding Assays Targeting the Receptor-Binding Domain. *Microbiol. Spectr.* **2022**, *10*, e0266922. [CrossRef]
14. Kates, O.S.; Haydel, B.M.; Florman, S.S.; Rana, M.M.; Chaudhry, Z.S.; Ramesh, M.S.; Safa, K.; Kotton, C.N.; Blumberg, E.A.; Besharatian, B.D.; et al. Coronavirus Disease 2019 in Solid Organ Transplant: A Multicenter Cohort Study. *Clin. Infect. Dis.* **2021**, *73*, e4090–e4099. [CrossRef]
15. Turtle, L.; Thorpe, M.; Drake, T.M.; Swets, M.; Palmieri, C.; Russell, C.D.; Ho, A.; Aston, S.; Wootton, D.G.; Richter, A.; et al. Outcome of COVID-19 in hospitalised immunocompromised patients: An analysis of the WHO ISARIC CCP-UK prospective cohort study. *PLoS Med.* **2023**, *20*, e1004086. [CrossRef]
16. Kwiatkowska, E.; Safranow, K.; Wojciechowska-Koszko, I.; Roszkowska, P.; Dziedziejko, V.; Myślak, M.; Różański, J.; Ciechanowski, K.; Stompór, T.; Przybyciński, J.; et al. SARS-CoV-2 mRNA Vaccine-Induced Cellular and Humoral Immunity in Hemodialysis Patients. *Biomedicines* **2022**, *10*, 636. [CrossRef]
17. Werbel, W.A.; Boyarsky, B.J.; Ou, M.T.; Massie, A.B.; Tobian, A.A.R.; Garonzik-Wang, J.M.; Segev, D.L. Safety and Immunogenicity of a Third Dose of SARS-CoV-2 Vaccine in Solid Organ Transplant Recipients: A Case Series. *Ann. Intern. Med.* **2021**, *174*, 1330–1332. [CrossRef]
18. Rincon-Arevalo, H.; Choi, M.; Stefanski, A.-L.; Halleck, F.; Weber, U.; Szelinski, F.; Jahrsdörfe, B.; Schrezenmeie, H.; Ludwi, C.; Sattler, A.; et al. Impaired humoral immunity to SARS-CoV-2 BNT162b2 vaccine in kidney transplant recipients and dialysis patients. *Sci. Immunol.* **2021**, *6*, 60. [CrossRef]
19. Longlune, N.; Nogier, M.B.; Miedougé, M.; Gabilan, C.; Cartou, C.; Seigneuric, B.; Del Bello, A.; Marion, O.; Faguer, S.; Izopet, J.; et al. High immunogenicity of a messenger RNA-based vaccine against SARS-CoV-2 in chronic dialysis patients. *Nephrol. Dial. Transpl.* **2021**, *36*, 1704–1709. [CrossRef]

20. Crespo, M.; Barrilado-Jackson, A.; Padilla, E.; Eguía, J.; Echeverria-Esnal, D.; Cao, H.; Faura, A.; Folgueiras, M.; Solà-Porta, E.; Pascual, S.; et al. Negative immune responses to two-dose mRNA COVID-19 vaccines in renal allograft recipients assessed with simple antibody and interferon gamma release assay cellular monitoring. *Am. J. Transpl.* **2022**, *22*, 786–800. [CrossRef]
21. Nithichanon, A.; Kamuthachad, L.; Salao, K.; Phoksawat, W.; Kamsom, C.; Wongratanacheewin, S.; Pipattanaboon, C.; Kanthawong, S.; Yordpratum, U.; Aromseree, S.; et al. A two-arm analysis of the immune response to heterologous boosting of inactivated SARS-CoV-2 vaccines. *Sci. Rep.* **2023**, *13*, 18762. [CrossRef]
22. Lagadinou, M.; Zareifopoulos, N.; Gkentzi, D.; Sampsonas, F.; Kostopoulou, E.; Marangos, M.; Solomou, E. Alterations in lymphocyte subsets and monocytes in patients diagnosed with SARS-CoV-2 pneumonia: A mini review of the literature. *Eur. Rev. Med. Pharmacol. Sci.* **2021**, *25*, 5057–5062.
23. Zhou, R.; To, K.K.-W.; Wong, Y.-C.; Liu, L.; Zhou, B.; Li, X.; Huang, H.; Mo, Y.; Luk, T.-Y.; Yeung, P.; et al. Acute SARS-CoV-2 Infection Impairs Dendritic Cell and T Cell Responses. *Immunity* **2020**, *53*, 864–877.e5. [CrossRef]
24. Park, J.; Dean, L.S.; Jiyarom, B.; Gangcuangco, L.M.; Shah, P.; Awamura, T.; Ching, L.L.; Nerurkar, V.R.; Chow, D.C.; Igno, F.; et al. Elevated circulating monocytes and monocyte activation in COVID-19 convalescent individuals. *Front. Immunol.* **2023**, *14*, 1151780. [CrossRef]
25. Cvetkovic, J.; Jacobi, R.H.J.; Miranda-Bedate, A.; Pham, N.; Kutmon, M.; Groot, J.; van de Garde, M.D.B.; Pinelli, E. Human Monocytes Exposed to SARS-CoV-2 Display Features of Innate Immune Memory Producing High Levels of CXCL10 upon Restimulation. *J. Innate Immun.* **2023**, *15*, 911–924. [CrossRef]
26. Liu, X.; Munro, A.P.S.; Wright, A.; Feng, S.; Janani, L.; Aley, P.K.; Babbage, G.; Baker, J.; Baxter, D.; Bawa, T.; et al. Persistence of immune responses after heterologous and homologous third COVID-19 vaccine dose schedules in the UK: Eight-month analyses of the COV-BOOST trial. *J. Infect.* **2023**, *87*, 18–26. [CrossRef]

vaccines

MDPI

Article

Long-Term Immune Consequences of Initial SARS-CoV-2 A.23.1 Exposure: A Longitudinal Study of Antibody Responses and Cross-Neutralization in a Ugandan Cohort

Gerald Kevin Oluka [1,2], Jackson Sembera [2], Joseph Ssebwana Katende [1,2], Violet Ankunda [1], Laban Kato [1], Ashwini Kurshan [3], Carl Graham [3], Jeffrey Seow [3], Katie J. Doores [3], Michael H. Malim [3], Julie M. Fox [3], Pontiano Kaleebu [1,2] and Jennifer Serwanga [1,2,*]

1 Viral Pathogens Research Theme, Medical Research Council, Uganda Virus Research Institute and London School of Hygiene & Tropical Medicine (MRC/UVRI & LSHTM) Research Unit, Entebbe 26, Uganda
2 Department of Immunology, Uganda Virus Research Institute, Entebbe 26, Uganda
3 Department of Infectious Diseases, School of Immunology & Microbial Sciences, King's College London, London SE1 9RT, UK
* Correspondence: jennifer.serwanga@mrcuganda.org

Abstract: Background: This study assessed the long-term dynamics of neutralizing antibodies in a Ugandan cohort primarily exposed to the A.23.1 SARS-CoV-2 variant, examining how this shaped immune breadth and potency against diverse strains following infection and prototype-based vaccination. **Methods:** We conducted a 427-day retrospective analysis of 41 participants across multiple SARS-CoV-2 waves, assessing binding and neutralizing antibody responses using in-house ELISA and pseudotyped virus neutralization assays. We quantified immune responses to key SARS-CoV-2 variants, A.23.1, D614G, Delta, and BA.4, capturing evolving immunity across the pandemic. **Results:** Neutralizing antibody titers against A.23.1 remained significantly higher than those against D614G, Delta, and BA.4, highlighting the solid immune memory following A.23.1 infection. Consistently lower titers were observed for BA.4 across all time points, aligning with its strong immune-evasion capability. Correlations between neutralizing titers and spike-directed IgG (S-IgG) concentrations were significantly stronger for A.23.1 than for D614G, with no correlation for BA.4. ChAdOx1-S vaccination substantially elevated the neutralizing titers across all variants, most notably BA.4, highlighting the essential role of vaccination in boosting immunity, even in individuals with initially low titers. **Conclusions:** Initial exposure to the A.23.1 variant triggered potent immune responses, shaping neutralizing antibody dynamics during subsequent exposures. These findings highlight the importance of accounting for early viral exposures in vaccine development and public health planning. The distinctly lower immune response to BA.4 highlights the need for continuous antigenic monitoring and timely vaccine updates for protection against emerging variants. Vaccination remains essential for reinforcing and sustaining immunity against evolving variants.

Keywords: immune imprinting; SARS-CoV-2 A.23.1 variant; cross-neutralization; antibody dynamics; neutralizing titers; antigenic surveillance; immune escape; variant-specific IgG immune responses

1. Introduction

Immune imprinting, first described by Thomas Francis, Jr. in the context of influenza over fifty years ago, refers to how the immune system's initial encounter with an antigen shapes future responses to future encounters with related antigens [1,2]. This con-

 https://doi.org/10.3390/vaccines13020143

cept has gained renewed interest in the study of emerging viral pathogens, including SARS-CoV-2 [3–6]. Research on variant-specific vaccines and successive epidemic waves has underscored the influence of initial immune priming on subsequent immune responses [5]. Understanding this phenomenon is essential for optimizing vaccine strategies and anticipating immune dynamics in response to evolving viral threats. Imprinting has been shown to have both beneficial [7–9] and detrimental effects [8,10]. Recent studies on SARS-CoV-2 variants show that initial immunization with multiple doses of the prototype mRNA-1273 vaccine effectively primes the immune system, enhancing broad cross-neutralizing antibody responses to subsequent Omicron-based boosters [11,12]. These findings underscore the critical role of early antigen exposure in shaping durable, broad-spectrum immunity against SARS-CoV-2.

Uganda confirmed its first COVID-19 case on 21 March 2020 [13] and launched its vaccination campaign on 10 March 2021 after receiving 864,000 doses of the AstraZeneca vaccine. In August 2020, initial SARS-CoV-2 genome sequences from infection clusters in Uganda were identified as lineage A.23, which is characterized by spike protein mutations R1021, F157L, V367F, Q613H, and P681R. These constituted 32% of viruses sequenced from June to August 2020, increasing to 50% from September to November 2020. By late October 2020, the A.23.1 variant with an additional spike mutation (P681R) emerged [14], and from December 2020 to January 2021, 90% of identified genomes (102 of 113) belonged to the A.23.1 lineage [15,16]. Uganda's Delta wave surged rapidly, rising from a daily average of 100 cases per day on 18 May 2021 to its peak at about 1800 cases per day by 12 June 2021, less than a month later. Between June and August 2021, the country recorded 2328 COVID-19 deaths, representing over half of its total mortality at the time. The Omicron wave, from December 2021 to January 2022, progressed even faster, peaking within just two weeks of onset at over 1800 cases per day [17], as summarized in Figure 1.

Our study uniquely investigated the A.23.1 variant, which constituted the primary antigenic exposure during Uganda's initial SARS-CoV-2 outbreak [15]. A.23.1 is slightly distinct from the Wuhan-1 strain used in the vaccines administered in this population, owing to the presence of both V367F and Q613H mutations that increase its infectivity over the Wuhan-1 strain [18]. This, combined with the NTD mutations, F157L and R102I, likely created a unique immunological imprint on the Ugandan population, with the long-term effects on subsequent immune responses to natural infection and vaccination remaining largely unexplored. We addressed this gap by analyzing immune responses in a Ugandan cohort initially exposed to the A.23.1 variant, determining antibody binding in response to SARS-CoV-2 natural infection [19] and vaccines [20] using Wuhan-1 strain antigens. The impact of A.23.1 on subsequent infections and vaccine responses remains uncertain, as does the specificity of serum-binding antibody titers in targeting A.23.1. It is also unclear how these antibody levels correlate with neutralization of A.23.1 and other SARS-CoV-2 variants. Clarifying these interactions is essential for understanding the broader immune landscape shaped by natural infection and vaccination.

This study investigated how primary infection with the A.23.1 SARS-CoV-2 variant shaped antibody responses to both subsequent natural infections and vaccinations with the ancestral strain. By longitudinally tracking immune responses, we aimed to provide critical insights into the dynamics of antibody evolution in this context. Specifically, we assessed (1) how primary infection with the A.23.1 SARS-CoV-2 variant influenced the magnitude and breadth of serum-neutralizing antibody responses, (2) the correlation between binding antibody levels and neutralizing capacity against A.23.1 and other SARS-CoV-2 variants, and (3) the implications for immune assessments in this cohort. This is the first analysis of immune responses to a non-Wuhan-1 primary SARS-CoV-2 variant infection in an African population, and it potentially has implications for tailored vaccine development.

2. Materials and Methods

2.1. Study Design and Population

This retrospective study, based on a well-characterized COVID-19 cohort [19], included 41 participants monitored through subsequent variant epidemic waves (Figure 1). SARS-CoV-2-positive participants were identified through rt-PCR testing as part of Uganda's national border surveillance, focusing on truck drivers who were essential to maintaining economic activity during the nationwide lockdown. This cohort provided a unique opportunity to study viral transmission in a high-risk, mobile population. During that period, all PCR-positive cases were mandatorily isolated at Masaka and Entebbe Regional Referral Hospitals until a confirmed PCR-negative result. This strict isolation policy was implemented to prevent further transmission. Infection onset (Day 0) was estimated using the initial rt-PCR confirmation documented in hospital records, as all PCR-positive truck drivers were mandatorily hospitalized. During follow-up, eight participants were vaccinated with the AstraZeneca ChAdOx1-S COVID-19 vaccine. Aligned with the emergence of COVID-19 variants and daily case counts (Figure 1), most samples collected between July 2020 and October 2021 primarily reflect immune responses to infections driven by the A.23.1 and Delta variants, which predominated during that period.

Of the 41 participants (median age: 29 years, IQR: 23–34), 78% were male. A majority (61%) were asymptomatic, 9.8% were symptomatic, and 29.3% had no symptom data (Table 1). Over a 427-day follow-up period (median 182.2 days, IQR 91.5–277.2), 156 plasma samples were collected at four intervals, which were 0–9, 92–182, 183–273, and 274–427 days post-PCR confirmation of infection. The study was approved by the Research and Ethics Committee of the Uganda Virus Research Institute (GC/127/833) and the Uganda National Council for Science and Technology (HS637ES). All participants provided written informed consent before their involvement.

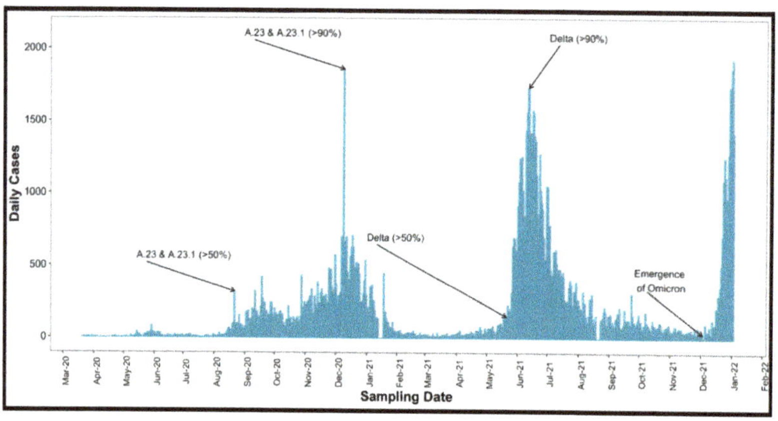

Figure 1. COVID-19 variant distribution and participant baseline characteristics. This figure shows the timeline of daily COVID-19 case counts and variant distribution from March 2020 to February 2022, indicating that samples collected between July 2020 and October 2021 are primarily linked to the A.23.1 and Delta variants. This figure is adapted and reused with permission from Bbosa et al. [21].

Table 1. Characteristics of study participants, $n = 41$.

Characteristics	n (%)
Total participants	41 (100)
Age, years (Median, IQR)	29.0 (23.0–34.0)
Gender	
Female	9 (22.0)
Male	32 (78.0)
Symptoms	
Yes *	4 (9.8)
No	25 (61.0)
Unknown	12 (29.3)

* Mild symptoms were chest pain and shortness of breath ($n = 1$), cough and runny nose ($n = 1$), fever ($n = 1$), and headache ($n = 1$).

2.2. Conventional In-House ELISA to Quantify Binding Antibody Concentrations

Anti-Spike-IgG antibodies were quantified using an optimized in-house ELISA protocol [22]. Briefly, 96-well flat-bottomed medium-binding plates (Greiner Bio-One, #655001, kremsmünster, Austria) were coated with 50 µL of recombinant wild-type spike-protein or nucleoprotein antigen (R&D Systems, #10474-CV-01M, #10474-CV-01M, Minneapolis, MN, USA) at 3.0 µg/mL and incubated overnight at 4 °C. The following day, plates were washed with PBS containing 0.05% Tween 20 (PBS-T) and blocked for 1 h at room temperature using PBS-T containing 1% BSA (Sigma, #A3803, Marlborough, MA, USA). Heat-inactivated plasma samples (56 °C for 30 min) were diluted 1:100 in PBS-T with 1% BSA and added in duplicate to the wells for 2 h of incubation at room temperature. After incubation, plates were washed five times with PBS-T, followed by one hour of incubation with 1:10,000 diluted horseradish peroxidase–conjugated goat anti-human IgG (γ-chain specific, Sigma, #A0170) in PBS-T with 1% BSA, at room temperature.

The assay included pre-determined negative and positive plasma samples, along with monoclonal antibodies CR3022 (0.1 µg/mL) targeting the spike protein and CR3009 (2 µg/mL) targeting nucleocapsid. Blank wells in duplicate served as controls. After washing, 50 µL of TMB substrate (Sera Care, #5120-0075, Milford, MA, USA) was added to each well and incubated for 3 min. The reaction was stopped by adding 50 µL of 1M hydrochloric acid (Sera Care, #5150-0021). Optical densities were measured at 450 nm, with blank well values subtracted to obtain net responses. Antibody concentrations were calculated using 4-parameter logistic standard curves and expressed in ng/mL, with values below the detection limit assigned 0 ng/mL. Longitudinal N-IgG concentrations were tracked to detect reinfection, defined by an 11-fold rise following the initial antibody peak, as previously reported [19].

2.3. Preparation of SARS-CoV-2 Pseudotyped Viruses and Assessment of Neutralizing Titers

Pseudotyped HIV-based viruses expressing SARS-CoV-2 spike variants D614G, B.1.617.2 (Delta), A.23.1, or Omicron (BA.4/5) were generated by culturing 3.5×10^6 HEK293T/17 cells in 10 mL of complete Dulbecco's Modified Eagle's Medium (supplemented with 10% FBS and 1% Pen/Strep). The cells were co-transfected with 15 µg of pHIV-Luciferase plasmid, 10 µg of HIV-Gag/Pol p8.91 plasmid, and 5 µg of SARS-CoV-2 variant spike protein plasmid using 90 µg of Polyethylenimine (PEI-Max, Polysciences, PA, USA) transfection reagent. After 18 h, the media were replaced, and the supernatant was collected 48 h post-transfection, filtered (0.45 µm), and stored at −80 °C. Heat-inactivated plasma samples were serially diluted five-fold starting at 1:25, in duplicates, using DMEM media with 10% FBS and 1% Pen/Strep. These were incubated with pseudotyped virus for 1 h at 37 °C in 96-well culture plates, followed by the addition of 12,500 HeLa cells stably expressing the human ACE-2 in 50 µL per well. The plates were incubated for 72 h at 37 °C with 5% CO_2 in a humidified incubator. Infection inhibition was assessed using Bright-Glo luciferase (Promega, Madison, WI, USA) and quantified on a Victor™ X3 multilabel reader (Perkin Elmer, Waltham, MA, USA). The ID50 values, representing the dilution required to achieve 50% neutralization, were calculated using curve fitting with the dose–response drc package in R software, v4.4.1.

2.4. Statistical Methods

Boxplots displayed the medians, means, and quartiles, while the Wilcoxon test, adjusted with Bonferroni correction for multiple comparisons, assessed significant differences in neutralization titers. Spearman rank correlation evaluated the relationship between neutralization titers and binding antibody responses. The significance threshold was $p \leq 0.05$.

3. Results

3.1. Longitudinal Analysis of Variant-Specific Neutralizing Antibody Responses Revealed Temporal Trends and Stability

We analyzed neutralizing antibody titers over time against several SARS-CoV-2 variants, A.23.1, D614G, Delta, and BA.4 (Figure 2). Neutralization against BA.4 remained consistently low across the study period (Figure 2A). To provide further insights, we segmented the study into four intervals of approximately 3 months each: 0–91 days, 92–182 days, 183–273 days, and 274–427 days. Boxplot comparisons across these intervals, using an unpaired Wilcoxon test to address missing data (Figure 2B), revealed significantly lower neutralizing titers against BA.4 compared to both A.23.1 and Delta at all time points. At the final time point (274–427 days), A.23.1 titers were significantly higher than those of the D614G variant ($p < 0.05$). The unpaired Wilcoxon test revealed no significant differences in neutralizing titers over time for any of the viral variants, indicating a consistent neutralization pattern throughout the study (Figure 2C). This consistency highlights uniform temporal dynamics of neutralizing antibody responses across intervals, irrespective of the viral variant. However, the boxplot analysis revealed significantly higher S-IgG concentrations against D614G compared to A.23.1 during the early phase of the study (Figure 2D), a trend that persisted even after stratifying the data by D614G responders and non-responders (Figure 2E). These results highlight the variability in neutralizing responses between viral variants and underscore the importance of analyzing immunogenicity in the context of dominant infection waves.

3.2. Limited Potency and Breadth of Neutralizing Antibody Responses Against Diverse SARS-CoV-2 Variants, with BA.4 Demonstrating the Highest Immune Evasion

Neutralizing antibody responses against diverse SARS-CoV-2 variants were limited in both potency and breadth over the 427-day observation period. As shown in the heatmap (Figure 3A), only a small subset of participants consistently maintained high neutralization titers across all variants and time points. Notably, BA.4 demonstrated the greatest resistance, with most participants exhibiting low neutralization titers, reflected by lighter heatmap cells. Only a few individuals achieved robust neutralization of this variant, underscoring the challenge of eliciting broad and durable immunity. These findings highlight the ongoing need for vaccines that provide more comprehensive protection against emerging variants.

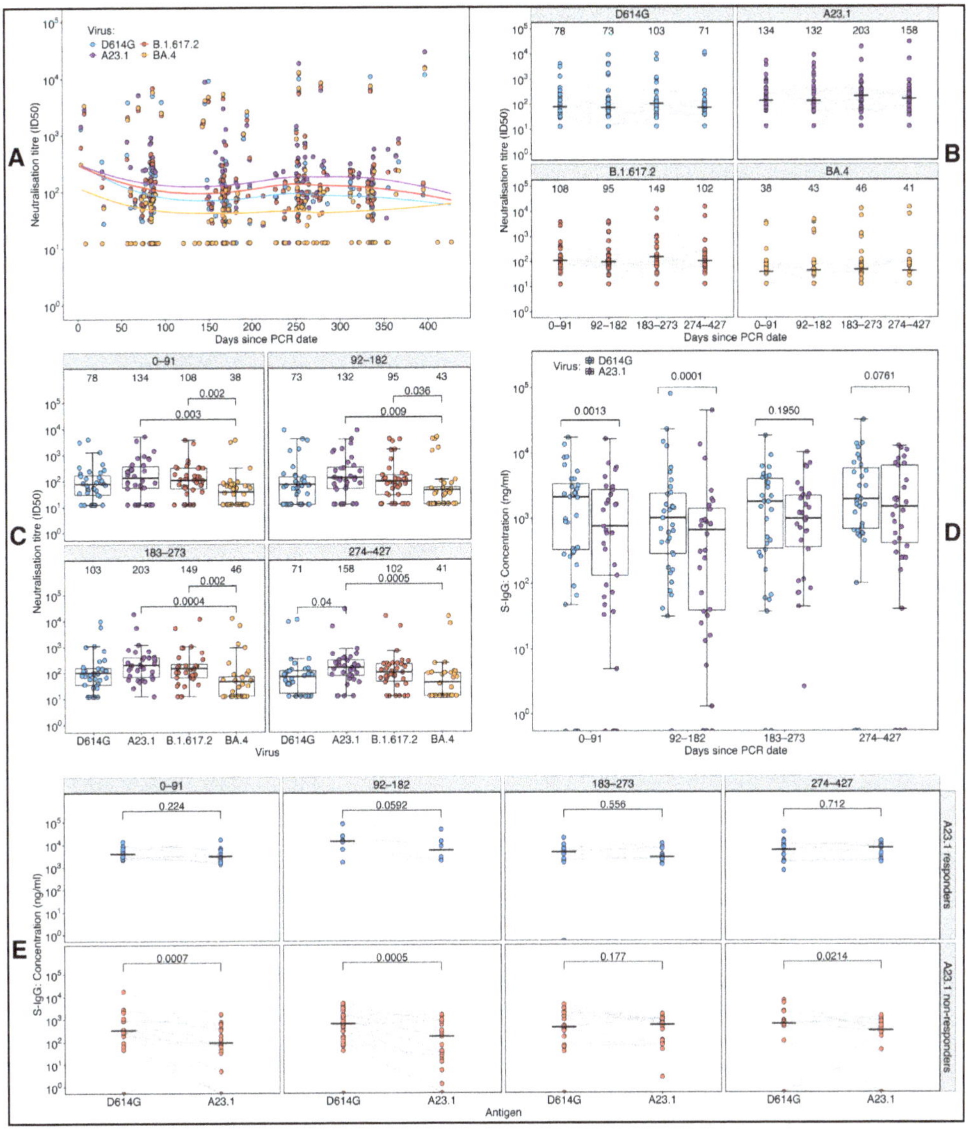

Figure 2. Longitudinal comparison of neutralizing titers and S-IgG levels across SARS-CoV-2 strains. This figure illustrates the longitudinal trends in neutralizing antibody titers and full spike (S)-IgG concentrations across SARS-CoV-2 variants. The line plots show neutralization titers over time for the D614G prototype and the A.23.1, Delta, and BA.4 variants, with the time categorized into four quarterly intervals, 0–91, 92–182, 183–273, and 274–427 days (**A**), and the median titers per quarter (**B**). Boxplots illustrate the distributions of antibody levels displaying medians (horizontal black line) and interquartile ranges (top and bottom of the box) across study groups. Boxplots depict the distribution of neutralizing titers for each virus variant across quarterly time intervals (**C**). Additionally, comparative boxplots illustrate S-IgG concentrations (ng/mL) across the D614G prototype and the A.23.1 variants, analyzed for all study participants (**D**). Using the D614G S-IgG cut-off of 0.432, the data were further stratified by D614G responders and non-responders at each quarterly time point (**E**). Statistical significance was determined at a threshold of $p \leq 0.05$. Significance bars indicate the p-values.

A stacked-bar graph analysis among participants revealed that neutralizing antibody geometric mean titers (GMTs) were mostly low (25–100) against D614G, while intermediate titers/GMTs (100–500) were more prevalent for A.23.1 across all time points (Figure 3B, Table 2). Delta variant responses primarily fell within the low (25–100) and intermediate (100–500) ranges, whereas BA.4 consistently showed low neutralization titers, highlighting its significant immune evasion compared to the other variants throughout the study period. Notably, only a small fraction of participants achieved high neutralization titers (>2000) across all variants, indicating a generally weak immune response, especially against the highly resistant BA.4 variant.

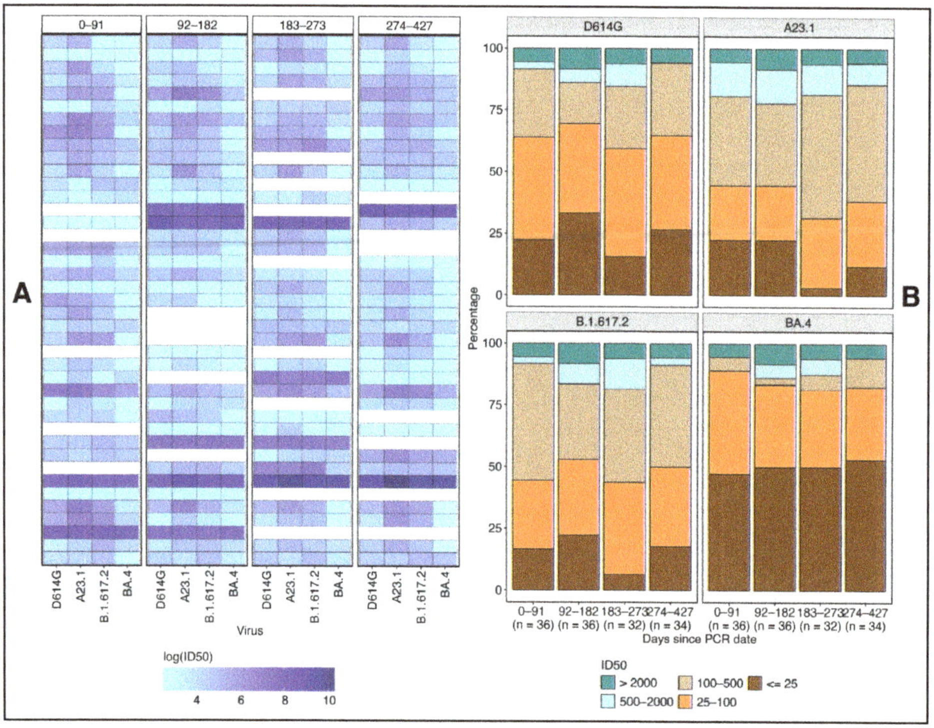

Figure 3. Longitudinal potency and breadth of neutralizing antibody responses against SARS-CoV-2 variants over 427 days. This figure shows a heatmap and bar graph illustrating the neutralizing antibody responses against various SARS-CoV-2 variants over 427 days. In the heatmap (**A**), darker cells represent higher neutralizing titers, while lighter cells indicate lower titers; white cells represent missing data. Each row corresponds to a participant's neutralization responses over time, highlighting that only a few participants maintained high neutralizing titers across all viruses and time points. The stacked bar graph (**B**) shows the proportion of participants within different neutralization titer groups over time for each variant. Most subjects displayed low (25–100) titers against D614G, intermediate (100–500) titers against A.23.1, and a mix of low and intermediate titers against the Delta variant.

These findings show the variability in neutralizing antibody potency across SARS-CoV-2 variants, with BA.4 showing the highest resistance to neutralization. The small number of participants exhibiting consistently high titers across all time points highlights the challenge of achieving broad, potent immunity, especially against immune-evasive strains, with implications for vaccine design and long-term immune assessment.

Table 2. Proportion of subjects neutralizing SARS-CoV-2 variants at various neutralizing titers over time.

Time Point (Days)		ID50 ≤ 25 Limited	25–100 Low	100–500 Intermediate	500–2000 High	ID50 > 2000 Robust
0–91	D614G	8 (22.2)	15 (41.7)	10 (27.8)	1 (2.8)	2 (5.6)
	A.23.1	8 (22.2)	8 (22.2)	13 (36.1)	5 (13.9)	2 (5.6)
	Delta	6 (16.7)	10 (27.8)	17 (47.2)	1 (2.8)	2 (5.6)
	BA.4	17 (47.2)	15 (41.7)	2 (5.6)	0 (0)	2 (5.6)
92–182	D614G	12 (33.3)	13 (36.1)	6 (16.7)	2 (5.6)	3 (8.3)
	A.23.1	8 (22.2)	8 (22.2)	12 (33.3)	5 (13.9)	3 (8.3)
	Delta	8 (22.2)	11 (30.6)	11 (30.6)	3 (8.3)	3 (8.3)
	BA.4	18 (50.0)	12 (33.3)	1 (2.8)	2 (5.6)	3 (8.3)
183–273	D614G	5 (15.6)	14 (43.8)	8 (25.0)	3 (9.4)	2 (6.3)
	A.23.1	1 (3.1)	9 (28.1)	16 (50.0)	4 (12.5)	2 (6.3)
	Delta	2 (6.3)	12 (37.5)	12 (37.5)	4 (12.5)	2 (6.3)
	BA.4	16 (50.0)	10 (31.3)	2 (6.3)	2 (6.3)	2 (6.3)
274–427	D614G	9 (26.5)	13 (38.2)	10 (29.4)	0 (0)	2 (5.9)
	A.23.1	4 (11.8)	9 (26.5)	16 (47.1)	3 (8.8)	2 (5.9)
	Delta	6 (17.6)	11 (32.4)	14 (41.2)	1 (2.9)	2 (5.9)
	BA.4	19 (55.9)	9 (26.5)	4 (11.8)	0 (0)	2 (5.9)

This table presents the number and corresponding proportions of subjects exhibiting varying levels of neutralizing titers against each SARS-CoV-2 variant over time. The table categorizes subjects into distinct neutralization levels, illustrating their distribution across distinct time intervals: 0–91 days, 92–182 days, 183–273 days, and 274–427 days. This breakdown provides an overview of the participants' responses at low, intermediate, and high neutralization titers for each virus variant, enabling the comparison of neutralization patterns throughout the study period.

3.3. Correlation Between Neutralization Titers and Spike-Specific IgG Binding Responses Across SARS-CoV-2 Variants

We assessed the correlation between neutralizing antibody titers (ID_{50}) and D614G as well as A.23.1 S-IgG concentrations across SARS-CoV-2 variants D614G, A.23.1, Delta, and BA.4 over time using Spearman rank correlation analysis. For the D614G variant, we observed a significant, moderate positive correlation between neutralizing titers (ID50) and S-IgG levels both in the early infection phase (0–91 days) and the later phase (274–427 days) (Figure 4A). Similar trends were noted for A.23.1 and Delta, reinforcing the consistency of the binding–neutralization relationship across these variants. Similarly, for A.23.1 and Delta, consistent correlations were noted at these time points, indicating robust alignment between binding and neutralizing responses. However, a lower correlation was detected during the intermediate phase (92–182 days) for D614G and A.23.1, suggesting a temporary decline in the binding–neutralization relationship (Figure 4B). No significant correlation was found for BA.4 at any time point, highlighting a distinct immune response to this variant.

These findings emphasize the temporal dynamics of antibody binding and neutralizing responses, highlighting the differential correlation between S-IgG levels and neutralization titers across various SARS-CoV-2 variants. The analysis underscores the pivotal role of spike-specific IgG antibodies in mediating protection, particularly against variants like D614G and A.23.1. The distinct lack of correlation observed for BA.4 further illustrates its unique immunogenic properties, suggesting potential immune evasion. This divergence has significant implications for vaccine development and future therapeutic strategies, particularly in addressing variants capable of escaping immune recognition.

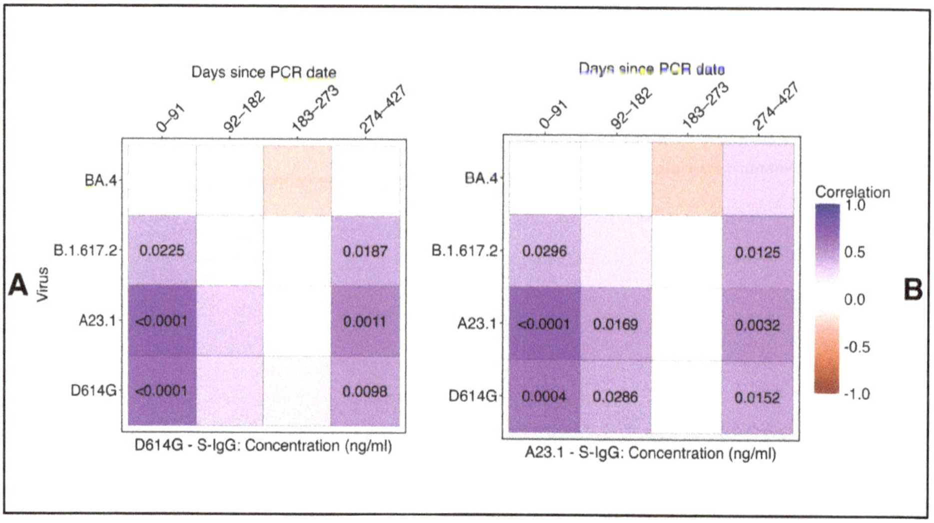

Figure 4. Correlation heat map of neutralizing antibody titers against SARS-CoV-2 variants and spike-directed IgG antibodies. This figure displays heat maps comparing the correlations between neutralizing antibody titers against SARS-CoV-2 variants D614G, A.23.1, Delta, and BA.4 and spike-directed IgG antibody levels for D614G (**A**) and A.23.1 (**B**). Positive correlations are indicated in purple, while negative correlations are shown in red. Statistical significance was determined at a threshold of $p \leq 0.05$; p-values are indicated in the heatmap.

3.4. Comparative Longitudinal Analysis of GMT Fold Changes and Neutralization Titers in Reinfected and Vaccinated Subjects

We performed a comparative analysis of geometric mean titer (GMT) fold changes relative to D614G and A.23.1 across all time points, as well as neutralizing titers for 13 reinfected subjects and pre- and post-vaccination titers in 8 ChAdOx1-S-vaccinated participants (Figure 5). At each time point, fold changes in neutralizing titers were calculated for each virus variant relative to D614G (Figure 5A) and A.23.1 (Figure 5B). A fold change greater than 0 indicated an increase in neutralizing titers, while a fold change below 0 represented a decrease. A fold change of 0 implied no change in titers. When neutralizing titers were compared to D614G, Delta exhibited a marginal increase across all time points, indicating a slight enhancement in the neutralizing response. Over time, A.23.1 demonstrated a gradual fold increase in neutralizing titers compared to D614G, signifying consistently higher titers for A.23.1. In contrast, BA.4 showed a consistent fold decrease relative to D614G, indicating lower neutralizing antibody responses for BA.4 at all time points.

Relative to A.23.1 (Figure 5B), all other virus variants showed a fold decrease across all time points, highlighting the superior neutralizing response elicited by A.23.1. This finding suggests that A.23.1 maintained a stronger neutralizing response compared to D614G, Delta, and BA.4 throughout the study period. Neutralizing titers for reinfected subjects, defined by an 11-fold or higher increase in N-IgG concentrations after the initial peak, were assessed (Figure 5C). A total of thirteen subjects met the reinfection criteria. For these individuals, neutralizing titers displayed a declining trend during the first 182 days post-primary infection, followed by a gradual increase between 183 and 273 days across all virus variants. In a separate analysis of eight participants who received both doses of the AZN vaccine, we compared neutralizing titers before and after vaccination (Figure 5D). BA.4 titers, which were initially low post primary infection, rose sharply by 15-fold after vaccination. Delta titers increased by nine-fold, D614G by six-fold, and A.23.1 by two-fold.

These results highlight the strong boosting effect of vaccination, enhancing neutralizing responses against all variants, including BA.4, which had exhibited persistently lower responses pre-vaccination.

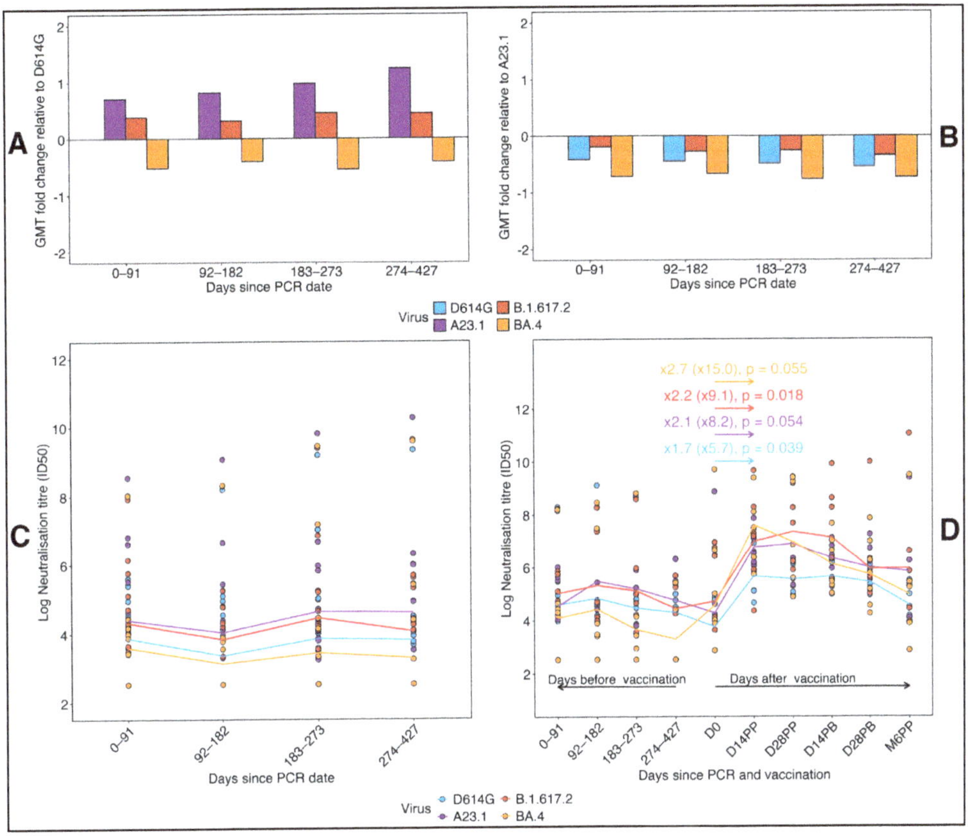

Figure 5. Fold changes in neutralizing titers relative to D614G and A.23.1 and neutralization patterns in re-infected and vaccinated Subjects. This figure shows the log-transformed geometric mean titer (GMT) fold changes in neutralizing antibody responses relative to D614G (**A**) and A.23.1 (**B**) across different time points in a cohort of 41 participants. A fold change above 0 indicates an increase, while a fold change below 0 indicates a decrease in neutralizing titers relative to the reference virus. Panel (**C**) displays the neutralizing titers of re-infected subjects over time, categorized by days post-infection, with a focus on variations in neutralization responses across different virus variants. (**D**) illustrates the neutralizing titers before and after vaccination in vaccinated subjects, showing the comparative changes in responses to each virus variant following vaccination. Horizontal lines represent the log-transformed geometric mean titers at each time point for each virus. Fold changes are presented as log-transformed values, with raw unlogged values in brackets. Statistically significant differences are indicated, marked by p-values ≤ 0.05, confirming a consistent rise in antibody titers across all variants following vaccination.

These findings highlight the dynamic nature of neutralizing antibody responses across SARS-CoV-2 variants, revealing significant variability in immune recognition. The analysis underscores the profound enhancement in immune responses following vaccination, particularly against variants with initially low neutralization profiles. The substantial post-vaccination increases in neutralizing titers against BA.4, Delta, and D614G demonstrate the critical role of vaccination in bolstering the breadth of neutralizing antibody responses. Furthermore, the consistently higher neutralizing titers observed against A.23.1, both before and after vaccination, reinforce the observed effect of immune imprinting from the primary A.23.1 SARS-CoV-2 infection in this population. These findings have important implications for understanding variant-specific immune responses and guiding future vaccination strategies.

4. Discussion

This study aimed to investigate the long-term dynamics of neutralizing antibody responses in a Ugandan cohort, with a specific focus on the influence of early exposure to the A.23.1 SARS-CoV-2 variant on subsequent immune responses to both natural infections and vaccinations with the wild-type prototype-based vaccines. Given the unique exposure history of this cohort, which first encountered the A.23.1 variant before the more globally dominant Delta and Omicron (BA.4) variants emerged, this study was justified by the need to explore the effects of immune imprinting in an African population and its broader implications for public health and vaccine design strategies. We hypothesized that initial infection with A.23.1 would leave an immunological imprint that could influence the magnitude, specificity, and durability of neutralizing responses to subsequent infections and vaccinations. Our primary finding was the sustained and robust neutralizing antibody response against the A.23.1 variant, which surpassed responses to D614G, Delta, and BA.4. This highlights the potential impact of initial antigenic exposure on shaping long-term immune responses and is supported by previous observations of preferential neutralization of the primary infecting variant over other variants [23]. Additionally, neutralizing responses to BA.4 were significantly weaker across all time points, underscoring the unique immune-evasive and antigenic divergence properties of this variant, consistent with findings from global studies on Omicron variants [24,25]. The higher neutralizing titers against A.23.1 throughout indicate a lasting imprint that may confer enhanced protection against this variant. These results align with the concept of immune imprinting, where the first antigen encounter primes the immune system in ways that influence responses to future exposures [26].

This study primarily investigates the A.23.1 variant, first identified in Uganda, and its impact on immune responses to subsequent variants, including Delta and Omicron (BA.4). While other early variants of concern (VOCs), such as Beta (B.1.351) and Gamma (P.1), possess the E484K mutation in the RBD and confer stronger immune evasion compared to Alpha (N501Y) [27], these variants did not play a significant roles in Uganda's early SARS-CoV-2 epidemic waves. Instead, lineage A.23 dominated the initial infections, evolving into A.23.1 before transitioning to Delta and, later, Omicron. Genomic surveillance data show that Alpha, Beta, and Gamma VOCs circulated at minimal circulation in Uganda [21], thus limiting the opportunity to assess immune responses to these variants in our cohort. Despite this, immune imprinting effects observed with A.23.1 are consistent with findings from other populations exposed to different primary variants. For example, research in South Africa showed that initial exposure to Beta influenced subsequent immune responses differently from those who first encountered the ancestral Wuhan-1 strain [28]. Similarly, studies in the UK and China demonstrated that early infection with specific SARS-CoV-2 variants shaped preferential neutralization patterns against related strains [29,30], a phenomenon also confirmed in controlled animal models [31]. These findings underscore the broader relevance of immune imprinting across diverse epidemiological settings, emphasizing the need for tailored vaccine strategies that consider early viral exposures. Understanding these dynamics is crucial for optimizing future vaccine formulations and ensuring robust protection against emerging variants.

Our findings revealed that despite prior imprinting by the A.23.1 variant, vaccination in previously infected individuals substantially increased neutralizing antibody titers and breadth across all tested variants. However, neutralizing antibody responses to A.23.1 remained higher than those against D614G, further highlighting the A.23.1 imprint. This suggests that prior exposure to A.23.1 did not diminish the potency and breadth of the vaccination response, even in the presence of a response favoring the primary infection variant over the variant of the vaccine antigen, thus highlighting the effectiveness of vaccines in enhancing and broadening immunity. This aligns with other studies showing that COVID-19 vaccines can elicit broad and potent neutralizing responses regardless of prior variant exposure [12]. Notably, our data also revealed a pronounced reduction in neutralizing capacity against the BA.4 variant at all time points, aligning with this variant's potential for immune evasion [32]. These results corroborate prior studies demonstrating diminished vaccine efficacy and reduced antibody neutralization against Omicron subvariants [33–35], underscoring the necessity for ongoing surveillance and potential vaccine updates to counter evolving viral threats. Our findings introduce a crucial dimension to the literature on immune imprinting and SARS-CoV-2. While previous studies focused on the priming effect of the original Wuhan-1 strain and subsequent variants of concern, the impact of early circulating variants, such as A.23.1, was overlooked. This study bridges the gap by examining the A.23.1 variant, revealing how other non-Wuhan-1 strains like A.23.1 influence long-term immune responses.

A key strength of this study was its longitudinal design, which allowed for extended assessment of immune responses, offering a dynamic view of antibody kinetics. The combined use of binding and neutralizing antibody assays, alongside multiple SARS-CoV-2 variants, enhanced the robustness and comprehensiveness of our findings. However, the relatively small sample size and the predominance of males and asymptomatic participants could introduce bias and limit generalizability. Nonetheless, these demographics accurately represent those most affected by COVID-19 in sub-Saharan Africa.

The differential neutralizing antibody responses observed against various SARS-CoV-2 variants suggest that the initial exposure to A.23.1 may have induced a unique immunological imprint, potentially through mechanisms like epitope specificity and B-cell memory formation [35]. The lack of a significant correlation between S-IgG concentrations and neutralizing titers for the BA.4 variant further highlights the evolving challenges posed by new SARS-CoV-2 strains [36]. Clinically, our results suggest that individuals initially exposed to the A.23.1 variant may have enhanced protection against similar variants but could be less protected against highly divergent strains like BA.4. This supports the need for variant-specific boosters to ensure broad and effective immunity. Moreover, the demonstrated boost in neutralizing antibodies following vaccination in previously infected individuals supports the continued use of vaccines to enhance and diversify immune responses in populations with prior SARS-CoV-2 exposure. The diminished sensitivity of the BA.4 Omicron variant was anticipated, as Omicron variants possess up to 15 mutations in the receptor-binding domain (RBD) [37,38]. Mutations in Omicron, such as K417N, G446S, E484A, and Q493R, have been shown to significantly compromise the neutralizing ability of RBD-binding antibodies whose epitopes overlap with the ACE2-binding motif.

5. Study Limitations

While this study provides valuable insights into the long-term immune consequences of initial SARS-CoV-2 A.23.1 exposure, several limitations should be acknowledged. First, the sample size of 41 participants, although carefully characterized and followed longitudinally, is relatively small, which may limit the generalizability of our findings. However, the depth of our immunological assessments across an extended period strengthens the interpretation of immune imprinting effects. While the sample size is modest, our approach ensures robust statistical comparisons by leveraging repeated measurements per participant over time, thus enhancing the statistical power of our analysis. To validate our findings, we applied stringent statistical corrections, including the Wilcoxon test with Bonferroni adjustments for multiple comparisons and Spearman correlation analyses to assess binding and neutralization relationships. Second, the cohort was predominantly comprised of young, male truck drivers who were asymptomatic or mildly symptomatic. This demographic representation, although reflective of Uganda's early outbreak dynamics, may not fully capture immune responses in older or more clinically severe cases. Future studies should expand to more diverse cohorts to validate these findings across broader populations. Third, while we analyzed neutralizing antibody responses against key SARS-CoV-2 variants (A.23.1, D614G, Delta, and BA.4), earlier VOCs, such as Alpha, Beta, and Gamma, were not included due to their low prevalence in Uganda at the time of study recruitment, potentially limiting direct comparisons with global immune imprinting patterns. Finally, while neutralizing antibodies are a critical correlate of protection, additional functional immune parameters, such as T-cell responses, were not assessed in this study. Future work incorporating cellular immunity will be essential to provide a more comprehensive understanding of immune imprinting and long-term immunity.

6. Conclusions

In conclusion, this study provides critical insights into the long-term immune consequences of primary SARS-CoV-2 A.23.1 exposure, demonstrating that early viral encounters shape the breadth, magnitude, and durability of neutralizing antibody responses to subsequent infections and vaccinations. Our findings highlight the persistence of strong neutralizing responses against A.23.1, contrasted by significantly reduced cross-neutralization against immune-evasive variants, such as Omicron BA.4. While vaccination effectively boosted immunity across all tested variants, the imprint of A.23.1 remained evident, reinforcing the role of early antigenic exposure in shaping long-term immune trajectories. These results underscore the necessity of continuous antigenic surveillance and periodic vaccine updates to address evolving variants with enhanced immune escape potential. Furthermore, this study emphasizes the importance of tailored immunization strategies that consider population-specific exposure histories to optimize vaccine effectiveness. Future research integrating cellular immunity and expanding cohort diversity will be crucial to fully unravel the complexities of immune imprinting and its implications for global SARS-CoV-2 vaccine and public health strategies.

Author Contributions: Conceptualization, J.S. (Jennifer Serwanga) and P.K.; methodology, G.K.O., J.S. (Jackson Sembera), J.S.K. and J.S. (Jennifer Serwanga); laboratory investigation, G.K.O., J.S. (Jackson Sembera), A.K., J.S.K., L.K., C.G., J.S. (Jeffrey Seow) and J.S. (Jennifer Serwanga); data curation and formal analysis, V.A., G.K.O., C.G. and J.S. (Jennifer Serwanga); resources, K.J.D., M.H.M., J.M.F., P.K. and J.S. (Jennifer Serwanga); writing—original draft preparation, J.S. (Jennifer Serwanga); writing—review and editing, G.K.O., J.S. (Jennifer Serwanga), P.K., J.M.F., M.H.M., K.J.D., C.G. and J.S. (Jeffrey Seow); supervision, K.J.D. and J.S. (Jennifer Serwanga); funding acquisition, J.M.F., K.J.D., M.H.M., P.K. and J.S. (Jennifer Serwanga). All authors have read and agreed to the published version of the manuscript.

Funding: This research was funded as part of the EDCTP2 program supported by the European Union and the Swedish International Development Cooperation Agency (Sida, Sweden) (grant number RIA2020EF-3008-COVAB). The work was conducted at the Uganda Virus Research Institute, King's College London, and the MRC/UVRI and LSHTM Uganda Research Unit, which is jointly funded by the UK Medical Research Council (MRC), which is part of UK Research and Innovation (UKRI) and the UK Foreign, Commonwealth, and Development office (FDCO) under the MRC/FDCO

Concordat agreement, and it is also part of the EDCTP2 program, supported by the European Union. The work was funded in part by the Government of Uganda under the Science, Technology, and Innovation Secretariat—Office of the President (STI-OP), grant number MOSTI-PRESIDE-COVID-19-2020/15. This publication is based on research funded in part by the Bill and Melinda Gates Foundation through the GIISER Uganda Grant Agreement, Investment ID INV-036306. The findings and conclusions contained within are those of the authors and do not necessarily reflect positions or policies of the Bill and Melinda Gates Foundation.

Institutional Review Board Statement: The study was conducted in accordance with the Declaration of Helsinki and approved by the Institutional Review Board (or Ethics Committee) of the Uganda Virus Research Institute (Ref: GC/127/833, 7 October 2020) and the Uganda National Council for Science and Technology (HS637ES, 22 January 2021).

Informed Consent Statement: Written informed consent was obtained from all participants involved in the study.

Data Availability Statement: The raw data supporting the conclusions of this article will be made available by the authors upon request from the corresponding author (JSer).

Acknowledgments: The authors are grateful to the study participants in the COVID-19 study cohort, who donated the specimens used in this study. The following reagent was produced under HHSN272201400008C and obtained through BEI Resources, NIAID, NIH: Monoclonal Anti-SARS Coronavirus Recombinant Human Antibody, Clone CR3022 (produced in HEK293 Cells), NR-52481. The following reagent was obtained through BEI Resources, NIAID, NIH: Monoclonal Anti-SARS Coronavirus Recombinant Human IgG1, Clone CR3022 (produced in Nicotiana benthamiana), NR-52392. The Nucleoprotein mAb CR3009 (NIBSC Repository, Product No. 101011) used as a positive control was obtained from the Centre for AIDS Reagents, NIBSC, UK.

Conflicts of Interest: The authors declare no conflicts of interest.

References

1. Monto, A.S.; Malosh, R.E.; Petrie, J.G.; Martin, E.T. The Doctrine of Original Antigenic Sin: Separating Good From Evil. *J. Infect. Dis.* **2017**, *215*, 1782–1788. [CrossRef]
2. Haaheim, L.R. Original antigenic sin. A confounding issue? *Dev. Biol.* **2003**, *115*, 49–53.
3. Rijkers, G.T.; van Overveld, F.J. The "original antigenic sin" and its relevance for SARS-CoV-2 (COVID-19) vaccination. *Clin. Immunol. Commun.* **2021**, *1*, 13–16. [CrossRef] [PubMed]
4. Zimmermann, P.; Curtis, N. Factors That Influence the Immune Response to Vaccination. *Clin. Microbiol. Rev.* **2019**, *32*, e00084-18. [CrossRef] [PubMed]
5. Tortorici, M.A.; Addetia, A.; Seo, A.J.; Brown, J.; Sprouse, K.; Logue, J.; Clark, E.; Franko, N.; Chu, H.; Veesler, D. Persistent immune imprinting occurs after vaccination with the COVID-19 XBB.1.5 mRNA booster in humans. *Immunity* **2024**, *57*, 904–911.e4. [CrossRef]
6. Johnston, T.S.; Li, S.H.; Painter, M.M.; Atkinson, R.K.; Douek, N.R.; Reeg, D.B.; Douek, D.C.; Wherry, E.J.; Hensley, S.E. Immunological imprinting shapes the specificity of human antibody responses against SARS-CoV-2 variants. *Immunity* **2024**, *57*, 912–925.e914. [CrossRef] [PubMed]
7. Bayas, J.M.; Vilella, A.; Bertran, M.J.; Vidal, J.; Batalla, J.; Asenjo, M.A.; Salleras, L.L. Immunogenicity and reactogenicity of the adult tetanus-diphtheria vaccine. How many doses are necessary? *Epidemiol. Infect.* **2001**, *127*, 451–460. [CrossRef]
8. Mugitani, A.; Ito, K.; Irie, S.; Eto, T.; Ishibashi, M.; Ohfuji, S.; Fukushima, W.; Maeda, A.; Hirota, Y. Immunogenicity of the trivalent inactivated influenza vaccine in young children less than 4 years of age, with a focus on age and baseline antibodies. *Clin. Vaccine Immunol.* **2014**, *21*, 1253–1260. [CrossRef]
9. Kanesa-Thasan, N.; Sun, W.; Ludwig, G.V.; Rossi, C.; Putnak, J.R.; Mangiafico, J.A.; Innis, B.L.; Edelman, R. Atypical antibody responses in dengue vaccine recipients. *Am. J. Trop. Med. Hyg.* **2003**, *69* (Suppl. S6), 32–38. [CrossRef] [PubMed]
10. Englund, J.A.; Walter, E.B.; Gbadebo, A.; Monto, A.S.; Zhu, Y.; Neuzil, K.M. Immunization with trivalent inactivated influenza vaccine in partially immunized toddlers. *Pediatrics* **2006**, *118*, e579–e585. [CrossRef]
11. Chibwana, M.G.; Moyo-Gwete, T.; Kwatra, G.; Mandolo, J.; Hermanaus, T.; Motlou, T.; Mzindle, N.; Ayres, F.; Chaponda, M.; Tembo, G.; et al. AstraZeneca COVID-19 vaccine induces robust broadly cross-reactive antibody responses in Malawian adults previously infected with SARS-CoV-2. *BMC Med.* **2022**, *20*, 128. [CrossRef] [PubMed]

12. Liang, C.-Y.; Raju, S.; Liu, Z.; Li, Y.; Asthagiri Arunkumar, G.; Case, J.B.; Scheaffer, S.M.; Zost, S.J.; Acreman, C.M.; Gagne, M.; et al. Imprinting of serum neutralizing antibodies by Wuhan-1 mRNA vaccines. *Nature* **2024**, *630*, 950–960. [CrossRef]
13. Bugembe, D.L.; Kayiwa, J.; Phan, M.V.T.; Tushabe, P.; Balinandi, S.; Dhaala, B.; Lexow, J.; Mwebesa, H.; Aceng, J.; Kyobe, H.; et al. Main Routes of Entry and Genomic Diversity of SARS-CoV-2, Uganda. *Emerg. Infect. Dis.* **2020**, *26*, 2411–2415. [CrossRef]
14. Lubinski, B.; Frazier, L.E.; Phan, M.V.T.; Bugembe, D.L.; Cunningham, J.L.; Tang, T.; Daniel, S.; Cotten, M.; Jaimes, J.A.; Whittaker, G.R. Spike Protein Cleavage-Activation in the Context of the SARS-CoV-2 P681R Mutation: An Analysis from Its First Appearance in Lineage A.23.1 Identified in Uganda. *Microbiol. Spectr.* **2022**, *10*, e01514-22. [CrossRef] [PubMed]
15. Bugembe, D.L.; Phan, M.V.T.; Ssewanyana, I.; Semanda, P.; Nansumba, H.; Dhaala, B.; Nabadda, S.; O'Toole, Á.N.; Rambaut, A.; Kaleebu, P.; et al. Emergence and spread of a SARS-CoV-2 lineage A variant (A.23.1) with altered spike protein in Uganda. *Nat. Microbiol.* **2021**, *6*, 1094–1101. [CrossRef]
16. Bugembe, D.L.; Phan, M.V.T.; Ssewanyana, I.; Semanda, P.; Nansumba, H.; Dhaala, B.; Nabadda, S.; O'Toole, Á.N.; Rambaut, A.; Kaleebu, P.; et al. A SARS-CoV-2 lineage A variant (A.23.1) with altered spike has emerged and is dominating the current Uganda epidemic. *MedRxiv* **2021**. [CrossRef]
17. Laing, N.; Mylan, S.; Parker, M. Does epidemiological evidence support the success story of Uganda's response to COVID-19? *J. Biosoc. Sci.* **2024**, 1–8. [CrossRef] [PubMed]
18. Li, Q.; Wu, J.; Nie, J.; Zhang, L.; Hao, H.; Liu, S.; Zhao, C.; Zhang, Q.; Liu, H.; Nie, L. The impact of mutations in SARS-CoV-2 spike on viral infectivity and antigenicity. *Cell* **2020**, *182*, 1284–1294.e9. [CrossRef] [PubMed]
19. Serwanga, J.; Ankunda, V.; Sembera, J.; Kato, L.; Oluka, G.K.; Baine, C.; Odoch, G.; Kayiwa, J.; Auma, B.O.; Jjuuko, M.; et al. Rapid, early, and potent Spike-directed IgG, IgM, and IgA distinguish asymptomatic from mildly symptomatic COVID-19 in Uganda, with IgG persisting for 28 months. *Front. Immunol.* **2023**, *14*, 1152522. [CrossRef] [PubMed]
20. Serwanga, J.; Baine, C.; Mugaba, S.; Ankunda, V.; Auma, B.O.; Oluka, G.K.; Kato, L.; Kitabye, I.; Sembera, J.; Odoch, G.; et al. Seroprevalence and durability of antibody responses to AstraZeneca vaccination in Ugandans with prior mild or asymptomatic COVID-19: Implications for vaccine policy. *Front. Immunol.* **2023**, *14*, 1183983. [CrossRef] [PubMed]
21. Bbosa, N.; Ssemwanga, D.; Namagembe, H.; Kiiza, R.; Kiconco, J.; Kayiwa, J.; Lutalo, T.; Lutwama, J.; Ssekagiri, A.; Ssewanyana, I.; et al. Rapid replacement of SARS-CoV-2 variants by delta and subsequent arrival of Omicron, Uganda, 2021. *Emerg. Infect. Dis.* **2022**, *28*, 1021–1025. [CrossRef] [PubMed]
22. Oluka, G.K.; Namubiru, P.; Kato, L.; Ankunda, V.; Gombe, B.; Cotten, M.; Team, C.-I.; Musenero, M.; Kaleebu, P.; Fox, J.; et al. Optimisation and Validation of a conventional ELISA and cut-offs for detecting and quantifying anti-SARS-CoV-2 Spike, RBD, and Nucleoprotein IgG, IgM, and IgA antibodies in Uganda. *Front. Immunol.* **2023**, *14*, 1113194. [CrossRef]
23. Bekliz, M.; Adea, K.; Vetter, P.; Eberhardt, C.S.; Hosszu-Fellous, K.; Vu, D.-L.; Puhach, O.; Essaidi-Laziosi, M.; Waldvogel-Abramowski, S.; Stephan, C. Neutralization capacity of antibodies elicited through homologous or heterologous infection or vaccination against SARS-CoV-2 VOCs. *Nat. Commun.* **2022**, *13*, 3840. [CrossRef]
24. Pastorio, C.; Noettger, S.; Nchioua, R.; Zech, F.; Sparrer, K.M.J.; Kirchhoff, F. Impact of mutations defining SARS-CoV-2 Omicron subvariants BA.2.12.1 and BA.4/5 on Spike function and neutralization. *iScience* **2023**, *26*, 108299. [CrossRef]
25. Wang, Q.; Guo, Y.; Iketani, S.; Nair, M.S.; Li, Z.; Mohri, H.; Wang, M.; Yu, J.; Bowen, A.D.; Chang, J.Y.; et al. Antibody evasion by SARS-CoV-2 Omicron subvariants BA.2.12.1, BA.4 and BA.5. *Nature* **2022**, *608*, 603–608. [CrossRef]
26. Reynolds, C.J.; Pade, C.; Gibbons, J.M.; Butler, D.K.; Otter, A.D.; Menacho, K.; Fontana, M.; Smit, A.; Sackville-West, J.E.; Cutino-Moguel, T.; et al. Prior SARS-CoV-2 infection rescues B and T cell responses to variants after first vaccine dose. *Science* **2021**, *372*, 1418–1423. [CrossRef]
27. Khateeb, J.; Li, Y.; Zhang, H. Emerging SARS-CoV-2 variants of concern and potential intervention approaches. *Crit. Care* **2021**, *25*, 244. [CrossRef]
28. Madhi, S.A.; Baillie, V.; Cutland, C.L.; Voysey, M.; Koen, A.L.; Fairlie, L.; Padayachee, S.D.; Dheda, K.; Barnabas, S.L.; Bhorat, Q.E.; et al. Efficacy of the ChAdOx1 nCoV-19 COVID-19 Vaccine against the B.1.351 Variant. *N. Engl. J. Med.* **2021**, *384*, 1885–1898. [CrossRef]
29. Seow, J.; Jefferson, G.C.E.; Keegan, M.D.; Yau, Y.; Snell, L.B.; Doores, K.J. Profiling serum immunodominance following SARS-CoV-2 primary and breakthrough infection reveals distinct variant-specific epitope usage and immune imprinting. *PLoS Pathog.* **2024**, *20*, e1012724. [CrossRef]
30. Jia, T.; Wang, F.; Chen, Y.; Liao, G.; Xu, Q.; Chen, J.; Wu, J.; Li, N.; Wang, L.; Yuan, L.; et al. Expanded immune imprinting and neutralization spectrum by hybrid immunization following breakthrough infections with SARS-CoV-2 variants after three-dose vaccination. *J. Infect.* **2024**, *89*, 106362. [CrossRef]
31. Degryse, J.; Maas, E.; Lassaunière, R.; Geerts, K.; Kumpanenko, Y.; Weynand, B.; Maes, P.; Neyts, J.; Thibaut, H.J.; Alpizar, Y.A.; et al. Antigenic Imprinting Dominates Humoral Responses to New Variants of SARS-CoV-2 in a Hamster Model of COVID-19. *Microorganisms* **2024**, *12*, 2591. [CrossRef] [PubMed]
32. Cao, Y.; Wang, J.; Jian, F.; Xiao, T.; Song, W.; Yisimayi, A.; Huang, W.; Li, Q.; Wang, P.; An, R.; et al. Omicron escapes the majority of existing SARS-CoV-2 neutralizing antibodies. *Nature* **2022**, *602*, 657–663. [CrossRef] [PubMed]

33. Guo, H.; Ha, S.; Botten, J.W.; Xu, K.; Zhang, N.; An, Z.; Strohl, W.R.; Shiver, J.W.; Fu, T.M. SARS-CoV-2 Omicron: Viral Evolution, Immune Evasion, and Alternative Durable Therapeutic Strategies. *Viruses* **2024**, *16*, 697. [CrossRef] [PubMed]
34. Mannar, D.; Saville, J.W.; Zhu, X.; Srivastava, S.S.; Berezuk, A.M.; Tuttle, K.S.; Marquez, A.C.; Sekirov, I.; Subramaniam, S. SARS-CoV-2 Omicron variant: Antibody evasion and cryo-EM structure of spike protein-ACE2 complex. *Science* **2022**, *375*, 760–764. [CrossRef] [PubMed]
35. Yisimayi, A.; Song, W.; Wang, J.; Jian, F.; Yu, Y.; Chen, X.; Xu, Y.; Yang, S.; Niu, X.; Xiao, T.; et al. Repeated Omicron exposures override ancestral SARS-CoV-2 immune imprinting. *Nature* **2024**, *625*, 148–156. [CrossRef]
36. Di, H.; Pusch, E.A.; Jones, J.; Kovacs, N.A.; Hassell, N.; Sheth, M.; Lynn, K.S.; Keller, M.W.; Wilson, M.M.; Keong, L.M.; et al. Antigenic Characterization of Circulating and Emerging SARS-CoV-2 Variants in the U.S. throughout the Delta to Omicron Waves. *Vaccines* **2024**, *12*, 505. [CrossRef] [PubMed]
37. Starr, T.N.; Greaney, A.J.; Addetia, A.; Hannon, W.W.; Choudhary, M.C.; Dingens, A.S.; Li, J.Z.; Bloom, J.D. Prospective mapping of viral mutations that escape antibodies used to treat COVID-19. *Science* **2021**, *371*, 850–854. [CrossRef] [PubMed]
38. Jawad, B.; Adhikari, P.; Podgornik, R.; Ching, W.Y. Impact of BA.1, BA.2, and BA.4/BA.5 Omicron mutations on therapeutic monoclonal antibodies. *Comput. Biol. Med.* **2023**, *167*, 107576. [CrossRef]

MDPI AG
Grosspeteranlage 5
4052 Basel
Switzerland
Tel.: +41 61 683 77 34

Vaccines Editorial Office
E-mail: vaccines@mdpi.com
www.mdpi.com/journal/vaccines

www.ingramcontent.com/pod-product-compliance
Lightning Source LLC
Chambersburg PA
CBHW061601210926
51850CB00009B/2178
9783725868308